Psychological Assessment and Treatment of Older Adults

Psychological Assessment and Treatment of Older Adults

Nancy A. Pachana, PhD
Victor Molinari, PhD, ABPP
Larry W. Thompson, PhD, ABPP
Dolores Gallagher-Thompson, PhD, ABPP

hogrefe

Library of Congress of Congress Cataloging in Publication information for the print version of this book is available via the Library of Congress Marc Database under the Library of Congress Control Number 2021934339

Library and Archives Canada Cataloguing in Publication

Title: Psychological assessment and treatment of older adults / Nancy A. Pachana, PhD, Victor Molinari, PhD, ABPP, Larry W. Thompson, PhD, ABPP, Dolores Gallagher-Thompson, PhD, ABPP.

Names: Pachana, Nancy A., editor. | Molinari, Victor, 1952- editor. | Thompson, Larry W., editor. | Gallagher-Thompson, Dolores, editor.

Description: Edited by Nancy A. Pachana, Victor Molinari, Larry W. Thompson, and Dolores Gallagher-Thompson. | Includes bibliographical references.

Identifiers: Canadiana (print) 20210152192 | Canadiana (ebook) 20210152362 | ISBN 9780889375710 (softcover) | ISBN 9781616765712 (PDF) | ISBN 9781613345719 (EPUB)

Subjects: LCSH: Older people—Mental health. | LCSH: Older people—Psychology. | LCSH: Geriatric psychiatry.

Classification: LCC RC451.4.A5 P79 2021 | DDC 618.97/689—dc23

www.hogrefe.com

PUBLISHING OFFICES

USA:	Hogrefe Publishing Corporation, 361 Newbury Street, 5th Floor, Boston, MA 02115 Phone (857) 880-2002; E-mail customerservice@hogrefe.com
EUROPE:	Hogrefe Publishing GmbH, Merkelstr. 3, 37085 Göttingen, Germany Phone +49 551 99950-0, Fax +49 551 99950-111; E-mail publishing@hogrefe.com

SALES & DISTRIBUTION

USA:	Hogrefe Publishing, Customer Services Department, 30 Amberwood Parkway, Ashland, OH 44805 Phone (800) 228-3749, Fax (419) 281-6883; E-mail customerservice@hogrefe.com
UK:	Hogrefe Publishing, c/o Marston Book Services Ltd., 160 Eastern Ave., Milton Park, Abingdon, OX14 4SB Phone +44 1235 465577, Fax +44 1235 465556; E-mail direct.orders@marston.co.uk
EUROPE:	Hogrefe Publishing, Merkelstr. 3, 37085 Göttingen, Germany Phone +49 551 99950-0, Fax +49 551 99950-111; E-mail publishing@hogrefe.com

OTHER OFFICES

CANADA:	Hogrefe Publishing, 82 Laird Drive, East York, Ontario M4G 3V1
SWITZERLAND:	Hogrefe Publishing, Länggass-Strasse 76, 3012 Bern

Printed and bound in the USA

ISBN 978-0-88937-571-0 (print) • ISBN 978-1-61676-571-2 (PDF) • ISBN 978-1-61334-571-9 (EPUB)
http://doi.org/10.1027/00571-000

Acknowledgments

Tell me with whom you associate, and I will tell you who you are.

Johann Wolfgang von Goethe

We would like to thank our colleagues, mentors, and friends, past, present, and future, in the Society of Clinical Geropsychology, for their passion for the profession and their commitment to early career clinicians and researchers.

Contributors

Rebecca S. Allen, PhD, ABPP
Department of Psychology
Alabama Research Institute on Aging
The University of Alabama
Tuscaloosa, AL, USA

Sherry A. Beaudreau, PhD, ABPP
Sierra Pacific Mental Illness Research and Clinical Center
VA Palo Alto Health Care System
Palo Alto, CA, USA

Department of Psychiatry and Behavioral Sciences
Stanford University School of Medicine Stanford, CA, USA

School of Psychology (honorary)
The University of Queensland
Brisbane, QLD Australia

Danielle N. Berkel, M.A.
Department of Psychology
University of Colorado at Colorado Springs
Colorado Springs, CO, USA

Shane S. Bush, PhD, ABPP
Long Island Neuropsychology, PC
Lake Ronkonkoma, NY, USA

University of Alabama
Tuscaloosa, AL, USA

Brian D. Carpenter, PhD
Department of Psychological and Brain Sciences
Washington University
St. Louis, MO, USA

Dolores Gallagher-Thompson, PhD, ABPP
Department of Psychiatry and Behavioral Sciences (Emeritus)
Stanford University School of Medicine Stanford, CA, USA

School of Psychology (honorary)
The University of Queensland
Brisbane, QLD Australia

Laura Gallego-Alberto, PhD
Universidad Autónoma de Madrid
Facultad de Psicología
Madrid, Spain

Alisa O'Riley Hannum, PhD, ABPP
PFC Floyd K. Lindstrom Outpatient Clinic
VA Eastern Colorado Healthcare System
Colorado Springs, CO, USA

Gregory A. Hinrichsen, PhD, ABPP
Icahn School of Medicine at Mount Sinai
New York, NY, USA

Lindsey Jacobs, PhD, MSPH, ABPP
Department of Psychiatry
Harvard Medical Center
VA Boston Healthcare System
Boston, MA, USA

Julia Kasl-Godley, PhD
Adjunct Faculty, Doctoral Program in Clinical Psychology Program, the Wright Institute

Berkeley Cognitive Behavioral Therapy Clinic, the Wright Institute
Berkeley, CA, USA

VA Hospice and Palliative Care Center, VA Palo Alto Health Care System
Palo Alto, CA, USA

Andrés Losada, PhD
Universidad Rey Juan Carlos
Facultad de Ciencias de la Salud
Madrid, Spain

Julie Lutz, PhD
Center for the Study and Prevention of Suicide
University of Rochester Medical Center
Rochester, NY, USA

María Márquez-González, PhD
Universidad Autónoma de Madrid
Facultad de Psicología
Madrid, Spain

Victor Molinari, PhD, ABPP
University of South Florida
Tampa, FL, USA

Nancy A. Pachana, PhD
School of Psychology
The University of Queensland
Brisbane, QLD, Australia

Kyle S. Page, PhD, ABPP
Edward Hines, Jr. VA Hospital
Hines, IL, USA

María S. Pedroso-Chaparro, MA
Universidad Autónoma de Madrid
Facultad de Psicología
Madrid, Spain

Matthew Picchiello, BA
Department of Psychological & Brain Sciences
Washington University
St. Louis, MO, USA

Candice D. Reel, MA
Department of Psychology
Alabama Research Institute on Aging
The University of Alabama
Tuscaloosa, AL, USA

Hillary J. Rouse, M.A.
University of South Florida
Tampa, FL, USA

Viktoriya Samarina, PhD
Sierra Pacific Mental Illness Research and Clinical Center
VA Palo Alto Health Care System
Palo Alto, CA, USA

Rachael Spalding, MS
Department of Psychology
West Virginia University
Morgantown, WV, USA

Ann M. Steffen, PhD, ABPP
Department of Psychological Sciences
University of Missouri – St. Louis
St. Louis, MO, USA

Madhuvanthi Suresh, MS
Palo Alto University
Palo Alto, CA, USA

Larry W. Thompson, PhD, ABPP
Department of Psychiatry and Behavioral Sciences (emeritus)
Stanford University School of Medicine Stanford, CA, USA

School of Psychology (honorary)
The University of Queensland
Brisbane, QLD, Australia

Stacey Wood, PhD, ABPP
Department of Psychology, Scripps College
Claremont, CA, USA

Nabeel T. Yehyawi, PsyD, ABPP
VA Central Iowa Health Care System
Des Moines, IA, USA

Preface

In this work, we have assembled experts in the field of clinical geropsychology to provide key theoretical constructs across a range of interventions and disorders. The chapters offer key readings on the topics covered, and copious case examples are offered. The text assumes a basic literacy with respect to psychological diagnosis, assessment, and intervention paradigms. Each chapter also addresses the cultural implications of the topic at hand, and how such considerations translate into practice.

Chapter 2 tackles the important subject of clinical assessment of older adults, including the clinical interview and a variety of common validated assessment tools for use with frequently presented syndromes such as depression and cognitive syndromes. The chapter emphasizes careful consideration of the unique circumstances and context of the older person, as variables such as having English as a second language, an earlier history of head trauma, or a recent loss may all affect the way a person presents and reacts to testing. It is easy to say this in a textbook; much harder to ferret out useful background information from a client who lacks any relatives or friends, or whose medical chart is complex and contradictory. But the effort to understand the person as fully as possible leads to the most useful and complete clinical picture.

Cognitive behavioral therapy (CBT), the most common and widely researched intervention in older populations, is discussed regarding its application to depression, again one of the most common presentations of older adults to mental health services, in Chapter 3. Conceptualizing depression in older adults and working through the therapeutic process are reviewed. Chapter 3 also discusses how positive psychology principles and strategies of change can be integrated into existing CBT interventions with older adults.

Chapter 4 brings together Case-Based Approaches With Older Adults: Acceptance and Commitment Therapy, Interpersonal Psychotherapy, and Dialectical Behavior Therapy with older adults. For each type of intervention, its condensed background theory and basic principles of its application are given, and illustrated with an expanded case example. Modifications of approaches with older adults are highlighted.

Anxiety symptoms and disorders, although highly prevalent among older populations, are often not given as much attention across clinical settings. In Chapter 5, diagnosis, assessment, and treatment approaches for anxiety disorders are described. Key issues to keep in mind to avoid diagnostic and assessment misdirections are given. Posttraumatic stress disorder is also discussed in this chapter, with a detailed case discussion presented.

Working with older persons living with dementia and those who care for them is the topic of Chapter 6. A brief overview of dementia is followed by recommendations. Finally, lifestyle interventions to reduce the likelihood of dementia are discussed. The last are an important growth area in research as well as in practical applications when working with older persons.

Long-term care (LTC) settings are one of the richest and most fulfilling environments for psychologists to work in. Why is this? LTC interventions (and often assessments) must take a systems perspective, and often a systems approach to implementation, if they are to be successful. While demanding, such an approach can also yield gains across the entire facility. Chapter 7 covers theoretical models of care, as well as practical intervention strategies, in LTC settings.

Especially for early career psychologists, determining decisional capacity in older adults can be daunting. Chapter 8 discussed key issues in determining capacity, including issues of culture and family dynamics. Ethical and legal considerations are detailed, and the process of undertaking capacity assessments is laid out in detail, with a complex medicolegal case example presented to highlight key issues in practice.

Chapter 9 addresses the underresearched but incredibly clinically important topic of elder abuse, with particular emphasis on identifying and acting on risk. Culturally specific conceptualizations of abuse are offered. Strategies for screening for elder abuse are described, and issues arising in the reporting of abuse are detailed.

Psychological interventions developed for use in palliative care contexts are described in Chapter 10. Palliative care practice guidelines are discussed; the interventions are informed by developmental theory. Advance care planning and common issues arising in the last phase of life are also covered here.

The psychological sequelae of grief and loss, as well as death and dying, are covered in Chapter 11. A variety of interventions are described, including the use of acceptance and commitment therapy and mindfulness interventions in palliative care contexts. Factors affecting bereavement in care partners, and appropriate interventions in these circumstances, are also discussed. The case examples in Chapters 10 and 11 are linked to illustrate end-of-life complexities.

Understanding the context and application of assessment and intervention strategies with older persons is useful both for established practitioners encountering increasing numbers of older adults in their practice and for young professionals entering a field where the likelihood of seeing older adults professionally is ever-increasing. For practitioners who have not seen a large number of older clients, irrespective of their maturity within general professional practice, treating older clients can be daunting. Medical illnesses, unfamiliar medications and their side effects, and complex sociodemographic histories can seem bewildering. We have pitched the text to make sense of these complexities and contextualize them without diminishing the importance of a thorough understanding of older persons themselves.

The importance of understanding specific ethical and systemic issues in working with older persons is highlighted across chapters. Case examples or vignettes are given in each chapter to bring the work to life. Please note that significant details about all cases described in this work have been changed to maintain confidentiality and privacy. Recommended readings are provided at the end of each chapter.

Where to go for further information on working with older adults? A great place to start is the Council of Professional Geropsychology Training Programs (CoPGTP) [https://copgtp.org/] and GeroCentral [https://gerocentral.org/], both excellent online resources. The top professional organizations such as the Society of Clinical Geropsychology (APA Division 12/ii), Psychologists in Long-Term Care (PLTC), the International Psychogeriatric Association (IPA), and the Gerontological Society of America are well worth exploring for the value of their networking and informational resources; all are easily findable online.

If this volume inspires interest in readers who may desire to gain advanced expertise in clinical geropsychology, the authors hope that they will consider becoming certified as specialists. The American Board of Professional Psychology (ABPP) is the major credentialing organization in the US that certifies specialists, and since 2014 there has been a specialty board in geropsychology (American Board of Geropsychology; ABGERO). Certification requires not only specialized education and supervised training, but also demonstration of competence in assessment, intervention, and consultation with older adults, by oral examination. Such a process allows the public and other health care professionals to identify those who have been designated to be competent in professional geropsychology. For more information, please go to the ABGERO website (https://abgero.org/).

Nancy A. Pachana
Victor Molinari
Larry W. Thompson
Dolores Gallagher-Thompson

Contents

Chapter 1
Introduction to Working With Older Adults

Nancy A. Pachana
Larry W. Thompson

Introduction

Working with people from a psychological perspective increasingly focuses on the individual and their needs. The field of psychology is becoming less concerned with testing the dogmas of schools of thought and more focused on what interventions work for which people, under which circumstances. One group for whom the focus of psychological enquiry has increased is older adults, who represent an increasing proportion of the population across the globe (see Figure 1.1).

Figure 1.1 is worth keeping in mind for psychologists, as demographics play an important part in government and private sector planning, innovation, and spending for health care. As clinicians, we also find that demographics play a key role in how we envision the clinical populations we serve, and how these populations are changing over time. Changing demographics around age are not a temporary state of affairs, but rather represent the state of the globe for the foreseeable future. And it is also not simply the number of older adults that is increasing worldwide; lifespan is also increasing around the globe (see Figure 1.2).

However, perhaps the key to clinical gerontology is the ability to recognize the individuality of the patient, and hence the wide varieties of thinking and behaviors that this age group can demonstrate. As people age, they become more and more heterogeneous (Pachana, 2016). This is due to the accumulation of everything from life experiences, positive and negative, to life choices, including lifestyle choices as they relate to health. This then means that a person in later life is a unique combination of past medical, social, physical and psychological health and well-being, as well as a complex amalgamation of beliefs, preferences, and goals. This complexity presents itself daily in clinical practice. Cohort effects are important here, as the formative experiences of older persons earlier in life will have lasting impacts on all aspects of functioning, as well as approaches to their own problem solving and belief systems (including views on self-efficacy and buying into ageist stereotypes). This is another important issue in clinical practice, where the therapist and the client often come from different cohorts, and will have to work together to come to a

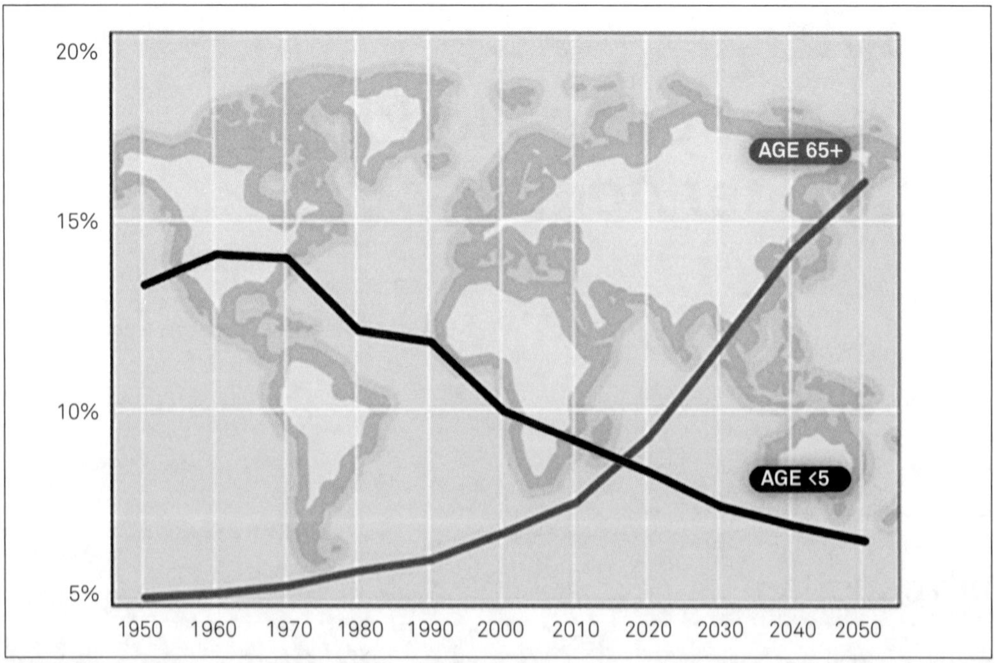

Figure 1.1 Demographic changes in aging: 1950-2050
Note. Reprinted with permission from *World Population Prospects: The 2004 Revision*, by United Nations, 2005.

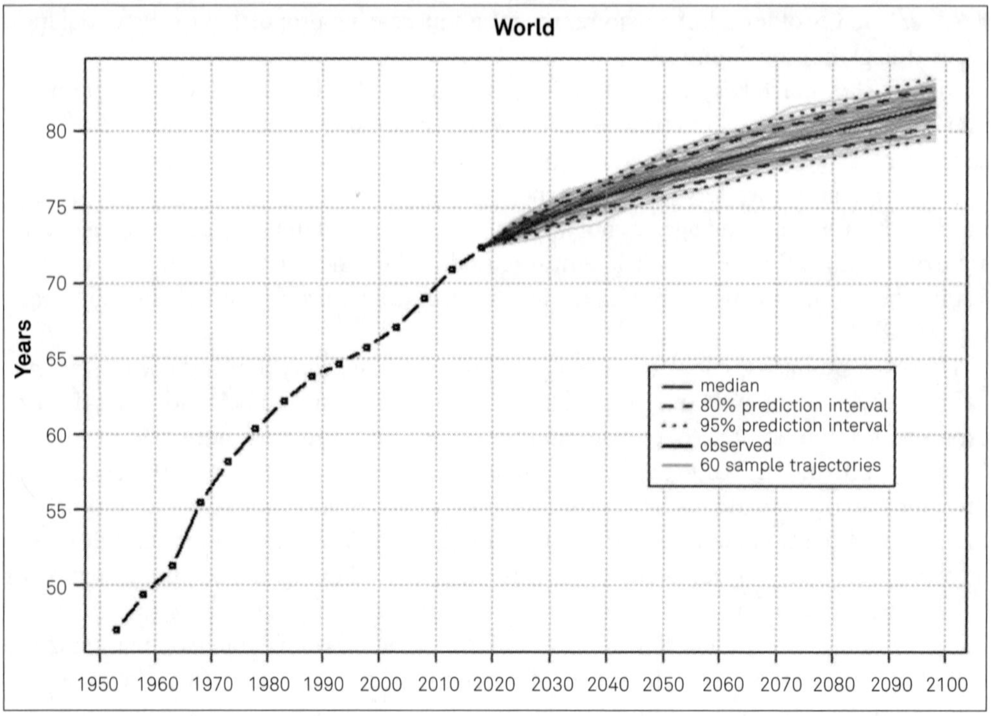

Figure 1.2 Increasing lifespan worldwide
Note. From World Population Prospects 2019, by DESA, Population Division, United Nations, (http://population.un.org/wpp/).

mutual understanding. Recognition of this multifactorial presentation is required of clinicians not just to get a good clinical history, but also to develop real rapport and a solid working relationship with their clients.

In an era of precision medicine, with its promise of molecularly tailored solutions to diseases, informed by genetics, psychology may look distinctly "old school" in its reliance on paper and pencil tests and face-to-face conversations to deliver person centered care. Yet a strength of psychology is its adaptation to current technological and measurement advances (e.g., telehealth and functional magnetic resonance imaging) in continuing to pursue the quest for the relief of symptoms of distress, and the fostering of skills to assist coping and flourishing with respect to mental well-being. The forward direction of psychology appears to be in entertaining less concern for particular assessment and intervention techniques that are effective across all populations, and more emphasis on discovering which approaches are most effective for persons from particular age cohorts, cultural backgrounds, and individual contexts. The field is also increasingly interested in the most effective procedures which can translate into real-world health care systems and communities of practice. Implementation science is still in many ways in its infancy, but in terms of building best practice models, such approaches are extremely important.

Changes in health globally also demonstrate that in most countries, increased lifespan has been matched with increasing health span. The US has seen some sliding on mortality and morbidity, mainly due to uninsured persons and the opioid crisis. However, globally, many countries are experiencing real gains in active health span, as well as in older adults working longer. It is important for clinical geropsychologists, particularly those in training or early in their professional careers, to recognize the changes across cohorts in terms of health, employment, and social and financial expectations, so that connections with older clients are not clouded by stereotypes or outmoded expectations (Laidlaw & Pachana, 2009). It is also increasingly clear that health solutions, particularly for older adults, will often have to occur in a multidisciplinary context. Many of the chapters in this book speak to the need to understand and work with other disciplines to achieve optimal outcomes.

As a field, clinical geropsychology has been sensitive to the training implications of demographic imperatives worldwide. All of the chapters in this work reference the Pikes Peak geropsychology competencies for trainees and psychologists (Knight et al., 2009). These competencies (which can be found listed in Appendix 1) include attitudinal, knowledge, and skills competencies for practice in professional geropsychology. Additionally, the Pikes Peak model requires familiarity with the importance of using a multimethod and interdisciplinary approach, and of clinical work that is sensitive to cultural differences and diversity. The Pikes Peak Knowledge and Skills Assessment Tool (Appendix 2; Karel et al., 2012) should be considered an important tool for informing clinical geropsychology practice; ratings as novice, intermediate, advanced, proficient, and expert, based on anchor items reflecting the various competencies can help guide continuing education as well as matching current skill levels to changing clinical demands in the workplace. The Pikes Peak competencies speak to a desire both to inform early career psychologists about the breadth and depth of knowledge required for competence in the field, and to provide a similar service to more mature practitioners wishing to shift their practices to serve more older adults. Increasingly, clinicians will wish to increase their skills in treating older adults, and we are hoping this text helps to meet those needs.

Age-Related Changes – The Big Picture

The following represents a brief overview of common age-related changes that one can expect to encounter when assessing and treating an older adult. The interested reader seeking further information is referred to any of the more comprehensive texts listed at the end of this chapter in the section Suggested General Resources for Clinical Gerontology.

The World Health Organization (WHO) definition of health states that health goes beyond simple physical health to embrace "a complete state of physical, mental, and social well-being, and not merely the absence of disease or infirmity" (WHO, 1948). Thus, when considering age-related changes, such physical, mental, and social changes should be considered together, with the understanding, as stated above, that older adults are heterogeneous and are not all aging in the same way (Pachana, 2016). Indeed, various parts of the brain and body within a single person do not all age at the same rate; likewise, aspects of psychological and social functioning may be more or less well-preserved. Finally, acute illnesses such as delirium may diminish functioning, particularly cognitive functioning, for a short time, but treatment can (and very often does) restore functioning. This is particularly important to note in determining capacity. Similarly, changes in lifestyle can improve health and well-being. Aging should not be thought of as linear decline; it is a dynamic, responsive process. For example, for many years, personality was seen to be set in stone quite early in adulthood; now we know that personality shifts occur over the entire lifespan (Schwaba & Bleidorn, 2018) and are also linked with culture and ethnicity (Chopik & Kitayama, 2018).

Important health conditions associated with increasing age include chronic obstructive pulmonary disease, cancer, osteoarthritis, macular degeneration, type 2 diabetes, hypertension, and Alzheimer's and Parkinson's diseases; these conditions often share underlying basic biological mechanisms (such as inflammation) but are also greatly impacted by sociodemographic and lifestyle factors (Franceschi et al., 2018). Older adults over age 65 generally have at least one chronic illness for which they are taking a regular medication. All of the diseases listed here, along with others that may be encountered by clinicians, have the potential to negatively impact cognition and mental health, as well as to cause functional limitations (e.g., instrumental activities of daily living, or IADLs). Understanding the impact both of common medical conditions as well as medication side effects, on cognitive and emotional function is very important, as polypharmacy is also an issue among older persons. Between 1988 and 2010, the median number of prescription medications used among adults aged 65 and older in the US doubled from two to four, while the proportion taking five or more medications tripled from 12.8% to 39.0% (Charlesworth et al., 2015). Medication side effects may often underpin changes in cognition or affect. Here again, the point should be underlined about the importance of collaborative work and good communication channels with other health care professionals.

Cognitive changes with aging involve the interplay between changes in the brain and physical and psychological health, as well as lifestyle behaviors (O'Hara, 2020; Pachana, 2016). Important brain changes with increasing age include declines in production of neurotransmitters and of the sensitivity of neuroreceptors, which can influence mood and behavior, as well as cognitive functioning. Cumulative small changes in brain structures, such as minor vascular events which can negatively impact the white matter connective fibers in the brain, may contribute to slower speeds of physical reaction times and of cognitive processing speed, and slower word or memory retrieval. Age-related changes, as mentioned, can vary across individuals, particularly impacted by prior levels of education, occupational history, and social factors such as isolation. Older adults can also compensate for decrements in cognitive functioning by recruiting more intact portions of the brain, a process Park and colleagues call *scaffolding* (Reuter-Lorenz & Park, 2014).

Typically, normal, expected age-related changes in cognition include declines in memory and executive functioning; these changes are commonly of a magnitude that might be characterized as annoying without significantly affecting daily functioning. There are several types of memory: short-term and working memory (information we are currently using, like remembering a telephone number in order to dial it), episodic memory (memory for past events, i.e., autobiographical memories as well as more recent experiences), semantic memory (memory for facts), and procedural memory (memory for skills and tasks, such as how to ride a bike or swing a tennis racquet). The greatest declines in later life are seen in episodic memory, followed by short-term memory, while procedural memory is relatively preserved.

Similarly, executive functioning encompasses a broad suite of skills including planning, emotional regulation, and goal directed activities. Again, older adults may find declines in their abilities to plan or in goal-directed activities, while because of changes in neurotransmitter functioning, emotional regulation is actually better later than earlier in life (Lantrip & Huang, 2017).

Thus, multiple factors can influence the cognitive changes seen in later life, and clinicians need to be inclusive in their formulations and strategies for intervention when faced with such changes. While many of these are due to physiological changes in the brain, many may be minimized or even corrected with proper attention and healthy lifestyle change. Moreover, and critically, involvement of the older adult in understanding their goals for both assessment and intervention is critical, and their views should directly inform interventions (Pachana et al., 2010).

Older adults value their independence, which is why functional limitations may cause more distress than physical or even psychiatric symptoms. Functional declines such as muscle weakness, gait instability, and limitations in *activities of daily living* (ADLs) and *instrumental activities of daily living* (IADLs) are not only tied to medical conditions but are also related to lifestyle behaviors such as excessive alcohol consumption (León-Muñoz et al., 2017) and sleep difficulties (Stone et al., 2018), and have been shown in some studies to differ between ethnic groups (McGrath et al., 2017).

An understanding of dementia is crucial for clinicians working with older persons. Alzheimer's disease and vascular dementia are among the most common forms of dementia, all of which include family history of the illness as a nonmodifiable risk factor (Pachana, 2016). Potentially modifiable risk factors for increased risk of dementia of these types include high blood pressure and high serum cholesterol, presence of diabetes and stroke, and incidence of head injury; protective factors include a diet low in fat and regular consumption of fish, and a nonsedentary lifestyle, with avoidance of smoking particularly associated with lower risk of Alzheimer's disease (Patterson et al., 2007). The impact of sleep disturbance on both risk of dementia as well as its symptoms, particularly memory and behavioral sequelae, is a growing area of research, which also holds some promise for symptom amelioration (Shi et al., 2018). Thus, positive lifestyle interventions should be considered, along with more specific psychological and behavioral interventions when treating persons living with dementia.

Culture plays an important role in beliefs and attitudes toward dementia, risk factors for dementia, and the impact of dementia upon caregivers of those living with the disease. In both assessment and treatment, it is best practice for psychologists to be aware of the impact of culture and ethnicity on tests, assessment results, intervention strategies, and available collateral and community support for both persons living with dementia and those who care for them (American Psychological Association [APA], 2012). An often-overlooked cultural population with respect to dementia is Indigenous peoples. Dementia is the most common age-related cognitive condition among Aboriginal peoples (Bennett, 2008). Culture-based public health system approaches have produced positive health outcomes in American Indian, Alaska Native, and Native Hawaiian populations and have implications for research and practice in the dementia context, but this remains an underresearched area (Browne et al., 2017).

The topics covered above are expanded on and linked with case examples in the following chapters; the above is just a brief overview. Whenever one is writing a text, one is conscious of how research and practice may be evolving, and there is a recent development that bears mentioning here. It is impossible for us not to mention the significant global impact of the disease caused by a novel coronavirus, referred to as COVID-19, on both the global human population in general, and older adults specifically. In the course of writing this text, there have occurred epic shifts in medical and psychological service delivery (via telehealth), the rise of awareness of ageism in framing the impact of the virus, and an understanding of how social distancing has impacted care, particularly for those in nursing homes and palliative care settings. We believe that the material covered in this text is relevant in guiding a professional and empathic response to the mental health aspects of this crisis. Social distancing may have profound effects on older populations for whom it is known that social isolation negatively impacts health and well-being. Gaps in the availability of everything from elective surgery to primary care consultations to certain medications may be an additional source of morbidity and mortality for older persons. This book will go to press as many of these situations in the world are evolving, and particularly impacting front-line clinicians. The best advice at this stage is to be guided by best-practice approaches for scientist-practitioners: Be aware of the clinical research (as described above and illustrated in the following chapters) as well as the major psychological theories of aging, which take into account critical factors such as cohort effects, coping and adaptive strategies, and resilience.

Important Overarching Psychological Theories of Aging

One of the most important theories of adaptation in later life is Paul Baltes's *selective optimization with compensation* theory of successful aging (Baltes & Baltes, 1990). This theory suggests that individuals who age successfully actively use three strategies to make this transition into later life possible: selection, optimization, and compensation. *Selection* includes identifying relevant goals, prioritizing them, and recognizing when they have been achieved. *Optimization* refers to the use of strategies to facilitate successful achievement of set goals. *Compensation* refers to the individual adapting to limitations (perhaps due to aging processes) that interfere with getting to their goal.

With regard to the example of COVID-19, how can older adults successfully adapt to these unprecedented circumstances? First, older adults might select the things that are most important to them; since isolation from family, particularly grandchildren, is viewed as a major source of distress, overcoming this isolation may be prioritized as a goal. This goal perhaps in the current circumstances takes precedence over lesser goals (meeting friends, going out for dinner). Optimization refers to a strategy to achieve the goal; potentially here it is setting up regular daily short sessions over the telephone or internet. Compensation involves problem solving about what might interfere with goal attainment, and here this might include buying the older adult (or the children!) a mobile device or computer to facilitate the maintenance of social contact.

Social support and social networks are increasingly recognized as having positive benefits for everything from brain health to positive aging (Pachana, 2016). The finding that older individuals report equal, if not greater, levels of social support than do younger age groups intrigued Stanford University researcher Laura Carstensen (Carstensen et al., 1999), who developed *socioemotional selectivity theory* to make sense of how growing older shifts how people view their friendship networks. The key lies in perception of time – as we age, we recognize that we have lived more of our lives than we have left to live, and this leads us to prioritize those relationships from which the greatest meaning and satisfaction are derived. In later life, the number of people in one's social network declines, and this was thought to be due passive attrition due to death or incapacity. Carstensen demonstrated that older adults selectively prune their social networks to include those who offer the strongest social support, moving away from sources of unsatisfactory or unreliable support (English & Carstensen, 2014). The sense of having limited time left also drives people toward activities which are more meaningful, and leads to greater generativity, a feature of Gene Cohen's complimentary theory of phases of human potential (Cohen, 2005). Cohen proposes a series of human potential phases, which "reflect evolving mental maturity, ongoing human development, and psychological growth as we age" (Cohen, 2005, p. 7).

In a period when many people, not just older adults, have a feeling of a potentially foreshortened future, Carstensen's and Cohen's theories are apt for those working with this population. Cartensen's theory proposes that individuals cultivate networks that give maximal support; many older persons have found increased social supports online in response to COVID-19, but those left on the wrong side of the so-called digital divide require increased support and attention. The confines of various forms of lockdown can be reframed as time to focus on meaningful activities, and for many older adults this involves reaching out in terms of volunteering or otherwise making use of personal resources. Both theories underscore the drive for meaningful connection in later life, which is often associated with resilience.

Resilience, meaning broadly an individual's adaptation to stress and adversity, is a construct which has been researched throughout the lifespan, including later life. Resilience is usually studied at the individual level, but it can also operate at a group level, and can be measured at the level of households, families, neighborhoods, communities, and societies.

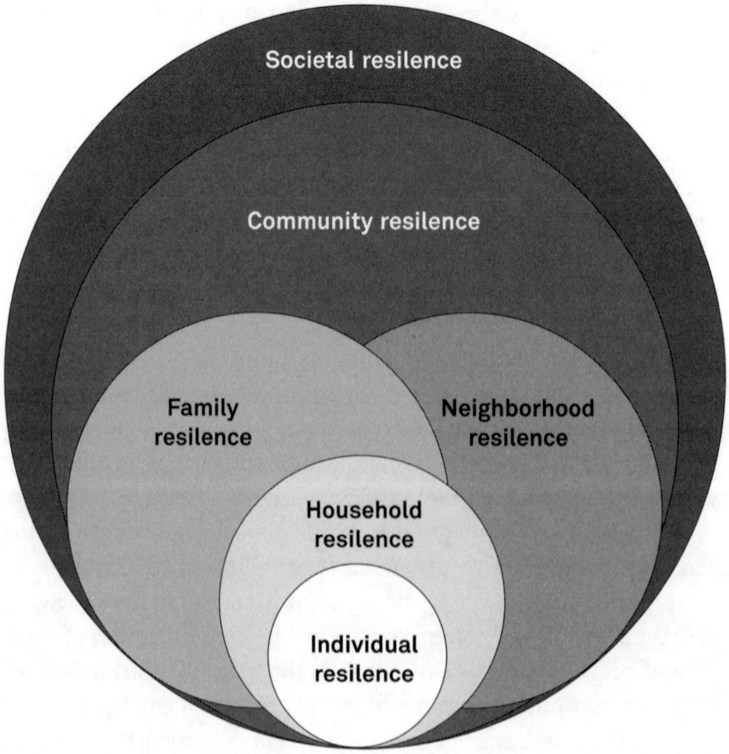

Figure 1.3 Model of resilience

Note. Reprinted with permission from "Resilience: Thoughts on the Value of the Concept for Critical Gerontology," by K. Wild et al., 2013. *Ageing & Society, 33*, p. 137–158. © Ageing and Society, 2013.

In Figure 1.3, Wild and colleagues (2013) highlight not only these conceptualizations of resilience but also the differing scales of resilience that impact older adults' ability to cope with adverse circumstances.

Clinical psychologists also often conceptualize resilience as an individual trait, but the experience to date with COVID-19 shows the value of all levels of resilience, from household "bubbles" where people shelter in place, to societal and national levels of resilience, in everything from health care services to supply chains. For older adults, these ties have been severely tested, with everything from lack of family at the bedside while dying, to nursing home lockdowns causing huge distress to families and residents alike (Pachana et al., 2020). Research pre-dating COVID-19 demonstrates the range of factors associated with resilience in later life. In the large US Successful Aging Evaluation (SAGE) study, after adjusting for age, a higher self-rating for successful aging was associated with higher education levels, better cognitive functioning, better perceived physical and mental health, a reduced amount of depression, and greater optimism and resilience (Jeste et al., 2012). These same factors may be associated with resilience during the COVID-19 global pandemic, and clinical geropsychologists will have an important role to play in advocating for mental health services for older adults.

Lastly, immigration and acculturation are tied to mental health in older adults. Worldwide, the median age of international migrants is 38.4 years, almost a decade older than the median global age of 29.2 years, with international migrants in particular suffering increased mental health problems coupled with increased barriers to accessing mental health services (Pachana, 2016). This is particularly true in the US for recent older immigrants (Choi et al., 2016). Values and beliefs about aging, roles and responsibilities (often gendered) in later life, and what is a good death, are all shaped by one's cultural values, and often thrown into turmoil for immigrants. In some studies, immigrants have been shown to have a higher prevalence of dementia compared with their US-born counterparts (Moon et al., 2019).

In the current COVID-19 crisis, ageism and xenophobia have both left older immigrants feeling rejected by their societies. Older immigrants may be more likely to experience both loneliness and social isolation, due to language barriers and lack of acculturation, especially among recent immigrants. First-generation immigrants also have lower rates of health service utilization for both mood and anxiety disorders (Bauldry & Szaflarski, 2017). Asian immigrants of all ages have experienced increased stigma globally due to the virus possibly originating in China. While communities and governments have sought to encourage support for immigrants and discourage stigma against older adults as well as Asian immigrants, older migrants will no doubt still be very vulnerable to psychological distress in the current crisis.

Globally, we are in a time of transition, one that includes a heightened awareness of the value of social contact, and the necessity of strong societal supports for all citizens. Older adults and their resilience as well as vulnerabilities have also been spotlighted. Those working to restore and maintain the wellbeing of the older members within our communities should be inspired to redouble efforts to ensure this group is well understood, and receives the highest standard of clinical care.

Suggested Resources for Clinical Gerontology

Bush, S., Allen, R., & Molinari, V. (2016). *Ethical practice in geropsychology.* American Psychological Association.

Fingerman, K., Berg, C., Antonucci, T., & Smith, J. (Eds.). (2011). *Handbook of lifespan development*. Springer.

Knight, B. (Ed.). (2020). *Encyclopedia of clinical geropsychology*. Oxford University Press.

Lichtenberg, P. A., & Mast, B. T. (Eds.). (2015). *APA handbook of clinical geropsychology: Vol. 1. History and status of the field and perspectives on aging, and Vol. 2. Assessment, treatment, and issue of later life*. American Psychological Association.

Mehrotra, C., & Wagner, L. S. (2019). *Aging and diversity: An active learning experience* (3rd ed.). Routledge.

O'Hara, R. (Ed.). (2020). *Handbook on mental health and aging.* Elsevier.

Pachana, N. A. (2016). *Very short introduction to aging*. Oxford University Press.

Pachana, N. A., & Laidlaw, K. (Eds.). (2014). *Oxford handbook of clinical geropsychology: International perspectives.* Oxford University Press.

Sue, D. W., Sue, D., Neville, H. A., & Smith, L. (2019). *Counseling the culturally diverse: Theory and practice.* Wiley.

Whitfield, K., & Baker, T. (Eds.). (2013). *Handbook of minority aging.* Springer. https://doi.org/10.1891/9780826109644

References

American Psychological Association. (2012). Guidelines for the evaluation of dementia and age-related cognitive change. *American Psychologist, 67*(1), 1–9. https://doi.org/10.1037/a0024643

Baltes, P. B., & Baltes, M. M. (1990). Psychological perspectives on successful aging: The model of selective optimization with compensation. In P. B. Baltes & M. M. Baltes (Eds.), *Successful aging: Perspectives from the behavioral sciences* (pp. 1–34). Cambridge University Press. https://doi.org/10.1017/CBO9780511665684.003

Bauldry, S., & Szaflarski, M. (2017). Immigrant-based disparities in mental health care utilization. *Socius, 3*. https://doi.org/10.1177/2378023116685718

Bennett, D. A. (2008). Cognitive health in indigenous peoples. *Neurology*, 71, 1466–1467. https://doi.org/10.1212/01.wnl.0000326063.56822.22

Browne, C. V., Ka'opua, L. S., Jervis, L. L., Alboroto, R., & Trockman, M. L. (2017). United States Indigenous populations and dementia: Is there a case for culture-based psychosocial interventions? *The Gerontologist, 57*(6), 1011–1019. https://doi.org/10.1093/geront/gnw059

Carstensen, L. L., Isaacowitz, D. M., & Charles, S. T. (1999). Taking time seriously: A theory of socioemotional selectivity. *American Psychologist, 54*(3), 165–181. https://doi.org/10.1037/0003-066X.54.3.165

Charlesworth, C. J., Smit, E., Lee, D. S., Alramadhan, F., & Odden, M. C. (2015). Polypharmacy among adults aged 65 years and older in the United States: 1988-2010. Journals of Gerontology. *Series A, Biological Sciences and Medical Sciences, 70*(8), 989–995. https://doi.org/10.1093/gerona/glv013

Choi, S., Kim, G., & Lee, S. (2016). Effects of nativity, length of residence, and county-level foreign-born density on mental health among older adults in the US. *Psychiatric Quarterly, 87*(4), 675-688. https://doi.org/10.1007/s11126-016-9418-2

Chopik, W. J., & Kitayama, S. (2018). Personality change across the life span: Insights from a cross-cultural, longitudinal study. *Journal of Personality, 86*(3), 508-521. https://doi.org/10.1111/jopy.12332

Cohen, G. D. (2005). *The mature mind: The positive power of the aging brain.* Basic Books.

English, T., & Carstensen, L. L. (2014). Selective narrowing of social networks across adulthood is associated with improved emotional experience in daily life. *International journal of behavioral development, 38*(2), 195–202.

Franceschi, C., Garagnani, P., Morsiani, C., Conte, M., Santoro, A., Grignolio, A., Monti, D., Capri, M., & Salvioli, S. (2018). The continuum of aging and age-related diseases: Common mechanisms but different rates. *Frontiers in Medicine, 5*, 61. https://doi.org/10.3389/fmed.2018.00061

Jeste, D. V., Savla, G. N., Thompson, W. K., Vahia, I. V., Glorioso, D. K., Martin, A. S., Palmer, B. W., Rock, D., Golshan, S., Kraemer, H. C. & Depp, C. A. (2012). Association between older age and more successful aging: Critical role of resilience and depression. *American Journal of Psychiatry, 170*(2), 188–96. https://doi.org/10.1176/appi.ajp.2012.12030386

Karel, M. J., Holley, C. K., Whitbourne, S. K., Segal, D. L., Tazeau, Y. N., Emery, E. E., Molinari, V., Yang, J., & Zweig, R. A. (2012). Preliminary validation of a tool to assess knowledge and skills for professional geropsychology practice. *Professional Psychology: Research and Practice, 43*(2), 110–117. https://doi.org/10.1037/a0025788

Knight, B. G., Karel, M. J., Hinrichsen, G. A., Qualls, S. H., & Duffy, M. (2009). Pikes Peak model for training in professional geropsychology. *American Psychologist, 64*(3), 205–214. https://doi.org/10.1037/a0015059

Laidlaw, K., & Pachana, N. A. (2009) Aging, mental health, and demographic change. *Professional Psychology: Research and Practice, 40*(6), 601–608. https://doi.org/10.1037/a0017215

Lantrip, C., & Huang, J. H. (2017). Cognitive control of emotion in older adults: A review. *Clinical psychiatry (Wilmington, Del.), 3*(1), 9. https://doi.org/10.21767/2471-9854.100040

León-Muñoz, L. M., Guallar-Castillón, P., García-Esquinas, E., Galán, I., & Rodríguez-Artalejo, F. (2017). Alcohol drinking patterns and risk of functional limitations in two cohorts of older adults. *Clinical Nutrition, 36*(3), 831–838. https://doi.org/10.1016/j.clnu.2016.05.005

McGrath, R. P., Ottenbacher, K. J., Vincent, B. M., Kraemer, W. J., & Peterson, M. D. (2017). Muscle weakness and functional limitations in an ethnically diverse sample of older adults. *Ethnicity & Health,* 1-12. https://doi.org/10.1080/13557858.2017.1418301

Moon, H., Badana, A. N., Hwang, S. Y., Sears, J. S., & Haley, W. E. (2019). Dementia prevalence in older adults: variation by race/ethnicity and immigrant status. *American Journal of Geriatric Psychiatry, 27*(3), 241–250. https://doi.org/10.1016/j.jagp.2018.11.003

O'Hara, R. (Ed.). (2020). *Handbook on mental health and aging.* Elsevier.

Pachana, N. A. (2016). *Very short introduction to aging.* Oxford University Press.

Pachana, N. A., Beattie, E., Byrne, G., & Brodaty, H. (2020). COVID-19 and psychogeriatrics: The view from Australia. *International Psychogeriatrics, 32*(10), 1135–1141. https://doi.org/10.1017/S1041610220000885

Pachana, N. A., Paton, H., & Squelch, N. (2010). The importance of feedback and communication strategies with older adults: Therapeutic and ethical considerations. In N. A. Pachana, K. Laidlaw, & B. G. Knight (Eds.), *Casebook of clinical geropsychology: International perspectives on practice* (pp. 155–177). Oxford University Press. https://doi.org/10.1093/med/9780199583553.003.0010

Patterson, C., Feightner, J., Garcia, A., & MacKnight, C. (2007). General risk factors for dementia: A systematic evidence review. *Alzheimer's & Dementia, 3*(4), 341-347. https://doi.org/10.1016/j.jalz.2007.07.001

Reuter-Lorenz, P. A., & Park, D. C. (2014). How does it STAC up? Revisiting the scaffolding theory of aging and cognition. *Neuropsychology review, 24*(3), 355–370. https://doi.org/10.1007/s11065-014-9270-9

Schwaba, T., & Bleidorn, W. (2018). Individual differences in personality change across the adult life span. *Journal of personality, 86*(3), 450–464. https://doi.org/10.1111/jopy.12327

Shi, L., Chen, S. J., Ma, M. Y., Bao, Y. P., Han, Y., Wang, Y. M., . . . Lu, L. (2018). Sleep disturbances increase the risk of dementia: A systematic review and meta-analysis. *Sleep Medicine Reviews, 40,* 4–16 https://doi.org/10.1016/j.smrv.2017.06.010

Stone, K. L., Blackwell, T., Ancoli-Israel, S., Ensrud, K. E., Kado, D. M., Wallace, M. L., Cawthon, P. M., & Buysse, D. J. (2018). Sleep health and functional limitations in older adults. *Innovation in Aging, 2*(Suppl 1), 548. https://doi.org/10.1093/geroni/igy023.2024

United Nations, Department of Economic and Social Affairs, Population Division. (2019). *World population prospects 2019: Volume 2: Demographic profiles.*

United Nations, Department of Economic and Social Affairs, Population Division. (2004). *World population prospects: The 2004 revision.*

Wild, K., Wiles, J. L., & Allen, R. E. (2013). Resilience: Thoughts on the value of the concept for critical gerontology. *Ageing & Society, 33*(1), 137–158. https://doi.org/10.1017/S0144686X11001073

World Health Organization. (1948). Preamble to the Constitution of WHO as adopted by the International Health Conference, New York, 19 June–22 July 1946; signed on 22 July 1946 by the representatives of 61 States and entered into force on 7 April 1948. *Official Records of WHO,* no. 2, p. 100.

Chapter 2

Assessment Approaches for Psychiatric and Cognitive Syndromes

Viktoriya Samarina
Madhuvanthi Suresh
Matthew Picchiello
Julie Lutz
Brian D. Carpenter
Sherry A. Beaudreau

Introduction

Competent assessment is an essential functional skill for working with older adults. The following chapter describes basic principles for assessing an older population and serves as a primer for students or clinicians with limited experience in assessing older adults. Moreover, experienced geropsychology specialists may find this chapter useful when reviewing cases and working with patients.

One of the most important considerations in assessing late-life mental health is the ubiquity of co-occurring psychiatric and cognitive syndromes. On the one hand, older adults with psychiatric disorders often show signs of cognitive impairment, particularly executive dysfunction or memory deficits (Beaudreau & O'Hara, 2009; O'Hara, 2012). On the other hand, many older adults with cognitive syndromes have psychiatric symptoms or disorders, often termed "neuropsychiatric symptoms" based on the assumption that the mental health syndrome is part of a larger neurocognitive process (Taragano et al., 2008). Determining whether symptoms warrant a psychiatric diagnosis, cognitive diagnosis, or both is a common question for geropsychological assessment, as illustrated in the following case example referral:

> Mr. J. is a 75-year-old African-American man, recently widowed from his wife of 55 years, Jean, who died 9 months ago of cancer. Mr. J.'s oldest daughter, Janelle, lives in the nearby town and has been worried about her father's health over the last couple months due to his difficulty with activities of daily living, managing his chronic medical issues (e.g., type 2 diabetes mellitus), memory problems, motivational issues, and his recent comments about death while denying any plan to harm himself. His family have been thinking about moving Mr. J. to an assisted living facility, but he refuses. Mr. J.'s primary care physician recommended further testing by a geropsychologist to assess for possible depression and dementia, and to advise the patient and his family's in their decisions about his need for support services.

This referral includes several complex assessment issues regarding possible psychiatric and cognitive difficulties, interacting psychosocial and medical etiologies, and concerns about functional impairment and safety. Such complex issues are frequently encountered in assessing older adults.

The overarching goals of a competent geropsychology assessment are to

> conduct clinical assessment leading to DSM diagnoses and other clinically relevant problems, formulation of treatment plans and, specifically, differential diagnosis (common problems and issues include but are not limited to depression, anxiety, grief, delirium, dementia; and medication and physical disorders and their effects on functioning). (American Board of Geropsychology [ABGERO], 2017, p. 32)

Also, clinicians need to demonstrate an ability to select and administer evidence-based measures and appropriate techniques for the evaluation of psychiatric, cognitive, decision-making, functional ability, and safety and risk issues in older adults (ABGERO, 2017). This chapter surveys information about basic geropsychological assessment methods as outlined in the Pikes Peak functional competencies for trainees and psychologists (Appendix 1; Knight et al., 2009). These competencies include knowledge of the theory and current conceptualizations that inform geropsychology assessment and the psychometric properties of tests used with older adults. Additionally, the Pikes Peak model requires familiarity with the importance of using a multimethod and interdisciplinary approach, and appropriate integration of collateral information from family, friends, or caregivers during the assessment.

After reviewing these general assessment issues, we review available evidence-based assessment measures, including how best to assess mental health and cognition in older adults with varying levels of cognitive functioning, from no impairment to dementia. Throughout the chapter, we also discuss diversity issues and how they may impact the overall assessment process. It is important to recognize that aging is a diversity variable and that many older adults also have unique backgrounds and identities that intersect with their status as an older adult. These intersecting identities include, but are not limited to, disability status, culture, race, ethnicity, sexual minority status and gender identity, religious background, native language, immigration status, and veteran status.

Basic Assessment Principles in Older Adults

A good psychological assessment involves gathering information from multiple sources to respond to a referral question. Referrals come from a variety of sources and may differ depending on the setting in which the clinician practices. Common referral sources include neurologists, psychiatrists, primary care providers, neurosurgeons, nurse practitioners, social workers, or other psychologists. Family members or the older adult may also self-refer if they have concerns about the older patient's cognitive functioning or mental health. In many cases, it is necessary to reach out to the referring provider to clarify the referral question and goals of the assessment, and to confirm that as a clinician you are able to address the question and concerns appropriately and competently (Hinrichsen, 2019).

Generally, the purpose of geropsychological assessments is to determine the presence or absence of psychiatric diagnoses and cognitive disorders. The clinician synthesizes the patient's medical, cognitive, and psychiatric history to form hypotheses about the etiology of the presenting problem. This information guides recommendations for further treatment or services to address any psychiatric and cognitive syndromes and related concerns. Referrals are often triggered by concerns about an older adult's safety, including, but not limited to, an ability to function independently while performing specific instrumental activities of daily living (IADLs; e.g., driving) or more general activities of daily living (ADLs; e.g., attending to basic hygiene). Other typical referral questions include differentiating between a mood disorder (e.g., depression) and dementia, or assessing capacity to make decisions. Unresolved diagnostic questions or issues raised during the evaluation often lead the clinician to recommend further specialized assessments from another professional.

Regarding the case example of Mr. J., it will be important to determine which diagnoses should be ruled out (e.g., dementia or depression), assess for suicide risk, and choose which measures can be used to assess these areas of concern. This information will help guide Mr. J. and his family's decision about his future living situation and potential need for additional care. Thus, the assessment recommendations often inform critical decisions of the older adults and their family members regarding housing, issues with autonomy, and the need for an additional evaluation of competency. These recommendations can include the need for further testing of medical or neurological issues through referral to a primary care or specialty provider, or an occupational or physical therapist, or a referral for a driving evaluation.

Mr. J.'s referral source is concerned that he might not be fit to live on his own. An older adult's safety and well-being should be routinely assessed, including any signs of elder abuse. Elder abuse includes not only physical and sexual abuse, in which there may be physical or other interpersonal warning signs observed with family members or caregivers, but also self-neglect and financial abuse which may not be as readily identified (for information about signs of elder abuse, see Acierno et al., 2010). If Mr. J. is unable to meet his basic needs – for instance, he does not meet general dietary guidelines and has poor hygiene – this could be an instance of self-neglect. Observations regarding whether Mr. J. behaves differently when his family is present (e.g., fearful, nervous, and quiet) compared with when he is alone with the clinician, can indicate the potential for other physical or emotional abuse by family. The concerns Mr. J. has about missing money from bank accounts or potential mismanagement by family should be assessed for potential financial abuse. In some cases, older adults with significant memory concerns will report that their checkbook, money, or purse was stolen in the absence of financial abuse – either because they have forgotten that someone else is managing their money or due to confusion if they have been misplacing important financial items. The source of any such financial concerns should be clarified and reported as required for licensed professionals in the state in which the geropsychologist practices.

Sources of Information

Prior to the in-person assessment, a medical chart review is often conducted. This review can alert the clinicians to diagnoses or issues that will need to be considered in addressing referral questions. Medical chart reviews can provide crucial information about the older adult's past psychiatric diagnoses and history of treatment, medical history, current medications and hospitalizations, previous cognitive and neuropsychological testing results, previous psychiatric or psychosocial assessments, and previous family involvement in their treatment. For Mr. J., the following information was gathered during a medical chart review to inform his assessment:

> According to his medical record, at his last appointment with his primary care physician, Mr. J. had lost 10 pounds (4.5 kg), explaining, "There's just me, and my wife did all the cooking. Sometimes I don't feel like eating so I have a bowl of cereal." He also acknowledges that he has not been checking his blood glucose levels for his type 2 diabetes, though he reports taking his diabetes medication as directed. His physician has known Mr. J. for many years and has been treating his hypertension and high cholesterol with several medications. In total, Mr. J. takes four medications and a daily multivitamin. Mr. J. also has sleep apnea, though he doesn't use his continuous positive airway pressure (CPAP) regularly, despite his physician's urging that he is depriving his brain of oxygen and that he may feel more rested and alert after using it. Early signs of a cataract have reduced Mr. J.'s visual acuity, making it harder for him to see clearly at night because of the increased glare. This has made him reluctant to drive at night.

The clinician follows up on this information during a clinical interview. This additional preparation can increase the focus of a clinical interview on pertinent questions about the patient's history. In this case example of Mr. J., questions about the management of his health conditions, such as his diabetes, which can affect mood and cognition, should be discussed during the clinical interview. The astute clinician will further consider the potential for malnourishment and any gross mismanagement of his medical conditions and thus the need to rule out self-neglect.

The Clinical Interview

A flexible, semistructured clinical interview lasting 30–90 minutes is used to gather information about the older adult's background such as social, educational, developmental, familial, medical, psychiatric, and psychological history, and available brain neuroimaging or other critical medical test results (e.g., blood tests). The clinician may also add informal questions about local current events or television shows to test the patient's orientation and memory, potentially informing the level of cognitive impairment and selection of cognitive tests the clinician will administer. Information collected during the clinical interview will assist the clinician in formulating appropriate diagnoses and treatment plans. Collateral informants often provide beneficial information to help with diagnoses and treatment planning (Allen & Becker, 2019). For older adults with cognitive impairment, who may have difficulty providing an accurate timeline of events or for whom insight may be limited, collateral information can be useful in providing observations about changes in the older adult's behavior, functioning, mood, or cognitive status, and a more complete history of problems. The use of collateral sources, with the older adults' assent, can be integral to the assessment. However, clinicians must be cautious about collateral informants who may have motives to gain information (e.g., financial information) or to minimize the patient's symptoms.

Behavioral observations provide context to the older adult's current symptoms and functioning, which will help with diagnosis. The clinician should observe the older adult's level of consciousness (e.g., lethargic, hyperactive), overall appearance (e.g., tone of voice, eye contact, facial expressions, hygiene, weather appropriate attire), motor activity (e.g., tics, tremors, hyperkinesia or hypokinesia, hemiplegia), mood and affect (e.g., depressed, anxious, happy, tearful, etc.), level of cooperativeness and motivation, and any difficulties with language, prosody, thinking, judgment, and memory (Strauss et al., 2006). Lack of motivation observed during testing can be psychiatric or related to medical conditions (e.g., history of stroke or other neurological diseases).

For Mr. J., the clinician will need to consider how involvement of his family can facilitate the assessment. This assessment will then need to address the following: (a) whether any cognitive symptoms are due to bereavement-related depression; (b) if Mr. J. had any previously undetected signs of dementia only obvious in the absence of the support provided by his now-deceased wife; (c) any recent changes in his health status; and (d) other acute issues that could impact both his cognition and mood, such as malnutrition or deviations from his usual medical care management. The clinician will also consider how his age, sex, educational status, race and ethnicity, and rural-dwelling status influence test selection and interpretation.

Competent assessment in geropsychology also requires clinician knowledge and skills indicative of late-life cultural competence. To familiarize the reader with the scope of the importance of cultural competence for geropsychological assessment, the next section briefly discusses assessment considerations and resources for culturally diverse assessment.

Cultural Considerations

The proportion of older ethnic and racial minorities in the US, especially Latinx, African-American, and Asian and Pacific Islander adults has surged and is projected to rise over the next 30 years (Talamantes & Sanchez-Reilly, 2010). These projections further signal the public health need for culturally competent geropsychologists (American Psychological Association, 2009). Many recommendations of the cultural competence in neuropsychology model are relevant to culturally competent mental health and cognitive assessment of older adults (Rivera Mindt et al., 2010), including (1) seeking competency through additional training if the clinician determines their cultural competence is limited (e.g., continuing education courses or specific seminars or workshops), (2) reading materials which focus on practicing with different ethnic minorities, and (3) consulting colleagues familiar with the ethnic minority population of interest. Readings and continuing education courses on assessment with cross-cultural populations are often offered through the American Psychological Association.

If the clinician determines they cannot ethically evaluate the patient due to lack of competence with the specific ethnic minority and is unable to obtain appropriate training due to either language restrictions or other factors, it is recommended they refer the patient to another appropriate clinician. If that is not possible, the clinician may use an interpreter or obtain supervision from another colleague who is culturally competent in working with the specific ethnic minority. In an emergency situation, a family member may be asked to help with the interview and translation if the older adult's primary language differs from the primary language of the clinician, although some older adults may not be as forthcoming with information when a family member is present.

The use of interpreters, though beneficial, can also cause biases in an evaluation. They may unintentionally or intentionally change the clinician's questions or the patient's responses. It may also be challenging to translate certain tests directly, or the interpretation may change the way the test is administered, which may result in inappropriate understanding of the findings (Fernández & Abe, 2018). The clinician should ensure that the interpreters with whom they work are highly trained in test interpretation, remain objective throughout the entire evaluation, and who will sign a confidentiality agreement and interpret exactly what both the clinician and the patient say (Gerolimatos et al., 2015). Whenever possible, it is best to refer the older adult to a provider who is fluent in the same language.

Culturally competent assessment with older adults also means that the geropsychologist considers how the cultural background of the older adult could potentially impact the validity of the assessment, and subsequently makes efforts to increase the validity of the assessment. For older adults from diverse cultural backgrounds, the culturally competent geropsychologist thoughtfully plans how the clinical interview is to be conducted, how the tests are selected and interpreted, and acknowledges the limits of tests in the final report. During the clinical interview, the clinician remains mindful of their level of formality, power, eye contact, and personal space, as these factors can differ among different ethnical backgrounds and cultures. Specific verbal and nonverbal communication cues from the clinician can also impact rapport building as it can demonstrate respect toward the patient.

It is critical to use appropriate nonbiased measurements when available. One cross-cultural screening measure of dementia is the Rowland Universal Dementia Assessment Scale (RUDAS; Storey et al., 2004). It has six items focusing on memory, planning and praxis, language, judgment, and drawing and body orientation. Administration takes about 10 minutes, and it can be translated into 30 languages without changing the format of the test. Another measure of general cognitive abilities is the Cognitive Abilities Screening Instrument (CASI; Teng et al., 1994). This measure has been culturally validated in Japan, China, and the US. The resulting score ranges from 0 to 100 and focuses on assessing attention, concentration, orientation, short- and long-term memory, language, visuospatial skills, fluency, judgment, and abstraction. This measure has been found helpful in screening for dementia and monitoring disease course, and takes about 15–20 minutes to administer. The Cross-Cultural Cognitive Examination (CCCE; Glosser et al., 1993) was developed for cross-cultural epidemiological dementia research with participants from Guam and the US. The measure evaluates attention, language, visuospatial skills, verbal and visual memory, short-term memory, abstraction, and psychomotor speed. The diagnosis of dementia is given if three or more of these areas are impaired. This test may be useful if administered to people with lower literacy skills. Another cross-cultural measure is the Mini-Cog (Borson et al., 2000). It can be administered in 3 minutes and contains a brief memory task (three items) and a clock-drawing task, and was developed to differentiate between culturally, linguistically, and educationally different patients with dementia versus nondementia.

Using neuropsychological tests and norms meant for a different age, gender, or race group than that being evaluated may lead to invalid results and possible misdiagnoses (Fernández & Abe, 2018). Psychiatric and psychosocial measures may not have norms for older adults from diverse backgrounds, particularly those from different ethnic, racial, and cultural groups than the dominant cultural group. In addition, unless education-adjusted norms are available, older adults with fewer years of education should have their cognitive and neuropsychological tests interpreted with caution (Gross et al., 2015). Also, older adults for whom English is not a first language may have difficulty completing questionnaires or responding to cognitive or psychosocial questions due to lack of language proficiency.

In addition to culture, ethnicity, race, and language, other aspects of diversity to consider includes lesbian, gay, bisexual, transgender, queer or questioning, and other (LGBTQ+) status, sex and gender identity, religious affiliation, disability status, and veteran status. This information can be obtained during an intake questionnaire, interview, or both. The intersectionality of diverse identities within the same person means that no single prescriptive approach should be assumed in interacting with older adults from diverse backgrounds. Consideration of the impact of internalized stigma is important and may keep some older adults from being forthcoming with information during the interview or in completing questionnaires, due to mistrust of the clinician or the institution.

Clinicians should use neutral terms such as "partner" when referring to an older adult's married or romantic partner. During the assessment, obtaining information about the patient's unique life history and identity provides an important context to the presenting problems and factors impacting current functioning. For example, older adults who indicate they are veterans may also share that they have had previous Agent Orange exposure or have experienced combat trauma, all of which can impact their current well-being and the interpretation of both cognitive and mood assessments. Also, diversity status can inform the selection of measures, such as the decision to use veteran-normed measures when working with an older veteran or large-print questionnaires and primarily auditory measures of cognitive status with a visually impaired older adult.

The older adult's unique multicultural and identity characteristics often impact on assessment recommendations. For instance, professionals working with older adults who identify as LGBTQ+, have to consider what kind of services are available in the community and whether they are LGBTQ+-friendly. Veteran status could expand an older adult's resources to the Veterans health care system in which they would be entitled to services. With regard to sex, older women especially, face financial struggles (Gamache et al., 2003), particularly if they also identify as an ethnic or a racial minority, which may factor into the recommendations. Providers also should have a basic understanding of the older adult's values and religious affiliation, to inform treatment recommendations including any potential for connecting with church or other religion-based services that could fulfill a need as determined by the assessment (e.g., instrumental services, social support).

Applying these principles to Mr. J., the clinician may learn that he grew up in the American Midwest and that he speaks English as his first language. Cultural considerations, however, including his comfort working with a White provider are important. Current and past experiences with institutionalized racism, including, but not limited to, educational inequalities due to segregation, can factor into the assessment. It is important for the clinician to create a safe space for older adults to express these concerns, which can be accomplished by being open and attentive to what the patient has to say and to address any concerns the patient may have. Matching of clinicians to the older adult's background is not always possible, which can be a limiting factor for some older patients – such as Mr. J. if he is guarded and the clinician is unable to build good rapport with him due to an inability to gain his trust.

An additional cultural difference is age itself. Age differences between the clinician and the older adult can sometimes raise concerns on the part of the older adult regarding the competency of a younger provider. If raised as an issue by someone like Mr. J., open communication about the clinician's expertise in working with other older adults can often alleviate this concern.

General Considerations for the Evaluation

The clinician first obtains the older adult's consent or their assent if a family member has power of attorney. Because Mr. J. gave permission for his family to be involved in his assessment, and cognitive impairment needs to be ruled out, the inclusion of his family is especially important. It is not known if he is aware of the purpose of his visit and the referral question. Understanding what he hopes to gain from the assessment and to address any misconceptions about the assessment will be key. Mr. J. might have concerns about what the evaluation will find and the potential loss of his independence, such as fear that memory problems detected by the evaluation will mean he must move to a nursing care facility. Older adults who drive may have concerns that their driver's license will automatically be taken away from them. Clarifying the purpose and limits of the overall assessment will ensure that the older adult's evaluation provides the most accurate information.

Some older adults believe they are seeing a physician and not a mental health provider, either because they misunderstood the referral or a family member misrepresented the reason for the evaluation to ensure the older adult kept the appointment. It is important to spend alone time with the patient to attain consent or assent for the evaluation, and build rapport with them (Hinrichsen, 2019). Before starting testing with Mr. J., who had already assented to his family being present, the clinician could explain that the family's participation would be requested for the clinical interview portion, but they will be asked to sit in the waiting area while the patient completes the other tests with the clinician.

The clinician should discuss limits of confidentiality. The patient is informed that the clinician has a duty to break confidentiality and report information as required by state licensing regulations to state agencies (e.g., Adult Protective Services) or local law enforcement if the patient reports intent to harm themselves or others, or if there is suspected child, dependent, or elder abuse. At the end of the interview, the clinician should review the information with the older adult and family to verify details and chronology of the events and to address the patient's questions or concerns.

Common Late-Life Functional Issues and Psychiatric Syndromes

Functional Status

Evaluations of older adults should include an assessment of functional status. Reviewing the older adult's ability to complete ADLs and IADLs is important not only in making an appropriate diagnosis (e.g., Alzheimer's disease) but also in understanding whether their physical impairments are due to cognitive changes or some other disease process. ADLs are self-care activities, such as dressing, eating, bathing, toileting, and controlling bladder and bowel functions. IADLs are activities that allow the individual to live independently and be involved in such activities as doing housework, prepping meals, managing finances, taking medications independently, or using a telephone (Tatum et al., 2018). Typically, two brief self-report measures are used to assess ADLs and IADLs – the Katz ADL scale (Katz et al, 1970) and the Lawton IADL scale (Lawton & Brody, 1969). Each of these two measures can be completed by the older adult or administered by the clinician, and together take 5–10 minutes to complete. Additional follow-up questions about problematic ADLs and IADLs can be part of the assessment to gain a more complete picture regarding the older adult's strengths and limitations.

Psychiatric Syndromes

Common psychiatric issues to rule out in an older adult include anxiety disorders, trauma and stressor-related disorders, mood disorders (depression and bipolar disorder), and suicide risk. In Mr. J.'s case, several issues related to his psychiatric health and well-being included ruling out many of these issues, particularly depression and suicide risk.

Late-Life Anxiety Assessment

A brief introduction to anxiety symptoms and their impact on cognition is given in Chapter 5. Anxiety disorders are the most prevalent class of late-life mental health disorders (Byers et al., 2010). While assessing for anxiety disorders, other common comorbidities such as depression and medical illness must be considered.

There are many options for late-life anxiety measures. Two self-report questionnaires developed for use with older adults are the Geriatric Anxiety Inventory (GAI; Pachana et al., 2007) and the Geriatric Anxiety Scale (GAS; Segal et al., 2010). Other measures that have adequate or better validity and reliability with older populations and can be used to screen for anxiety include the Generalized Anxiety Disorder–7 item (GAD-7; Spitzer et al., 2006) scale and the Rating Anxiety in Dementia Scale (RAID; Shankar et al., 1999). This is not an exhaustive list but covers the most common measures in clinical practice and in some research.

The GAI is a dimensional assessment of common anxiety symptoms in older adults (Pachana et al., 2007). The scale has 20 agree or disagree items covering clinical and subsyndromal anxiety symptoms. The GAI can be administered through self-report or by a clinician and takes up to 10 minutes. A score of 10 or higher on the GAI indicates significant anxiety symptoms. The GAI has been translated into over 20 languages, which can be useful when working with older adults whose first and preferred language is not English. Further, GAI scores share a unidimensional structure across older adults from different cultural backgrounds, based on a cross-national validation study, suggesting that the GAI scores of older adults from different cultural backgrounds can be compared (Molde et al., 2019). The short-form version of the GAI (GAI-SF) exhibits good psychometric properties in clinical and nonclinical geriatric populations (Johnco et al., 2015). The GAI-SF has five items, and a score of 3 or higher is considered a positive screen for generalized anxiety disorder (GAD; Byrne & Pachana, 2011).

The GAS is a 30-item self-report measure used for assessing anxiety symptoms in older adults in the past week (Segal et al., 2010). A benefit of the GAS is that it assesses anxiety symptoms on three subscales: somatic, cognitive, and affective symptoms. Two studies have supported the GAS's psychometric properties in community and clinical geriatric samples (Gould et al., 2014; Segal et al., 2010), and initial validation of the GAS has been established in Chinese, Italian, and Iranian populations (Gatti et al., 2018; Lin et al., 2017; Bolghan-Abadi et al., 2013).

The Geriatric Anxiety Scale–10 item (GAS-10) is a short version of the GAS and is used as a screening measure for anxiety symptoms in older adults. The GAS-10 shows good psychometric properties in older adults, including the initial validation of a German version of the GAS-10 (Gottschling et al., 2019; Mueller et al., 2015).

Another measure, the GAD-7 scale, screens for anxiety symptoms (Spitzer et al., 2006). Respondents assign a severity rating for each item in the past 2 weeks. The GAD-7 scale has demonstrated strong psychometric properties in primary care and community settings (Kroenke et al., 2007; Löwe et al., 2008). The Generalized Anxiety Disorder–2 item (GAD-2) scale is a brief screener of anxiety symptoms in the past 2 weeks and uses the first two items from the GAD-7 scale (Kroenke et al., 2007). Both the GAD-7 and GAD-2 scales exhibit strong psychometric properties in older adult community samples (Wild et al., 2014).

To assess anxiety in patients with dementia, the Rating Anxiety in Dementia (RAID) scale can be used (Shankar et al., 1999). The RAID is an 18-item clinician-rated instrument completed through direct observation, informant report, and patient interview. Each item is assigned a severity rating on a 4-point Likert scale. A score of 11 or higher on the RAID scale indicates significant symptoms of anxiety, and the scale takes 20 minutes to administer.

Late-Life Depression Assessment

Depressive disorders and symptoms are the second most commonly occurring late-life psychiatric illness (Panza et al., 2010). Similar to anxiety symptoms, depressive symptom severity occurs on a spectrum, from subsyndromal, to minor, to major depression, and all levels of the spectrum are associated with significant psychosocial impairment across the lifespan (Judd et al., 2002). Depression and anxiety symptoms frequently occur concurrently in late life (Byers et al., 2010). When coupled with anxiety, late-life depression is more severe, chronic, and difficult to treat (Andreescu et al. 2007).

Assessment of depressive symptoms can include self-report or semistructured clinical interviews. Two common self-report measures are the Geriatric Depression Scale (GDS) and Beck Depression Inventory–II (BDI-II). The GDS screen for depression was developed and normed for older adults. It is a self-report measure with 30 yes-or-no items that can take up to 10 minutes to administer (Yesavage et al., 1982). Score ranges include 0–9 (*normal*), 10–19 (*mildly depressed*), and 20–30 (*severe depression*). The GDS has minimal items examining somatic symptoms to minimize confusion between depression symptoms and symptoms of medical illness and reduce the likelihood of false positives in a geriatric population. The short-form version of the GDS (GDS-SF; Sheikh & Yesavage, 1986) exhibits good psychometric properties in clinical and nonclinical geriatric populations (Burke et al., 1991; Herrmann et al., 1996). The GDS-SF has 15 items, and a score of 5 or more is considered a positive screen for depression disorder (Herrmann et al., 1996). The utility of the GDS among older adults with mild cognitive impairment has been established, but the GDS is not a reliable screening instrument in patients with Alzheimer's disease (Debruyne et al., 2009).

The BDI-II assesses depression severity in clinical and general patient populations, aged 13 to 80 years (Beck et al., 1996). The measure has 21 items, and respondents assign a severity rating for each item in the past 2 weeks. The BDI-II can be self-report or clinician administered and takes 10 minutes.

In older adults, the presence of clinically significant depressive symptoms has been associated with accelerated cognitive decline (Köhler et al., 2010). Executive function, episodic memory, visuospatial skills, verbal fluency, and psychomotor speed are cognitive domains that are particularly affected in late-life depression (Morimoto et al., 2015). Comorbidity of depression and cognitive impairment is associated with greater functional decline (Mehta et al., 2002). For older adults with a known diagnosis of dementia or other significant cognitive impairment, the Cornell Scale for Depression in Dementia (CSDD) can be used. The CSDD is a 19-item clinician-administered screening tool developed to assess depression severity in patients with dementia (Alexopoulos et al., 1988). Through semistructured interviews, the clinician gathers information from both the patient and an informant, and assigns a severity rating for each item on a 3-point Likert scale. Severity ratings from the interviews and direct observation reflect the rater's clinical impression. The CSDD takes 20 minutes to administer, and a score of 18 or more indicates significant symptoms of depression (Alexopoulos et al., 1988).

In the case of Mr. J., the clinician administers the GDS, on which the patient reports a moderate level of depression, which is considered clinically significant. This information is evaluated in light of the time course of his symptoms and the history of his depression (in which the patient and his family deny that Mr. J. ever had any issues with depression prior to his wife's death). The clinician examines Mr. J.'s responses to individual items on the GDS. Of concern, he endorses items for feelings of worthlessness and that life is not worth living. This leads to further assessment of suicide risk and resiliency factors.

Suicidal Risk in Older Adults

In the US and around the globe, suicide rates are elevated in later life (World Health Organization, 2014). Older adults are markedly more likely to die from a suicide attempt, with one death for every four suicide attempts in late life, compared with one death for every 25 attempts in the general population, and one death for every 100 to 200 attempts in younger adults (Drapeau & McIntosh, 2018). Further, older adults are more likely to have been in contact with a primary health care provider in the year and month prior to death by suicide (Stene-Larsen & Reneflot, 2019). These facts point to a critical need for valid and reliable assessment of suicidal ideation and behaviors among older adults. However, there is a paucity of suicide risk assessment measures developed and validated among older adults.

Only two measures assessing suicide risk have been developed especially for older adults. The Geriatric Suicide Ideation Scale (GSIS) assesses suicide ideation, death ideation, loss of personal and social worth, and perceived meaning in life, and has demonstrated good reliability and validity in samples of community-dwelling older adults, nursing home residents, and medical and psychiatric patients (Heisel & Flett, 2006, 2016). The Reasons for Living–Older Adults (RFL-OA) scale assesses protective factors against attempting suicide among older adults, and it has demonstrated good reliability and validity among community-dwelling older adults (Edelstein et al., 2009). A shortened version of the RFL-OA scale is available, as the original scale contains 69 items (Lutz et al., 2019). Other measures, both scales with multiple items (e.g., Suicide Behaviors Questionnaire-Revised [SBQ-R], Beck Scale for Suicide Ideation [BSS]) as well as single items from depression scales (e.g., Patient Health Questionnaire [PHQ-9], Beck Depression Inventory [BDI-II] suicide item), primarily developed and validated among younger adults are also frequently used to assess suicide risk among older adults. However, there is little evidence regarding the validity of these measures for use among older adults. In Veterans Health Administration (VHA) settings, items from the Columbia Suicide Severity Rating Scale (C-SSRS; Posner et al., 2008) are the required suicide screen for veterans of all ages. In non-VHA settings, geriatric measures of suicide risk and resiliency (e.g., GSIS and RFL-OA scale) would be preferred over other suicide screens or measures which have not been thoroughly investigated in older adults.

These measures have primarily been developed and validated among those without cognitive impairment. While mild cognitive impairment or early-stage dementia are associated with increased risk of suicide, severe or later-stage cognitive impairment is associated with reduced risk (e.g., Conejero et al., 2018; Haw et al., 2009; Serafini et al., 2016). No measures have been developed to assess suicide risk specifically among those with cognitive impairment. Clinicians should use their best judgment in the assessment of suicide risk among cognitively impaired older adults. Assessment of suicide risk among individuals with cognitive impairment may include the use of collateral sources and behavioral signs of depression. In general, clinical suicide risk assessments with older adults should not depend solely upon any one self-report measure, and instead involve a comprehensive assessment involving a clinical interview (e.g., see Bryan & Rudd, 2006).

With the case of Mr. J., suicide risk is a concern given that his responses on the GDS are indicative of thinking about being dead (death ideation) and worries of being a burden on his family (perceived burdensomeness), and his provider, and thoughts of worthlessness and that life is not worth living. It will be important to rule out whether he has additional thoughts of wanting to harm himself. In older adults, those with passive suicidal ideation (thoughts of being better off dead but no thoughts of harming oneself) should be taken seriously and screened. Mr. J. completes the GSIS which, consistent with his prior comments, indicates slightly elevated levels of death ideation and feelings of loss of worth, but no current active suicide ideation. In addition, he completes the RFL-OA measure, and endorses multiple reasons for living related to his family (his daughter) and faith. It is determined that he does not need emergency services, because he does not have current active suicidal ideation, intent, or plan, and he endorses reasons for living. However, a plan might be recommended for monitoring his suicide risk given his death ideation (e.g., to include ongoing assessment of his mood and reassessment for changes in suicidal ideation at his regular primary care check-ups), and interventions may be recommended to address his feelings of burdensomeness and worthlessness, both risk factors for suicide.

Alcohol and Substance Use Disorders in Older Adults

During the interview, the clinician should also focus on the potential for an alcohol or substance use disorder. In the case of Mr. J., it might be incorrectly assumed that such issues are not present, because they were not raised by him or his family. Another reason that older adults might not be assessed for alcohol or substance use disorders is the stereotypes about older adults not using drugs, or being less likely to benefit from interventions if such a disorder is present. As a result, practitioners may not do a thorough screening, or any screen for that matter, of alcohol, nicotine, and substance use in their older patients, thus missing a critical issue for the older patient.

Alcohol is one of the more common substances used among older adults, with harmful or hazardous drinking estimated in as many as 35–40% of middle-aged and older adults (Fink et al., 2002; Towers et al., 2018). If Mr. J. were to report alcohol consumption, it is important to find out what type of alcohol, how much of it he is consuming, and over what time period. Depending on the amount of alcohol in that drink, it may be considered several. The National Institute on Alcohol Abuse and Alcoholism suggest "adults over age 65 who are healthy and do not take medications should not have more than: 3 drinks on a given day or 7 drinks in a week" (National Institute on Alcohol Abuse and Alcoholism, 2019). Given reduced ability to metabolize alcohol with age and the potential for alcohol to interact with medications, older adults can be at risk for poor mental health or negative functional outcomes.

Another common issue can be medication misuse, given that many older adults also take one or more prescribed psychotropic medications to aid with anxiety, sleep, and pain, or powerful medications to help with chronic medical problems (e.g., heart or thyroid problems, and diabetes). Medication misuse can be intentional or not, and may include taking another person's medicine, taking the wrong dose or taking it for longer than medically required, or using the medication inappropriately, such as for recreational or nonmedical needs (Satre & Wolf, 2015). Patients may also accidentally misuse medications because they have misunderstood the directions given by their doctor, due to cognitive impairment or unclear directions. Some clinicians may not screen for illicit drug use, due to erroneous beliefs that illicit drug use is not an issue in older adults or because of concerns about how an older adult will react to questions about illicit drug use (Hinrichsen, 2019). A screen of illicit drug use should be included, particularly in light of more prevalent use of marijuana since its legalization, the epidemic of opioid addiction, and the potential for illicit use of any illicit drug at any age.

Physical, mental health, and social risk factors are related to an increased risk for alcohol problems and misuse of psychoactive substances in later life. Physical factors in older adults include characteristics such as being a White male, life transitions, health-related problems, chronic pain, disability, and polypharmacy. Mental health factors may include history of alcohol use, use of multiple substances, and prior or current mental health problems. Social risk factors in older adults include higher socioeconomic status, social isolation, grief, and unplanned or forced retirement (Kuerbis et al., 2014). General understanding and knowledge of why older adults often use or abuse alcohol or other substances, including nicotine, especially if they have multiple risk factors, should prompt the practitioner to do a more careful and detailed assessment if deemed appropriate.

To assess for hazardous drinking and medication misuse, there are several behavioral warning signs in older adults. For hazardous drinking, warning signs can include mood swings, falls, bruises, headaches, sleep problems, memory difficulties, poor hygiene, poor nutrition, and social isolation. Medication misuse warning signs can also include strong preference for specific medications and detailed knowledge about the medication, complaints about doctors who will not prescribe the medicines, anxiety or stress about the medication running low, poor hygiene, and social isolation (Barry & Blow, 2010).

Several alcohol screening measures are recommended for use with older adults who are at risk for alcohol use problems; several of these have been specifically validated for older adults. These alcohol screens include the CAGE (Ewing, 1984), Alcohol Use Disorders Identification Test–Concise (AUDIT-C; Bush et al., 1998), Michigan Alcoholism Screening Test–Geriatric Version (MAST-G; Blow et al., 1992), and Short-MAST-G (Blow et al., 1998). The CAGE–Adapted to Include Drugs (CAGE-AID; Brown & Rounds, 1995) and Drug Abuse Screen Test (DAST-10; Skinner, 1982) are brief screening instruments for drug and alcohol use.

With Mr. J., he reports chewing tobacco and smoking cigarettes starting in his early 20s and quitting all use in his 30s with the arrival of his first child. There is no indication of substance abuse or misuse of medications. He also reported "rarely drinking" during the clinical interview. However, on the AUDIT-C, his total score indicates likely hazardous drinking. When asked more specific questions about his drinking habits as a follow-up to the AUDIT-C, we learn that he drinks "one to two drinks" every night with each drink consisting of three shots of whiskey mixed with cola. He reports having started drinking this amount since his wife died, due to "boredom" and because it "helps calm my nerves."

The full assessment is not complete without an evaluation of Mr. J.'s cognitive functioning. This next section delves into cognitive screens and assessments, with a focus on memory and executive functioning.

Cognitive Screens and Assessments

Assessment of cognition

Cognition is assessed with standardized measures as part of the evaluation, and behavioral observations provide the necessary context to the assessment. The clinical interview helps determine approximately when cognitive problems began, whether some or all cognitive abilities have changed, and to what extent the cognitive changes impair functioning. Neuropsychological measures allow clinicians to establish a baseline and detect possible cognitive changes, propose a possible etiology, and implement a plan to help improve cognitive functioning or teach the patient compensatory strategies to help maintain or improve their cognitive functioning (Fernandez-Ballesteros et al., 2015). Multiple instruments can be used to assess cognitive functioning, including cognitive screens. These different screening measures can help differentiate individuals with no cognitive impairment, mild cognitive impairment, and dementia. Depending on the patient's performance, additional cognitive measures can be used to determine a patient's cognitive baseline.

One screening measure that is widely used is the Mini-Mental State Examination (MMSE; Folstein et al., 1975), composed of 11 items (orientation, immediate and delayed recall, working memory, language, and visuospatial skills), which has validity for use in screening White, African-American, and Latinx older adults for possible cognitive impairment (Rideaux et al., 2012). Though the MMSE is widely used, other screens may be preferred due to their having better sensitivity and specificity for detecting mild cognitive impairment, and because other cognitive screens are available for public use, whereas the MMSE is copyrighted and has a fee for use.

The Montreal Cognitive Assessment (MoCA; Nasreddine et al., 2005) is another brief paper-and-pencil screening tool used to detect mild cognitive impairment. This screen includes attention, concentration, executive functioning, memory, language, visuospatial skills, abstraction, calculation, and orientation domains. The test has been translated into 36 languages and is widely used. It is scored out of 30 points and takes about 10 minutes to administer. The MoCA is freely available and does not require permission for clinical or educational use. In contrast to the MMSE, the MoCA demonstrates good sensitivity for identifying mild cognitive impairment (90% for MoCA vs. 18% for MMSE) and Alzheimer's disease (100% for MoCA vs. 78% for MMSE) individuals. With regard to specificity, which is the percentage of normal controls that scored at or above 26 (the cutoff score), the MMSE correctly determines 100% of the normal controls, and MoCA determines 87% of the controls (Nasreddine et al., 2005). It is recommended to administer the MoCA to adults who are presenting with cognitive complaints but who do not display functional difficulties with their ADLs. Older adults who are displaying cognitive complaints and functional difficulties may benefit from first being assessed by the MMSE, and then the MoCA if their MMSE performance is in the normal range (Chertkow et al., 2007).

The Short Portable Mental Status Questionnaire (SPMSQ; Pfeiffer, 1975) was designed for use with older adults. It consists of 10 questions, is scored out of 10 points, and has a stronger emphasis on orientation than the MMSE. The SPMSQ includes seven questions focused on orientation, two questions test memory for current and past US presidents, and one question examines concentration and mental tracking with serial threes. Because it is focused mostly on orientation questions, the SPMSQ is not reliable for identifying mildly impaired or early dementia individuals (Pfeiffer, 1975). Rather, based on several studies (Moritz et al., 1995; Sands et al., 2003), this screener is better used to identify adults at risk for experiencing difficulties with basic ADLs, who can then be closely monitored.

Two other popular cognitive screens include the Saint Louis University Mental Status (SLUMS) exam (Morley & Tumosa, 2002), and the Short Blessed Test (SBT; Katzman et al., 1983). The SLUMS tests for orientation, short-term memory, calculations, confrontation naming, visuospatial skills, executive functioning abilities, and recognition of certain geometric figures. It takes about 7 minutes to administer, and scores range between 0 and 30 points. A score in the range 0–20 suggests dementia, 21–26 suggests a mild cognitive impairment, and between 27 to 30 is considered within normal limits for individuals with a high school education. In comparison with the MMSE, SLUMS is found to do a better job at identifying individuals with a mild cognitive impairment (Cruz-Oliver et al., 2012), as well as identifying early stages of dementia (Szcześniak & Rymaszewska, 2016). The SBT, also known as the Orientation-Memory-Concentration Test, is intended to identify dementia. It consists of six items and includes questions about orientation, saying months backward, remembering a name and an address, and counting from 20 down to 1 (Katzman et al., 1983).

Premorbid cognitive abilities can be measured with the Wechsler Adult Intelligence Scale, 4th edition (WAIS-IV; Wechsler, 2008) or the Wechsler Abbreviated Scale Intelligence, 2nd edition (WASI-II; Wechsler, 2011), which can be crucial in understanding the patient's possible cognitive impairment. WAIS-IV is a measure of overall cognitive functioning from patients aged 16 to 90 years. With multiple subtests and composite scores, this measure indicates individual strengths and weaknesses in multiple cognitive areas and emphasizes fluid reasoning, working memory, and processing speed (Lichtenberger & Kaufman, 2009). WAIS-IV provides a *full scale intelligence quotient* (FSIQ). The test consists of 10 core subtests and five supplemental subtests. The supplemental subtests can be administered if a core subtest is invalidated. The subtests make up the four indices: the Verbal Comprehension Index (VCI), Perceptual Reasoning Index (PRI), Working Memory Index (WMI), and Processing Speed Index (PSI). The General Ability Index can be calculated for individuals with specific neuropsychological problems, such as attention-deficit/hyperactivity disorder or neurodegenerative disease, as it is not heavily impacted by working memory and processing speed abilities (Climie & Rostad, 2011).

WASI-II is an abbreviated measure of cognitive intelligence and can be administered to individuals 6 to 90 years of age. It consists of four subtests: Vocabulary, Similarities, Block Design, and Matrix Reasoning. Vocabulary and Similarities make up the Verbal Comprehension Index (VCI), and Block Design and Matrix Reasoning make up the Perceptual Reasoning Index (PRI). When combined, the four subtests form the Full-Scale IQ-4 (FSIQ-4). Vocabulary and Matrix Reasoning, when combined, make up the Full-Scale IQ-2 (FSIQ-2). The WASI-II provides the examiner with the option of choosing a brief measure of intelligence if they are limited for time or if there are patient factors preventing a more comprehensive administration. The WASI-II is fairly simple to administer and takes significantly less time than the WAIS-IV. There are several limits to the WASI-II, including the fact that it is less comprehensive than the WAIS-IV and does not include measures of working memory and processing speed, which both contribute to overall intellectual functioning (McCrimmon & Smith, 2013).

Assessments of Memory

Memory complaints by an individual tend to be the most common reasons for a referral to a neuropsychologist. When a patient says they have "memory difficulties," it can mean multiple things. Some patients report memory problems when they have trouble coming up with the right word or cannot recall proper names, although they can easily recall short-term and long-term events. Others may indicate memory problems when they have trouble focusing on a task. Overall, memory impairment can be impacted by deficits in other cognitive areas, such as attention, processing speed, and executive functioning. Understanding different aspects of memory and other factors which can impact it is important in conceptualizing the case.

A comprehensive memory assessment evaluates the individual's orientation to time and place; learning and retention of meaningful structured information (e.g., Logical Memory I and II subtests from the Wechsler Memory Scale, 4th editon [WMS-IV]; Wechsler, 2009); rote learning, which allows the patient to learn information over several trials, provides data such as a learning curve, and tests free recall and recognition (e.g., Auditory Verbal Learning Test [AVLT]; Rey, 1941; or the California Verbal Learning Test [CVLT-II]; Delis et al., 2000); visuospatial memory (Visual Reproduction Test [WMS-IV]; Wechsler, 2009; or the Rey-Osterrieth Complex Figure; Osterrieth & Rey, 1944); and remote memory; and autobiographical memory. Measures designed to test learning should include one or more trials and a delay period followed by free recall and recognition or cued recall tasks (Lezak et al., 2012). Please see Table 2.1 for further details regarding the memory tests.

Table 2.1. Summary of all measures presented in the chapter

Measure name	What it assesses
Katz ADL scale (Katz et al., 1970)	Brief self-report measure of ADLs assessing independence in six functions
Lawton IADL scale (Lawton & Brody, 1969)	Brief self-report measure of IADLs assessing ability to perform eight instrument tasks
Geriatric Anxiety Inventory (GAI) (Pachana et al., 2007)	Measures clinical and subsyndromal anxiety in older adults (20 items)
Geriatric Anxiety Inventory – Short Form (GAI-SF) (Byrne & Pachana, 2011)	Short form (5 items) of the GAI, which measures anxiety in older adults
Geriatric Anxiety Scale (GAS) (Segal et al., 2010)	Self-report measure of anxiety symptoms in older adults in the past week (30 items)
Geriatric Anxiety Scale – Short Form (GAS-10) (Mueller et al., 2015)	Short-form (10 items) measure of GAS, which measures anxiety symptoms in older adults
Generalized Anxiety Disorder–7 (GAD-7) scale (Spitzer et al., 2006)	Measure of anxiety severity in the past 2 weeks.

Table 2.1. continued

Measure name	What it assesses
Generalized Anxiety Disorder–2 (GAD-2) scale (Kroenke et al., 2007)	Brief screen of anxiety symptoms in the past 2 weeks; short form (2-items) of GAD-7
Rating Anxiety in Dementia (RAID) (Shankar et al., 1999)	Anxiety in patients with dementia
Geriatric Depression Scale (GDS) (Yesavage et al., 1982)	Depression screen (30 items) for older adults
Geriatric Depression Scale – Short Form (GDS-SF) (Sheikh & Yesavage, 1986)	Short-form (15 items) of the GDS, which measures depression in older adults
Beck Depression Inventory-II (BDI-II) (Beck et al., 1996)	Depression severity in clinical and general patient populations, aged 13 to 80 years
Cornell Scale for Depression in Dementia (CSDD) (Alexopoulos et al., 1988)	Depression in older adults with dementia or other cognitive impairment
Geriatric Suicide Ideation Scale (GSIS) (Heisel & Flett, 2006, 2016)	Assesses suicide ideation, death ideation, loss of personal and social worth, and perceived meaning in life
Reasons for Living – Older Adults (RFL-OA) (Edelstein et al., 2009)	Assesses protective factors against attempting suicide among older adults
Columbia Suicide Severity Rating Scale (C-SSRS) (Posner et al., 2008)	Suicide screen for veterans of all ages
CAGE (Ewing, 1984)	Alcohol screening measure recommended for use with older adults
Alcohol Use Disorder Identification Test – Concise (AUDIT-C) (Bush et al., 1998)	Alcohol consumption screening measure to identify patients who engage in hazardous drinking or have an alcohol use disorder
Michigan Alcoholism Screening Test – Geriatric Version (MAST-G) (Blow et al., 1992)	Alcohol dependence screening measure (24 items) in older adults
Short-MAST-G (Blow et al., 1998)	Short form (10 items) of MAST-G to screen for alcohol dependence in older adults
CAGE–Adapted to Include Drugs (CAGE-AID) (Brown & Rounds, 1995)	Alcohol and drug use screening measure (4-items) recommended for use with older adults
Drug Abuse Screen Test (DAST-10) (Skinner, 1982)	Drug screen (not including alcohol) measuring the degree of drug use-related consequences

Table 2.1. continued

Measure name	What it assesses
Rowland Universal Dementia Assessment Scale (RUDAS) (Storey et al., 2004)	Cross-cultural dementia screener, which can be translated into 30 languages
Cognitive Abilities Screening Instrument (CASI) (Teng et al., 1994)	Measures general cognitive abilities; culturally validated in Japan, China, and the US
Cross-Cultural Cognitive Examination (CCCE) (Glosser et al., 1993)	Cross-cultural measure for people with lower literacy skills
Mini-Cog (Borson et al., 2000)	Differentiates between culturally, linguistically, and educationally different patients with dementia versus nondementia
Mini–Mental State Examination (MMSE) (Folstein et al., 1975)	Cognitive screening measure (11 items)
Montreal Cognitive Assessment (MoCA) (Nasreddine et al., 2005)	Cognitive screening measure validated for adults aged 55 to 85 years; recommended for use with adults who perform in the normal range on the MMSE.
Short Portable Mental Status Questionnaire (SPMSQ) (Pfeiffer, 1975)	Cognitive screening measure (10 items)
Saint Louis University Mental Status (SLUMS) exam (Morley & Tumosa, 2002)	Cognitive screening measure (11 items). Comparable to MMSE and MoCA
Short Blessed Test (SBT) (Katzman et al., 1983)	Cognitive screening measure (6 items) of orientation, memory and concentration; demonstrated to discriminate among mild, moderate, and severe cognitive deficits
Wechsler Abbreviated Scale of Intelligence, 2nd edition (WASI-II) (Wechsler, 2011)	Measures premorbid cognitive abilities; short version of the WAIS-IV
Wechsler Adult Intelligence Scale, 4th edition (WAIS-IV) (Wechsler, 2008)	Measures premorbid cognitive abilities; 10 core subtests and five supplemental subtests
Auditory Verbal Learning Test (AVLT) (Rey, 1941)	List-learning verbal memory task with immediate and delayed recall

Table 2.1. continued

Measure name	What it assesses
California Verbal Learning Test (CVLT-II) (Delis et al., 2000)	List-learning verbal memory task with immediate and delayed recall
Logical Memory I and II (WMS-IV) (Wechsler, 2009)	Structured verbal memory test assessing immediate and delayed recall and recognition
Visual Reproduction Test (WMS-IV) (Wechsler, 2009)	Immediate and delayed visuospatial memory test
Rey-Osterrieth Complex Figure (Osterrieth & Rey, 1944)	Visual memory test assessing visuospatial construction ability, processing speed, and immediate and delayed visual memory (Shin et al., 2006)
Trail Making Test (TMT) Form B (Tombaugh, 2004)	Set-shifting executive functioning task
Verbal Fluency Test (FAS) (Tombaugh & Rees, 1999)	Executive functioning test of phonemic verbal fluency
Animal Category (Tombaugh & Rees, 1999)	Executive functioning test of category verbal fluency
Clock Drawing Test (Agrell & Dehlin, 1998)	Executive functioning test of visuospatial, visual construction, and planning abilities; can assess for spatial dysfunction and neglect
Digits Forward and Backward subtests (Wechsler, 1981; Wechsler, 1997)	Executive functioning test of attention and working memory
Stroop Test (Stroop, 1992)	Executive functioning test measuring selective attention and inhibition through cognitive interference tasks
Wisconsin Card Sorting Test (WCST) (Heaton, 1993)	Executive functioning test measuring attention, perseverance, working memory, and cognitive flexibility
Wechsler Reading Achievement Test (WRAT-4; Wide Range Achievement Test – 4, 2006)	Reading test measuring premorbid abilities

Note. ADL = activities of daily living; IADL = instrumental activities of daily living.

To gauge the strengths and weaknesses of the patient and provide appropriate recommendations for treatment or future planning, memory must be tested using immediate recall, an interference task during a delay period, and a recognition task or cued recall. Immediate recall will test for how an individual may encode information, but it does not provide information on how the patient learns or retains the information, or how efficient their memory is. A delay period is needed to test how well the individual has learned the information. Providing an interference task during a delay can prevent the patient from repeating information presented during the immediate recall. This allows the examiner to better differentiate whether the patient learned the information following a delay or if the information was rehearsed in temporary storage. If the patient had difficulty recalling or retrieving the initially learned information, it is sometimes hard to know if it was due to poor retention or difficulties with retrieval, which is an issue that can be solved by administering a recognition task or a task for use of cues to retrieve the information (Lezak et al., 2012).

Assessments of Executive Functioning

Another important domain of cognition is executive functioning. Executive functions are responsible for complex cognitive abilities, such as identifying goals, mental planning, organizing behavior, and ability to plan in order to accomplish set goals (Miyake et al., 2000). Executive functions "enable a person to engage successfully in independent, purposive, self-directed, and self-serving behavior" (Lezak et al., 2012). Executive functions also play a role in emotional, motivational, and social skills. Maintaining intact executive functions enables older adults to perform and troubleshoot daily, routinized tasks and engage in complex social and functional responsibilities.

Frontal lobe damage has been shown to impact executive functioning. More specifically, when a significant injury or disease impacts the orbital and/or medial structures of the frontal regions, patients are seen to have a change in their behavior and personality. However, damage to other parts of the brain, such as the parietal region, basal ganglia, thalamus, and cerebellum, can also impact executive functions (Rabinovici et al., 2015). Executive function deficits may cause difficulties with an older adult's performance of ADLs, which may in turn reduce independence and quality of life (Mograbi et al., 2014). Older adults with executive dysfunction may struggle with flexibility in their thought, working memory difficulties, solving novel problems, decreased behavioral initiation, perseverative errors, trouble planning, disinhibition, and maintaining adequate social relationships. Trouble with executive functioning may be witnessed in patients with mild cognitive impairment or be an early sign of dementia, such as frontotemporal dementia, dementia with Lewy bodies, Parkinson's disease, Alzheimer's disease, and many others (Espinosa et al., 2009). When conceptualizing the case and determining the level of executive dysfunction, it is important to consider other factors such whether any other cognitive domains are impacted, motor and psychiatric symptoms, comorbid medical problems, and medication use.

During a clinical evaluation, patients rarely report specific executive functioning problems. Rather, they may misinterpret executive dysfunction as memory problems. To differentiate between memory loss and executive deficits, the clinician should ask whether the patient has experienced difficulty with planning or organizing, multitasking, making appropriate decisions, impulsivity, attention and concentration, problem solving, and flexible thinking. It is also important to test all of these factors during the neuropsychological evaluation (Rabinovici et al., 2015). Of note, if using a brief screener, the MoCA is more sensitive to executive functioning deficits than the MMSE is (Lam et al., 2013). Based on a systematic review (Faria et al., 2015), the seven most common tests of executive function used include Trail Making Test (TMT) Form B (Tombaugh, 2004), Verbal Fluency Test (FAS; Tombaugh & Rees, 1999), Animal Category (Tombaugh & Rees, 1999), Clock Drawing Test (Agrell & Dehlin, 1998), Digits Forward and Backward subtests (Wechsler, 1981; Wechsler, 1997), Stroop Test, and the Wisconsin Card Sorting Test (WCST; Heaton, 1993). Table 2.1 summarizes these tests.

Indeed performance on various memory or executive functioning measures may depend on diverse factors, including demographic and social factors, and cultural backgrounds for which there may not be norms for adjusting scores, therefore making interpretation of scores more challenging. Variables such as education and language abilities may also impact how people learn and recall different information (Maruff & Darby, 2006).

Case Example Conclusions

A mainstay of clinical geropsychology is the valid and comprehensive assessment of older adults in the context of complex presenting symptoms and issues. In our case example of Mr. J., he was administered a battery of mood and cognitive measures to determine his level of cognitive functioning and risk factors for depression, anxiety, and alcohol use (see Table 2.1 for a list of all measures reviewed in the chapter). These measures helped the clinician determine whether Mr. J. had a neurocognitive disorder versus a psychiatric diagnosis or a combination of both issues.

After completing several tests of memory and executive functioning, Mr. J. was shown to have performed below expectation for his age and education on all measures. However, a reading test (Wechsler Reading Achievement Test; WRAT-4; Wide Range Achievement Test – 4, 2006) indicated that his educational attainment approximated 11 years, several years fewer than the actual number of years he had gone to school for his certification as a chemistry teacher. When the clinician used age-sex-education adjusted norms for 11 years of education, Mr. J. was found to be mildly impaired on executive function measures with a speed component (i.e., TMT Form B), but within normal limits on other assessments. His slow response on tests seemed attributable to his depression and drinking, which fit with his and his family's report that his cognitive issues had emerged only after his wife died. His final diagnoses included major depressive disorder, moderate due to bereavement and alcohol use disorder. Follow-up cognitive assessments will be needed to rule out mild neurocognitive disorder, which should be assessed after Mr. J. improves his diabetes management and is treated for depression and his alcohol use disorder.

The clinician's recommendations based on the assessment of Mr. J. encompassed several factors:

- A referral to a licensed clinical social worker or psychologist is warranted to address his loneliness, social isolation, alcohol use, and depression. Mr. J. could particularly benefit from adaptive coping strategies, such as behavioral activation, an empirically supported therapy for late-life depression that involves increasing the frequency of enjoyed activities. Because Mr. J. reported great enjoyment in social activities, his individualized behavioral activation plan could include scheduling activities that engage him with his family, community, and church.
- While also addressing mood, he is strongly encouraged to further address his diabetes management as this may be a significant contributor to his reduced executive functioning. A follow-up with his primary care physician and weekly visits by a nurse is recommended to review his medications and to monitor his blood glucose and diabetes management. The physician and nurse should also continue to monitor him for depression and suicide risk.
- Lastly, he is referred for further neuropsychological testing in 6–12 months to determine if his cognition is stable or declining, given he had no record of any previous cognitive screen or other cognitive testing to establish a baseline.

Mr. J. was not interested in moving into an assisted living facility at that time, but he agreed to more regular check-ins by his daughter, Janelle, and to hiring a weekly in-home aide to assist with cleaning and meals. If his functional status were to decline further, with concern for his health and safety, Janelle agreed that she would revisit other housing options with her father, including assisted living or living with Janelle and her family but with a part-time hired aide.

At a follow-up one year later, it was found that Mr. J.'s executive functioning had improved to within normal limits, likely due to better diabetes management and improved mood. He reported that he enjoyed reconnecting with his church, and by having Janelle bring him each week, he had also been reconnecting with her. He still had "some difficult days," but he no longer had any thoughts of death, and he found that doing things he enjoyed as part of the behavioral activation he learned in treatment really helped.

Conclusions and Implications

As illustrated with the case of Mr. J., a carefully planned assessment can have a significant, positive impact on the older patient's mood, cognition, and overall well-being. A thorough geriatric assessment considers many aspects of an older adult's life situation, their diverse characteristics including minority status, and their abilities in the context of medical and physical, cognitive, and mental health functioning. The treatment plan carefully weighs independence and autonomy with safety, and often includes multiple different referrals to providers or services to address the older adult's different needs. When done properly and thoughtfully, a well-executed geriatric assessment can lead to key treatment recommendations that lead to improvement or stabilization of older adults in their cognition, medical management, mood, and daily functioning, and improvement in their overall quality of life.

Suggested Resources for Assessment With Older Adults

Attix, D. K., & Welsh-Bohmer, K. A. (2005). *Geriatric neuropsychology: Assessment and intervention.* The Guilford Press.

Lichtenberg, P. A. (2010). *Handbook of assessment in clinical gerontology* (2nd ed.). Academic Press.

Tuokko, H. A., & Smart, C. M. (2018). *Neuropsychology of cognitive decline: A developmental approach to assessment and intervention.* Guilford Press.

References

Acierno, R., Hernandez, M. A., Amstadter, A. B., Resnick, H. S., Steve, K., Muzzy, W., & Kilpatrick, D. G. (2010). Prevalence and correlates of emotional, physical, sexual, and financial abuse and potential neglect in the United States: The National Elder Mistreatment Study. *American Journal of Public Health, 100*(2), 292–297. https://doi.org/10.2105/AJPH.2009.163089

Agrell, B., & Dehlin, O. (1998). The clock-drawing test. *Age and Ageing, 27*(3), 399–403. https://doi.org/10.1093/ageing/27.3.399

Alexopoulos, G. S., Abrams, R. C., Young, R. C., & Shamoian, C. A. (1988). Cornell scale for depression in dementia. *Biological Psychiatry, 23*(3), 271–284. https://doi.org/10.1016/0006-3223(88)90038-8

Allen, D. N., & Becker, M. L. (2019). Clinical interviewing. In G. Goldstein, D. N. Allen, & J. DeLuca (Eds.), *Handbook of psychological assessment* (4th ed., pp. 307–336). Academic Press. https://doi.org/10.1016/B978-0-12-802203-0.00010-9

American Board of Geropsychology. (2017). *Examination manual for specialty board certification in geropsychology.* https://abgero.org/wp-content/uploads/2017/02/ABGERO-Procedures-Manual.pdf

American Psychological Association, Committee on Aging. (2009). *Multicultural competency in geropsychology.*

Andreescu, C., Lenze, E. J., Dew, M. A., Begley, A. E., Mulsant, B. H., Dombrovski, A. Y., Pollock, B. G., Stack, J., Miller, M. D., & Reynolds, C. F. (2007). Effect of comorbid anxiety on treatment response and relapse risk in late-life depression: Controlled study. *British Journal of Psychiatry, 190*(4), 344–349. https://doi.org/10.1192/bjp.bp.106.027169

Barry, K. L., & Blow, F. C. (2010). Screening, assessing and intervening for alcohol and medication misuse in older adults. In P. Lichtenberg (Ed.), *Handbook of assessment in clinical gerontology* (pp. 307–330). Academic Press. https://doi.org/10.1016/b978-0-12-374961-1.10012-0

Beaudreau, S. A., & O'Hara, R. (2009). The association of anxiety and depressive symptoms with cognitive performance in community-dwelling older adults. *Psychology and Aging, 24*(2), 507–512. https://doi.org/10.1037/a0016035

Beck, A. T., Steer, R. A., & Brown, G. K. (1996). *Manual for the Beck Depression Inventory-II.* Psychological Corporation.

Blow, F. C., Brower, K. J., Schulenberg, J. E., Demo-Dananberg, L. M., Young, J. P., & Beresford, T. P. (1992). The Michigan Alcoholism Screening Test- Geriatric version (MAST-G): A new elderly-specific screening instrument. *Alcoholism: Clinical and Experimental Research, 16*(2), 372.

Blow, F. C., Gillespie, B. W., Barry, K. L., Mudd, S. A., & Hill, E. M. (1998). Brief screening for alcohol problems in elderly populations using the Short Michigan Alcoholism Screening Test-Geriatric Version (SMAST-G). *Alcoholism: Clinical and Experimental Research, 22*(3), 20–25.

Bolghan-Abadi, M., Segal, D. L., Coolidge, F. L., & Gottschling, J. (2013). Persian version of the Geriatric Anxiety Scale: Translation and preliminary psychometric properties among Iranian older adults. *Aging and Mental Health, 17*(7), 896–900. https://doi.org/10.1080/13607863.2013.788999

Borson, S., Scanlan, J., Brush, M., Vitaliano, P., & Dokmak, A. (2000). The mini-cog: A cognitive 'vital signs' measure for dementia screening in multi-lingual elderly. *International Journal of Geriatric Psychiatry, 15*(11), 1021–1027. https://doi.org/10.1002/1099-1166(200011)15:11<1021::AID-GPS234>3.0.CO;2-6

Brown, R. L., & Rounds, L. A. (1995). Conjoint screening questionnaires for alcohol and other drug abuse: Criterion validity in a primary care practice. *Wisconsin Medical Journal, 94*(3), 135–140.

Bryan, C. J., & Rudd, M. D. (2006). Advances in the assessment of suicide risk. *Journal of Clinical Psychology: In Session, 62,* 185–200. https://doi.org/10.1002/jclp.20222

Burke, W. J., Roccaforte, W. H., & Wengel, S. P. (1991). The short form of the Geriatric Depression Scale: A comparison with the 30-item form. *Topics in Geriatrics, 4*(3), 173–178. https://doi.org/10.1177/089198879100400310

Bush, K., Kivlahan, D. R., McDonell, M. B., Fihn, S. D., & Bradley, K. A. (1998). The AUDIT alcohol consumption questions (AUDIT-C): An effective brief screening test for problem drinking. *Archives of Internal Medicine, 158*(16), 1789–1795. https://doi.org/10.1001/archinte.158.16.1789

Byers, A. L., Yaffe, K., Covinsky, K. E., Friedman, M. B., & Bruce, M. L. (2010). High occurrence of mood and anxiety disorders among older adults: The National Comorbidity Survey Replication. *Archives of General Psychiatry, 67*(5), 489–496. https://doi.org/10.1001/archgenpsychiatry.2010.35

Byrne, G. J., & Pachana, N. A. (2011). Development and validation of a short form of the Geriatric Anxiety Inventory–the GAI-SF. *International Psychogeriatrics, 23*(1), 125–131.

Chertkow, H., Nasreddine, Z., Joanette, Y., Drolet, V., Kirk, J., Massoud, F., Belleville, S., & Bergman, H. (2007). Mild cognitive impairment and cognitive impairment, no dementia: Part A: Concept and diagnosis. *Alzheimer's & Dementia, 3*(4), 266–282. https://doi.org/10.1016/j.jalz.2007.07.013

Climie, E. A., & Rostad, K. (2011). Test Review: Wechsler Adult Intelligence Scale. *Journal of Psychoeducational Assessment, 29*(6), 581–586. https://doi.org/10.1177/0734282911408707

Conejero, I., Navucet, S., Keller, J., Olié, E., Courtet, P., & Gabelle, A. (2018). A complex relationship between suicide, dementia, and amyloid: A narrative review. *Frontiers in Neuroscience, 12,* 371. https://doi.org/10.3389/fnins.2018.00371

Cruz-Oliver, D. M., Malmstrom, T. K., Allen, C. M., Tumosa, N., & Morley, J. E. (2012). The Veterans Affairs Saint Louis University Mental Status Exam (SLUMS exam) and the Mini-Mental Status Exam as predictors of mortality and institutionalization. *Journal of Nutrition, Health & Aging, 16*(7), 636–641. https://doi.org/10.1007/s12603-012-0098-9

Debruyne, H., Van Buggenhout, M., Le Bastard, N., Aries, M., Audenaert, K., De Deyn, P. P., & Engelborghs, S. (2009). Is the geriatric depression scale a reliable screening tool for depressive symptoms in elderly patients with cognitive impairment? *International Journal of Geriatric Psychiatry, 24*(6), 556–562. https://doi.org/10.1002/gps.2154

Delis, D. C., Kramer, J. H., Kaplan, E., & Ober, B. A. (2000). *California Verbal Learning Test* (2nd ed.). Psychological Corporation.

Drapeau, C. W., & McIntosh, J. L., for the American Association of Suicidology. (2018). *U.S.A. suicide 2017: Official final data.* American Association of Suicidology. http://www.suicidology.org

Edelstein, B. A., Heisel, M. J., McKee, D. R., Martin, R. R., Koven, L. P., Duberstein, P. R., & Britton, P. C. (2009). Development and psychometric evaluation of the Reasons for Living–Older Adults scale: A suicide risk assessment inventory. *Gerontologist, 49,* 736–745. https://doi.org/10.1093/geront/gnp052

Espinosa, A., Alegret, M., Boada, M., Vinyes, G., Valero, S., Martínez-Lage, P., Peña-Casanova, J., Becker, J. T., Wilson, B. A., & Tárraga, L. (2009). Ecological assessment of executive functions in mild cognitive impairment and mild Alzheimer's disease. *Journal of the International Neuropsychological Society, 15*(5), 751–757. https://doi.org/10.1017/S135561770999035X

Ewing J. A. (1984). Detecting alcoholism. The CAGE questionnaire. *JAMA, 252*(14), 1905–1907.5 https://doi.org/10.1001/jama.252.14.1905

Faria, C. D. A., Alves, H. V. D., & Charchat-Fichman, H. (2015). The most frequently used tests for assessing executive functions in aging. *Dementia & Neuropsychologia, 9*(2), 149–155. https://doi.org/10.1590/1980-57642015DN92000009

Fernández, A. L., & Abe, J. (2018). Bias in cross-cultural neuropsychological testing: Problems and possible solutions. *Culture and Brain, 6*(1), 1–35. https://doi.org/10.1007/s40167-017-0050-2

Fernandez-Ballesteros, R., Marquez, M. O., & Santacreu, M. (2015). Geropsychological assessment. In N. A. Pachana & K. Laidlaw (Eds.), *Oxford handbook of clinical Geropsychology* (pp. 184–222). Oxford University Press.

Fink, A., Morton, S. C., Beck, J. C., Hays, R. D., Spritzer, K., Oishi, S., & Moore, A. A. (2002). The alcohol-related problems survey: Identifying hazardous and harmful drinking in older primary care patients. *Journal of the American Geriatrics Society, 50*(10), 1717–1722. https://doi.org/10.1046/j.1532-5415.2002.50467.x

Folstein, M. F., Folstein, S. E., & McHugh, P. R. (1975). "Mini-mental state": A practical method for grading the cognitive state of patients for the clinician. *Journal of Psychiatric Research, 12*(3), 189–198. https://doi.org/10.1016/0022-3956(75)90026-6

Gamache, G., Rosenheck, R., & Tessler, R. (2003). Overrepresentation of women Veterans among homeless women. *American Journal of Public Health, 93*(7), 1132–1136. https://doi.org/10.2105/AJPH.93.7.1132

Gatti, A., Gottschling, J., Brugnera, A., Adorni, R., Zarbo, C., Compare, A., & Segal, D. (2018). An investigation of the psychometric properties of the Geriatric Anxiety Scale (GAS) in an Italian sample of community-dwelling older adults. *Aging & Mental Health, 22*(9), 1176–1184. https://doi.org/10.1037/t71206-000

Gerolimatos, L. A., Ciliberti, C. M., Gregg, J. J., Nazem, S., Bamonti, P. M., Cavanagh, C. E., & Edelstein, B. A. (2015). Development and preliminary evaluation of the Anxiety in Cognitive Impairment and Dementia (ACID) scales. *International Psychogeriatrics, 27*(11), 1825–1838. https://doi.org/10.1037/t53464-000

Glosser, G., Wolfe, N., Albert, M. L., Lavine, L., Steele, J. C., Calne, D. B., & Schoenberg, B. S. (1993). Cross-Cultural Cognitive Examination: Validation of a dementia screening instrument for neuroepidemiological research. *Journal of the American Geriatrics Society, 41*, 931–939. https://doi.org/10.1111/j.1532-5415.1993.tb06758.x

Gottschling, J., Dörendahl, J., Prell, T., Karbach, J., Bunz, M., Kindermann, I., Moussaoui, J., Spinath, F. M., Wedegartner, S., Witte, O. W., Greiff, S., & Segal, D. L. (2019). Measuring anxiety in older adults: Development, diagnostic accuracy, and preliminary validation of a short-form of the German Geriatric Anxiety Scale (GAS-G-SF). *Journal of Personality Assessment, 102*(2), 196–204. https://doi.org/10.1080/00223891.2019.1677679

Gould, C. E., Segal, D. L., Yochim, B. P., Pachana, N. A., Byrne, G. J., & Beaudreau, S. A. (2014). Measuring anxiety in late life: A psychometric examination of the geriatric anxiety inventory and geriatric anxiety scale. *Journal of Anxiety Disorders, 28*(8), 804–811. https://doi.org/10.1016/j.janxdis.2014.08.001

Gross, A. L., Mungas, D. M., Crane, P. K., Gibbons, L. E., MacKay-Brandt, A., Manly, J. J., Mukherjee, S., Romero, H., Sachs, B., Thomas, M., Potter, G. G., & Jones, R. N. (2015). Effects of education and race on cognitive decline: An integrative study of generalizability versus study-specific results. *Psychology and Aging, 30*(4), 863–880. https://doi.org/10.1037/pag0000032

Haw, C., Harwood, D., & Hawton, K. (2009). Dementia and suicidal behavior: A review of the literature. *International Psychogeriatrics, 21*, 440–453. https://doi.org/10.1017/S1041610209009065

Heaton, R. (1993). *Wisconsin Card Sorting Test manual.*

Heisel, M. J, & Flett, G. L. (2006). The development and initial validation of the Geriatric Suicide Ideation Scale. *American Journal of Geriatric Psychiatry, 14*, 742–751. https://doi.org/10.1097/01.JGP.0000218699.27899.f9

Heisel, M. J., & Flett, G. L. (2016). Investigating the psychometric properties of the Geriatric Suicide Ideation Scale (GSIS) among community-residing older adults. *Aging & Mental Health, 20*, 208–221. https://doi.org/10.1080/13607863.2015.1072798

Herrmann, N., Mittmann, N., Silver, I. L., Shulman, K. I., Busto, U. A., Shear, N. H., & Naranjo, C. A. (1996). A validation study of the Geriatric Depression Scale short form. *International Journal of Geriatric Psychiatry, 11*(5), 457–460. https://doi.org/10.1002/(SICI)1099-1166(199605)11:5<457::AID-GPS325>3.0.CO;2-2

Hinrichsen, G. A. (2019). *Assessment and treatment of older adults: A guide for mental health professionals.* American Psychological Association. https://doi.org/10.1037/0000146-000

Johnco, C., Knight, A., Tadic, D., & Wuthrich, V. M. (2015). Psychometric properties of the Geriatric Anxiety Inventory (GAI) and its short-form (GAI-SF) in a clinical and non-clinical sample of older adults. *International Psychogeriatrics, 27*(7), 1089–1097. https://doi.org/10.1017/S1041610214001586

Judd, L. L., Schettler, P. J., & Akiskal, H. S. (2002). The prevalence, clinical relevance, and public health significance of subthreshold depressions. *Psychiatric Clinics, 25*(4), 685–698. https://doi.org/10.1016/S0193-953X(02)00026-6

Katz, S., Downs, T. D., Cash, H. R., & Grotz, R. C. (1970). Progress in development of the index of ADL. *Gerontologist, 10*(1), 20–30. https://doi.org/10.1093/geront/10.1_Part_1.20

Katzman, R., Brown, T., Fuld, P., Peck, A., Schechter, R., & Schimmel, H. (1983). Validation of a short orientation-memory concentration test of cognitive impairment. *American Journal of Psychiatry, 140,* 734–739. https://doi.org/10.1176/ajp.140.6.734

Knight, B. G., Karel, M. J., Hinrichsen, G. A., Qualls, S. H., & Duffy, M. (2009). Pikes Peak model for training in professional geropsychology. *American Psychologist, 64*(3), 205. https://doi.org/10.1037/a0015059

Köhler, S., van Boxtel, M. P., van Os, J., Thomas, A. J., O'Brien, J. T., Jolles, J., Verhey, F. R. J., & Allardyce, J. (2010). Depressive symptoms and cognitive decline in community-dwelling older adults. *Journal of the American Geriatrics Society, 58*(5), 873–879. https://doi.org/10.1111/j.1532-5415.2010.02807.x

Kroenke, K., Spitzer, R. L., Williams, J. B., Monahan, P. O., & Löwe, B. (2007). Anxiety disorders in primary care: Prevalence, impairment, comorbidity, and detection. *Annals of Internal Medicine, 146*(5), 317–325. https://doi.org/10.7326/0003-4819-146-5-200703060-00004

Kuerbis, A., Sacco, P., Blazer, D. G., & Moore, A. A. (2014). Substance abuse among older adults. *Clinics in Geriatric Medicine, 30,* 629–654. https://doi.org/10.1016/j.cger.2014.04.008

Lam, B., Middleton, L. E., Masellis, M., Stuss, D. T., Harry, R. D., Kiss, A., & Black, S. E. (2013). Criterion and convergent validity of the Montreal cognitive assessment with screening and standardized neuropsychological testing. *Journal of the American Geriatrics Society, 61*(12), 2181–2185. https://doi.org/10.1111/jgs.12541

Lawton, M. P., & Brody, E. M. (1969). Assessment of older people: Self-maintaining and instrumental activities of daily living. *Gerontologist, 9*(3), 179–186. https://doi.org/10.1093/geront/9.3_Part_1.179

Lezak, M. D., Howieson, D. B., Bigler, E. D., & Tranel, D. (2012). *Neuropsychological assessment* (5th ed.). Oxford University Press.

Lichtenberger, E. O., & Kaufman, A. S. (2009). *Essentials of WAIS-IV assessment.* John Wiley.

Lin, X. L., Lu, D. L., Gottschling, J., Segal, D. L., & Tang, S. Y. (2017). Validation of a Chinese version of the Geriatric Anxiety Scale among community-dwelling older adults in mainland China. *Journal of Cross-Cultural Gerontology, 32*(1), 57–70. https://doi.org/10.1007/s10823-016-9302-4

Löwe, B., Decker, O., Müller, S., Brähler, E., Schellberg, D., Herzog, W., & Herzberg, P. Y. (2008). Validation and standardization of the Generalized Anxiety Disorder Screener (GAD-7) in the general population. *Medical Care, 46*(3), 266–274. https://doi.org/10.1097/MLR.0b013e318160d093

Lutz, J., Edelstein, B., Katz, E., & Gallegos, J. V. (2019). A shortened version of the Reasons for Living–Older Adults scale for clinical and research utility. *Gerontologist, 59,* e241–e247. https://doi.org/10.1093/geront/gny009

Maruff, P., & Darby, D. (2006). Age-related memory impairment. In P. J. Snyder, P. D. Nussbaum, & D. L. Robins (Eds.), *Clinical neuropsychology: A pocket handbook for assessment* (2nd ed.) (p. 155–182). American Psychological Association. https://doi.org/10.1037/11299-007

McCrimmon, A. W., & Smith, A. D. (2013). Review of the Wechsler Abbreviated Scale of Intelligence, second edition (WASI-II). *Journal of Psychoeducational Assessment, 31*(3), 337–341. https://doi.org/10.1177/0734282912467756

Mehta, K. M., Yaffe, K., & Covinsky, K. E. (2002). Cognitive impairment, depressive symptoms, and functional decline in older people. *Journal of the American Geriatrics Society, 50*(6), 1045–1050. https://doi.org/10.1046/j.1532-5415.2002.50259.x

Miyake, A., Friedman, N. P., Emerson, M. J., Witzki, A. H., Howerter, A., & Wager, T. D. (2000). The unity and diversity of executive functions and their contributions to complex "Frontal Lobe" tasks: A latent variable analysis. *Cognitive Psychology, 41*(1), 49–100. https://doi.org/10.1006/cogp.1999.0734

Mograbi, D. C., de Assis Faria, C., Fichman, H. C., Paradela, E. M. P., & Lourenço, R. A. (2014). Relationship between activities of daily living and cognitive ability in a sample of older adults with heterogeneous educational level. *Annals of Indian Academy of Neurology, 17*(1), 71–76. https://doi.org/10.4103/0972-2327.128558

Molde, H., Nordhus, I. H., Torsheim, T., Engedal, K., Bendixen, A. B., Byrne, G. J., Márquez-González, M., Losada, A., Feng, L., Kuan Tai Ow, E., Pisitsungkagarn, K., Taephant, N., Jarukasemthawee, S.,

Champagne, A., Landreville, P., Gosselin, P., Ribeiro, O., Diefenbach, G. J., Blank, K., Beaudreau, S. A., ... Pachana, N. A. (2019). A cross-national analysis of the psychometric properties of the Geriatric Anxiety Inventory. Journals of Gerontology. Series B. *Psychological Sciences and Social Sciences, 75*(7), 1475–1483. https://doi.org/10.1093/geronb/gbz002

Morimoto, S. S., Kanellopoulos, D., Manning, K. J., & Alexopoulos, G. S. (2015). Diagnosis and treatment of depression and cognitive impairment in late-life. *Annals of the New York Academy of Sciences, 1345*(1), 36. https://doi.org/10.1111/nyas.12669

Moritz, D. J., Kasl, S. V., & Berkman, L. F. (1995). Cognitive functioning and the incidence of limitations in activities of daily living in an elderly community sample. *American Journal of Epidemiology, 141*(1), 41–49. https://doi.org/10.1093/oxfordjournals.aje.a117344

Morley, J. E., & Tumosa, N. (2002). Saint Louis University Mental Status examination (SLUMS). *Aging Successfully, 12*(1), 4. https://doi.org/10.1037/t27282-000

Mueller, A. E., Segal, D. L., Gavett, B., Marty, M. A., Yochim, B., June, A., & Coolidge, F. L. (2015). Geriatric Anxiety Scale: Item response theory analysis, differential item functioning, and creation of a ten-item short form (GAS-10). *International Psychogeriatrics, 27*(7), 1099–1111. https://doi.org/10.1017/S1041610214000210

Nasreddine, Z. S., Phillips, N. A., Bédirian, V., Charbonneau, S., Whitehead, V., Collin, I., Cummings, J. L., & Chertkow, H. (2005). The Montreal Cognitive Assessment, MoCA: A brief screening tool for mild cognitive impairment. *Journal of the American Geriatrics Society, 53*(4), 695–699. https://doi.org/10.1037/t27279-000

National Institute on Alcohol Abuse and Alcoholism. (2019). https://www.niaaa.nih.gov/alcohols-effects-health/special-populations-co-occurring-disorders/older-adults.

O'Hara, R. (2012). The reciprocal relationship of neurocognitive and neuropsychiatric function in late life. *American Journal of Geriatric Psychiatry, 20*(12), 1001–1005. https://doi.org/10.1097/JGP.0b013e318275d60f

Osterrieth, P. A., & Rey, A. (1944). Filetest de copie d'une figure complexe [The test of copying a complex figure]. *Archives de Psychologie, 30,* 206–356.

Pachana, N., Byrne, G., Siddle, H., Koloski, N., Harley, E., & Arnold, E. (2007). Development and validation of the Geriatric Anxiety Inventory. *International Psychogeriatrics, 19,* 103–114. https://doi.org/10.1017/S1041610206003504

Panza, F., Frisardi, V., Capurso, C., D'Introno, A., Colacicco, A. M., Imbimbo, B. P., Santamato, A., Vendemiale, G., Seripa, D., Pilotto, A., Capurso, A., & Solfrizzi, V. (2010). Late-life depression, mild cognitive impairment, and dementia: possible continuum? *American Journal of Geriatric Psychiatry, 18*(2), 98–116. https://doi.org/10.1097/JGP.0b013e3181b0fa13

Pfeiffer, E. (1975). A short portable mental status questionnaire for the assessment of organic brain deficit in elderly patients. *Journal of the American Geriatrics Society, 23*(10), 433–441. https://doi.org/10.1111/j.1532-5415.1975.tb00927.x

Posner, K., Brent, D., Lucas, C., Gould, M., Stanley, B., Brown, G., Fisher, P., Zelazny, J., Burke, A., Oquendo, M., & Mann, J. (2008). *Columbia-suicide severity rating scale (C-SSRS).* Columbia University Medical Center.

Rabinovici, G. D., Stephens, M. L., & Possin, K. L. (2015). Executive dysfunction. *Continuum (Minneapolis, Minn.), 21*(3 Behavioral Neurology and Neuropsychiatry), 646–659. https://doi.org/10.1212/01.CON.0000466658.05156.54

Rey, A. (1941). L'examen psychologique dans les cas d'encephalopathie traumatique. *Archives de Psychologie, 28*(21), 286–340.

Rideaux, T., Beaudreau, S. A., Fernandez, S., & O'Hara, R. (2012). Utility of the abbreviated Fuld Object Memory Evaluation and MMSE for detection of dementia and cognitive impairment not dementia in diverse ethnic groups. *Journal of Alzheimer's Disease, 31*(2), 371–386. https://doi.org/10.3233/JAD-2012-112180

Rivera Mindt, M., Byrd, D., Saez, P., & Manly, J. (2010). Increasing culturally competent neuropsychological services for ethnic minority populations: A call to action. *Clinical Neuropsychologist, 24*(3), 429–453. https://doi.org/10.1080/13854040903058960

Sands, L. P., Yaffe, K., Covinsky, K., Chren, M. M., Counsell, S., Palmer, R., Fortinsky, R., & Landefeld, C. S. (2003). Cognitive screening predicts magnitude of functional recovery from admission to 3 months after discharge in hospitalized elders. Journals of Gerontology. Series A. *Biological Sciences and Medical Sciences, 58*(1), 37–45. https://doi.org/10.1093/gerona/58.1.M37

Satre, D. D., & Wolf, J. P. (2015). Alcohol abuse and substance misuse in later life. In P. A. Lichtenberg, B. T. Mast, B. D. Carpenter, & J. Loebach Wetherell (Eds.), *APA handbook of clinical geropsychology: Vol. 2. Assessment, treatment, and issues of later life* (pp. 121–144). American Psychological Association. https://doi.org/10.1037/14459-005

Segal, D. L., June, A., Payne, M., Coolidge, F. L., & Yochim, B. (2010). Development and initial validation of a self-report assessment tool for anxiety among older adults: The Geriatric Anxiety Scale. *Journal of Anxiety Disorders, 24*(7), 709–714. https://doi.org/10.1016/j.janxdis.2010.05.002

Serafini, G., Calcagno, P., Lester, D., Girardi, P., Amore, M., & Pompili, M. (2016). Suicide risk in Alzheimer's disease: A systematic review. *Current Alzheimer Research, 13,* 1083. https://doi.org/10.2174/1567205013666160720112608

Shankar, K. K., Walker, M., Frost, D., & Orrell, M. W. (1999). The development of a valid and reliable scale for rating anxiety in dementia (RAID). *Aging & Mental Health, 3*(1), 39–49. https://doi.org/10.1080/13607869956424

Sheikh, J. I., & Yesavage, J. A. (1986). Geriatric Depression Scale (GDS): recent evidence and development of a shorter version. *Clinical Gerontology, 5,* 165–173. https://doi.org/10.1300/J018v05n01_09

Shin, M. S., Park, S. Y., Park, S. R., Seol, S. H., & Kwon, J. S. (2006). Clinical and empirical applications of the Rey-Osterrieth Complex Figure Test. *Nature Protocols, 1*(2), 892–899. https://doi.org/10.1038/nprot.2006.115

Skinner, H. A. (1982). The Drug Abuse Screening Test. *Addictive Behaviors, 7*(4), 363–371. https://doi.org/10.1016/0306-4603(82)90005-3

Spitzer, R. L., Kroenke, K., Williams, J. B., & Löwe, B. (2006). A brief measure for assessing generalized anxiety disorder: The GAD-7. *Archives of Internal Medicine, 166*(10), 1092–1097. https://doi.org/10.1001/archinte.166.10.1092

Stene-Larsen, K., & Reneflot, A. (2019). Contact with primary and mental health care prior to suicide: A systematic review of the literature from 2000 to 2017. *Scandinavian Journal of Public Health, 47,* 9–17. https://doi.org/10.1177/1403494817746274

Storey, J. E., Rowland, J. T., Basic, D., Conforti, D. A., & Dickson, H. G. (2004). The Rowland Universal Dementia Assessment Scale (RUDAS): A multicultural cognitive assessment scale. *International Psychogeriatrics, 16*(1), 13–31. https://doi.org/10.1017/s1041610204000043

Strauss, E., Sherman, E. M., & Spreen, O. (2006). *A compendium of neuropsychological tests: Administration, norms, and commentary.* American Chemical Society. https://doi.org/10.1080/09084280701280502

Stroop, J. R. (1992). Studies of interference in serial verbal reactions. *Journal of Experimental Psychology: General, 121*(1), 15–23. https://doi.org/10.1037/0096-3445.121.1.15

Szcześniak, D., & Rymaszewska, J. (2016). Przydatność testu SLUMS w diagnostyce łagodnych zaburzeń poznawczych i otępień [The usefulness of the SLUMS test for diagnosis of mild cognitive impairment and dementia]. *Psychiatria polska, 50*(2), 457–472. https://doi.org/10.12740/PP/OnlineFirst/43141

Talamantes, M., & Sanchez-Reilly, S. (2010). Health and health care of Hispanic/Latino American older adults. In V. S. Periyakoil (Ed.), *eCampus Geriatrics.* http://geriatrics.stanford.edu/ethnomed/latino/

Taragano, F. E., Allegri, R. F., & Lyketsos, C. (2008). Mild behavioral impairment: A prodromal stage of dementia. *Dementia & Neuropsychologia, 2*(4), 256–260 https://doi.org/10.1590/S1980-57642009DN2040000.

Tatum Iii, P. E., Talebreza, S., & Ross, J. S. (2018). Geriatric assessment: An office-based approach. *American Family Physician, 97*(12), 776–784.

Teng, E. L., Hasegawa, K., Homma, A., Imai, Y., Larson, E., Graves, A., Sugimoto, K., Yamaguchi, T., Sasaki, H., & Chiu, D. (1994). The Cognitive Abilities Screening Instrument (CASI): A practical test for cross-cultural epidemiological studies of dementia. *International Psychogeriatrics, 6*(1), 45–62. https://doi.org/10.1017/S1041610294001602

Tombaugh T. N. (2004). Trail Making Test A and B: normative data stratified by age and education. *Archives of clinical neuropsychology: the official journal of the National Academy of Neuropsychologists, 19*(2), 203–214. https://doi.org/10.1016/S0887-6177(03)00039-8

Tombaugh, T. N., Kozak, J., & Rees, L. (1999). Normative data stratified by age and education for two measures of verbal fluency: FAS and animal naming. *Archives of clinical neuropsychology : the official journal of the National Academy of Neuropsychologists, 14*(2), 167–177.

Towers, A., Sheridan, J., Newcombe, D, & Szabo, A. (2018). *The prevalence of hazardous drinking in older New Zealanders.* Health Promotion Agency.

Wechsler, D. (1981). *Wechsler Adult Intelligence Scale-Revised*. Psychological Corporation, New York.

Wechsler, D. (1997). *Wechsler Adult Intelligence Scale* (3rd ed). The Psychological Corporation, San Antonio.

Wechsler, D. (2008). *Wechsler Adult Intelligence Scale–Fourth Edition (WAIS–IV).* NCS Pearson.

Wechsler, D. (2009). *Wechsler Memory Scale* (4th ed). Pearson.

Wechsler, D. (2011). *WASI-II: Wechsler Abbreviated Scale of Intelligence*. Psychological Corporation.

Wide Range Achievement Test – 4. Manual. (2006). Odessa, FL: Psychological Assessment Resources.

Wild, B., Eckl, A., Herzog, W., Niehoff, D., Lechner, S., Maatouk, I., Schellberg, D., Brenner, H., Müller, H., & Löwe, B. (2014). Assessing generalized anxiety disorder in elderly people using the GAD-7 and GAD-2 scales: Results of a validation study. *American Journal of Geriatric Psychiatry, 22*(10), 1029–1038. https://doi.org/10.1016/j.jagp.2013.01.076

World Health Organization. (2014). *Preventing suicide: A global imperative.* http://www.who.int/mental_health/suicide-prevention/exe_summary_english.pdf

Yesavage, J. A., Brink, T. L., Rose, T. L., Lum, O., Huang, V., Adey, M., & Leirer, V. O. (1982). Development and validation of a geriatric depression screening scale: A preliminary report. *Journal of Psychiatric Research, 17*(1), 37–49. https://doi.org/10.1016/0022-3956(82)90033-4

Chapter 3
Theoretical Support and Practical Strategies for CBT With Depressed Older Adults

Ann M. Steffen
Dolores Gallagher-Thompson
Larry W. Thompson

Introduction

This is an exciting time to be a behavioral health professional working with older adults. Our understanding of how to address mental health problems across the lifespan is continuing to develop, including the treatment of depressive symptoms and disorders in later life. Cognitive behavior therapy (CBT) has strong support as an evidence-based treatment for depressive symptoms and syndromes and for major depressive disorder (MDD) in older adults (Braun et al., 2016; Conti et al., 2017; Cuijpers et al., 2014). Most older adults, however, do not experience depression by itself. Age-related chronic illnesses are common and often result in polypharmacy and associated risks. Thus, behavioral health clinicians have a key role to play in offering nonpharmacological interventions to this population (Arnold, 2008; Gallo et al., 2016), both on their own and within the context of interprofessional care (Zeiss, 2016). Research shows that antidepressant medications are typically more effective for severe rather than mild or moderate cases of depression – the latter being more common in clinical practice with older adults (American Psychological Association, 2019). There are also concerns about medication side effects and interactions. For these reasons, older adults generally indicate that they prefer psychotherapy to antidepressant medications, when they are asked (Gum et al., 2006; McHugh et al., 2012). Depression that includes co-occuring anxiety symptoms often includes more somatic symptoms, social and functional impairments, and higher suicide risk (Petkus et al., 2013), with implications for targetting these combined symptoms. Thus, most of us will work clinically with older adults who struggle with symptoms of depression in addition to other mental and physical health concerns. We have written this chapter with that reality in mind.

In this chapter, we provide a case example and discussion of key components of this theoretical conceptualization and therapy approach. As we apply CBT to the case of Mrs. J., we review key areas of conceptualization (the "why?" of treatments), planning (what happens in sessions?), and adaptations (how are strategies implemented?) for older adults. This case is also used to point out how psychological interventions with depressed older adults are continuing to evolve, due to advances in both the science and practice of CBT.

Case Example: Treatment of Depression in an Older Adult

Mrs. J. is a cisgender woman and heterosexually identified 78-year-old widow who lives alone in her apartment in an independent living community. She was referred for CBT by her primary care physician because of chronic back pain and depression – neither of which responded well to treatments he had already done with her. Mrs. J. is of western European background, having come to the US after World War II with a husband she met overseas. She graduated from high school in her native country but was not fluent in English. She eventually learned English well enough to be able to work in a midlevel clerical position at a large insurance company while raising two sons. The marriage was described as happy, although Mrs. J. expresses a great deal of sadness about her husband's final years, when he developed dementia, and she was his primary caregiver. One son lives nearby and tries to see her regularly and check in on her health status; the other lives several thousand miles away and phones her about every 2 weeks. She has a college-age granddaughter named Hannah with whom she is very close; when Mrs. J. stopped driving 2 years ago, she gifted her car to Hannah. The granddaughter drives Mrs. J. to most medical and therapy appointments and wants to be part of the care team. Hannah is studying nursing and believes that helping her grandmother with activities of daily living will help her be a better nurse. In addition to taking her to medical appointments, Mrs. J. depends on her granddaughter Hannah for help with paying bills, grocery shopping, and getting connected to resources on the internet that could help with both her pain and her depression. Mrs. J.'s primary care physician has said that because of multiple medications (needed for other health conditions), Mrs. J. is a poor responder to antidepressants and therefore he thinks that at least a trial of CBT was indicated.

Mrs. J.'s initial Patient Health Questionnaire-9 (PHQ-9) score is 24, indicating severe self-reported depression. At the initial interview, she says she is a "loner" and only occasionally has lunch with friends outside of her senior apartments or goes out to a local park to walk – both activities she enjoys but is not doing on a regular basis. She also discusses a variety of remedies that she has tried for her chronic pain (such as acupuncture and herbal supplements) and expresses discouragement that it would ever improve. Accordingly, we decide on two therapy goals: (1) increase engagement in positive activities (particularly with other people) in order to improve mood and (2) explore other avenues for pain mitigation. Mrs. J. agrees to a course of CBT with mutual review after 3 months to see if continuation was indicated.

In this chapter, we will address how CBT was implemented with Mrs. J., how she responded, and what plans were made for maintenance of gains.

Conceptualizing Depression in Older Adults

Chapter 2 of this book provides a summary of the prevalence and clinical presentation of depression in older adults. Considering the range of factors that predispose individuals to depressive symptoms during later life, it is very important for clinicians to use a unifying theory to guide assessment and treatment planning. The behavioral model of depression in late life (Fiske et al., 2009) is a helpful way of viewing how predisposing factors along with recent losses and illnesses can sometimes (but not always) lead to depressive symptoms, through reductions in activity and a lowered rates of positive outcomes. Even depressive symptoms with strong biological components due to an underlying medical condition may be reduced through behavioral activation (BA) and other CBT change strategies. This behavioral model also indirectly helps to remind us that the predominant symptom of depression in older adults may be *anhedonia* (i.e., perceived lack of enjoyment and pleasure on a daily basis) rather than *dysphoria* (i.e., overt indicators of sadness such as crying, sad facial expressions, or endorsement of the term "depressed" to describe their experience). This anhedonic presentation of depression in later life is one of many reasons that depression goes underrecognized and undiagnosed in older adults. Both medical and behavioral health providers are far more likely to recognize sadness than loss of interest as indicative of depression (Gregg et al., 2013). Thus, this model helps clinicians focus on the key role of rewarding activities in daily life and understand why BA is the front-line intervention strategy for many older adults.

As shown in Figure 3.1, reductions in rewarding daily activities are a primary way that different stressful life events and loss experiences can increase depressive symptoms in older adults. There is growing evidence to indicate that social isolation is particularly

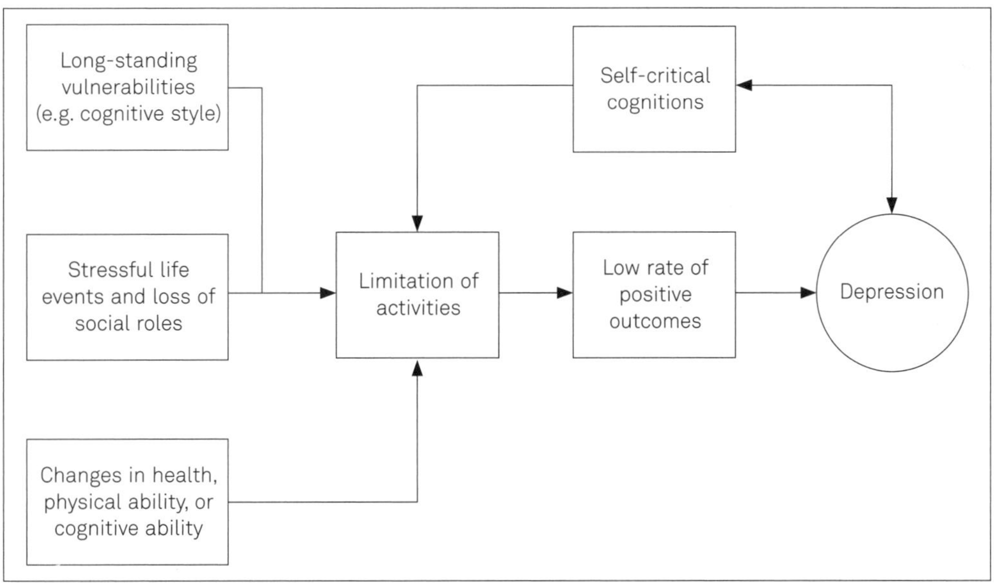

Figure 3.1 Behavioral model of depression

Note. Adapted with permission from "Depression in Older Adults," by A. Fiske et al., 2009, *Annual Review of Clinical Psychology, 5*, p. 369. © 2009 by Annual Review of Clinical Psychology.

important for depression in older adults, leading to a treatment focus on social and interpersonally engaging daily activities (Solomonov et al., 2019). In this model, the most important thoughts related to depression are self-referential, especially self-critical thoughts that continue to perpetuate the downward spiral of social isolation, reduced activity (especially social activities), and anhedonia.

> In the case of Mrs. J., we see that she has few positive activities in her daily life. Much of her time is spent at medical appointments, or reading alone in her apartment. She admits to feeling lonely and socially isolated (except for contact with her granddaughter, Hannah), despite having some activities (and people) she enjoys doing or being with. Clearly, her depressed mood is reinforced by the relative absence of positive reinforcement in her life.

Before we move into considering the treatment planning for this specific case, it is important to provide a brief overview of principles of CBT that are shared across problem areas. Although these principles are generalizable over the lifespan, our examples are specific to clinical work with older adults.

Cognitive Behavior Therapy With Older Adults

There are many excellent resources available to advance knowledge and skill development for readers interested in learning more about applying CBT to adults aged 65 years and older. Reviews of the principles, practices, and the strong evidence base for using CBT with older adults are available (Braun et al., 2016; Conti et al., 2017, Gallagher-Thompson & Thompson, 2010). In addition, we have included the section Suggested CBT Resources for Older Adults, at the end of this chapter.

CBT reflects a commitment to scientific evidence combined with a deeply humanistic approach to clinical work that emphasizes collaboration between the therapist and patient at every phase of treatment. Rather than considering CBT to be a range of specific therapeutic techniques to be used with older patients, clinicians are encouraged to view CBT as an orientation to therapy that applies a biopsychosocial conceptualization of problems and principles of change (Laidlaw et al., 2003, 2004). Individuals, and the problems they want help with, are always viewed within the context of their unique learning history as well as the social and physical environments that are present in their current lives. The problems that bring individuals into therapy, and well as their competencies and personal strengths, only make sense within the specific context of these life circumstances. Patients and therapists work together to identify patterns and develop new habits of behaving, thinking, and feeling that are a good fit for the patient's social and physical environments. Sometimes, however, the focus of CBT is on shaping the social and physical environments to be a better fit for the older adult's strengths and limitations. It is this focus on person–environment fit – along with the understanding of interactions among biological, emotional, behavioral, and cognitive processes – that drives specific CBT approaches to therapy with individuals across the lifespan. Therapists are encouraged to use a coherent conceptual framework in their work with patients, and have that framework be evident in the language they employ within therapy sessions. A good example of this applied to self-monitoring, activity scheduling, and cognitive change strategies is provided by Petrik et al. (2013). Because the science of change is constantly evolving, however, the specific theories and practices of CBT are also undergoing revision (Karpiak et al., 2016).

Remaining consistent over the past 30 years is CBT's focus on what Kanfer and Schefft (1988) called the six "think" rules: (1) *Think behavior* – help your older patients redefine the problem (and goals) in terms of concrete behaviors rather than in concepts like traits or abstract discussions of the problem "in general"; (2) *Think solution* – help your older patients ask continuously, "What might I be able to try out this week to improve the situation?"; (3) *Think positive* – have your older patients identify personal strengths and the positive aspects of any event or change effort; (4) *Think small steps* – help your older patients set limited goals to increase probability of some success and allow ongoing reevaluation of triggering situations; (5) *Think flexible* – help your older patients develop alternative ways of thinking and back-up plans so that they are prepared for the unexpected; and (6) *Think future* – focus on the time ahead rather than past events, and encourage your older patients to engage in planning and rehearsal. Thus, the theoretical foundations of CBT help clinicians and their older patients develop a shared conceptualization of factors that are maintaining the targeted problem, and together implement specific personal and environmental change strategies in a one-step-at-a-time manner.

Consistent with patient-centered care principles and practices, careful attention is paid to identifying a small number of problems (i.e., one or two) of most importance to the older adult, and developing specific treatment goals that are observable and measurable. It is important for each session to include a brief orientation with a reminder and assessment of those agreed-upon target problems and goals, so that the older patient can have concrete ways of seeing when they are improving. It is equally important for therapists to be able to track when the patient is not improving, so that troubleshooting can occur. As described in Chapter 2, group-level nomothetic methods are used for routinely monitoring therapy outcomes, such as the Geriatric Depression Scale (GDS; Yesavage et al., 1982; available in multiple languages at no cost) or the Beck Depression Inventory-II (BDI-II; Beck et al., 1996; which is now copyrighted and involves a fee). Some clinics treating older adults (particularly in primary care settings) use the PHQ-9 (Kroenke & Spitzer, 2002) for depression (which also is available in multiple languages at no cost) and the OQ-45 (Lambert, 2012; available for a licensing fee) for assessing subjective distress, life functioning, and social relationships.

CBT, however, also has a strong focus on identifying and routinely assessing individual-level (i.e., idiographic) concerns; clinicians are encouraged to help older patients track change each session by using assessment tools such as the Psychological Outcomes Profile (PSYCHLOPS; Sales & Alves, 2016; available at no cost) and/or single-item ratings developed together in session (i.e., "On a scale from 1 to 10, how connected did you feel with at least one person over the past week?" and "As you think about the past week, how would you describe your sense that life is meaningful, from 1–10?"). Most older adults have had experience with recovering from an illness or surgery in which they have been asked to use a 1–10 pain scale to rate their level of pain. Thus, single-item ratings in session are familiar, and 1–10 scales make intuitive sense. Asking for (and recording) a specific number to evaluate your older patient's experiences of target concerns is also an excellent strategy for maintaining focus from session to session.

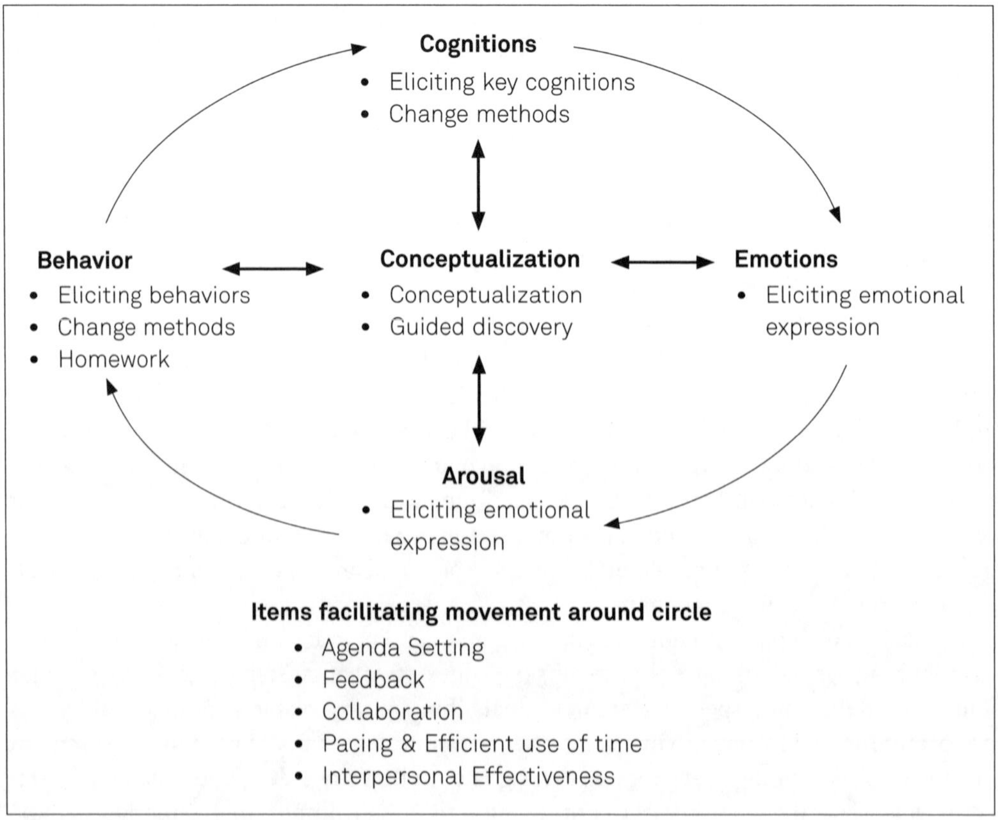

Figure 3.2 Therapeutic skills in CBT
Note. Reproduced with permission from *Manual of the Revised Cognitive Therapy Scale (CTS-R),* by I. A. James et al., 2001, unpublished manuscript, p. 2. © 2001 by James et al.

The Cognitive Therapy Rating Scale–Revised (James et al., 2001) has become a valuable way for trainees and clinicians to work on their development of CBT skills. As shown in Figure 3.2, CBT therapists are aware of and manage several processes throughout each therapy session, and across the course of therapy. Throughout this chapter, we will highlight skills and strategies that are especially important when applying CBT to the treatment of depression in older adults.

Early Phase of Therapy With Depressed Older Adults

Positive Psychology–Positive Aging

As mentioned earlier, CBT has emphasized a strengths-based perspective from its very beginnings, and previous generations of CBT therapists are well-acquainted with the importance of drawing upon patients' strengths within session and for treatment planning. There are also exciting new developments in the ways in which the science of positive psychology is being applied to clinical interventions with older adults. These applications of positive psychology coincide with antiageism campaigns happening across the globe. There is growing recognition of the significant harm and damage created by ageist attitudes, including those held by behavioral health providers and by patients. At the same time that positive psychotherapies continue to be developed and evaluated (Parks & Layous, 2016; Walsh et al., 2017), positive psychology principles and strategies of change have been integrated into existing cognitive and behavioral therapies with adults (Padesky & Mooney, 2012) and older adults (Bilbrey et al., in press; Hill, 2011).

In our case of Mrs. J., from the first session, the therapist worked to devote significant time to balancing the discussion of problems with identifying personal strengths and areas of life that were going well. When Mrs. J. was asked to provide recent examples of the issues that had brought her into therapy, the therapist would validate the difficulty of those: "I can hear the struggle you are having, as you talk about your pain and feeling lonely. At the same time..." The therapist noted past examples of Mrs. J. successfully managing other painful life experiences such as relocating to the US as an adult, having to learn English well enough to be able to be employed, and eventually nursing her husband through his Alzheimer's disease progression. When she became discouraged, the therapist would gently ask her if any part of her current challenges reminded her of other difficult phases in her life that she had successfully coped with. For example, when Mrs. J. cared for her husband she was often discouraged about the downhill course of his disease. She cried frequently and knew she was often close to "the limit" as far as how much stress she could handle as she dealt with all sorts of cognitive and behavior problems. However, she recognized that she DID manage her stress "somehow" (e.g., it turns out she listened to music often and watched certain favorite videos at home to relieve stress). She also called upon her two sons to help in whatever ways they could, and attended some of her granddaughter's school events (when she could find someone to stay with her husband). So, upon reflection, Mrs. J. saw that she did indeed have problem-solving skills and had some very adaptive ways to cope with stress. With a little direction from the therapist, she was able to see that these same strategies could be useful to her now in her current situation – although her experience of back pain kept coming up as a possible deterrent and needed to be addressed at the same time.

The therapist also listened for, and asked Mrs. J. to identify, words that she used for positive experiences (e.g., "satisfying," and "peaceful") and her feelings (e.g., "glad," and "pleased"). In the between-session mood-monitoring exercises discussed later, Mrs. J. specifically kept track of those positive experiences as well as recording levels of pain and negative thinking. By monitoring all three, she was able to see their interconnectedness and more clearly understand how one influenced the other.

Throughout all phases of therapy, therapists are encouraged to listen for and call attention to patients' personal strengths and signs of competence, while still validating current difficulties and painful experiences. Small signs of improvement are acknowledged as promising, while carefully judging how each patient responds to encouragement. This is modulated based on the degree of positive response versus signs of withdrawal due to too much "cheerleading" that may be experienced as invalidating by some patients. In those cases, clinicians can place comments about strengths and positive signs of improvement within the context of acknowledging difficulties. For example, they might say,

> This has been a really difficult time for you, and sometimes you wonder whether anything will get better. As I look over your scores from the past month, and as we talk through some of the efforts you've made in changing little things in your day, I see a lot of strength in you and much for us to be encouraged about. For example...

Explicit and implicit biases about aging influence older adults and their families (e.g., with internalized ageism shaping daily behaviors), professionals (e.g., career interests, expectations for different-aged patients, and discriminatory assessment and treatment practices), communities and national policies. Combating implicit ageist stereotypes *within therapists* involves both enhancing knowledge about aging and providing opportunities for contact with healthy older adults (Levy, 2018). A nice example of this is seen in the World Health Organization's antiaging initiatives (https://www.who.int/ageing/en/). In the case of Mrs. J.'s therapist, it was important that the clinician had experience with aging issues across a range of functioning, and was also involved in some community programs with older adults who were high functioning. This helped the clinician stay realistic (i.e., neither overestimating or underestimating what Mrs. J. was capable of). We are enthusiastic about the ways in which principles and strategies of positive psychology, along with attention to positive aging, will shape the future of professional training and behavioral health for older adults.

Attention to Emotions

Clinicians with only superficial exposure to CBT have wondered whether CBT allows for enough attention to the emotional experiences of patients within and outside of therapy. Because "emotion" does not appear alongside "cognitive" and "behavior" in the term "cognitive behavior therapy," it can appear to be neglected. As we will see throughout this chapter, it is simply impossible to deliver CBT without careful attention to emotions and emotional experiences of patients. Decisions about activity scheduling can only be made when the patient and therapist are aware of the ebb and flow of emotions related to different daily activities and events. Changing aspects of the physical and/or social environment is guided by assessing emotional experiences in those settings. Cognitive reappraisal strategies are only effective when the most current *and* emotionally loaded thoughts are identified, targeted, and modified. Additionally, the support of a warm and caring therapist is essential when patients are called upon to take the many risks involved in change.

For these reasons, the beginning phase of therapy will commonly involve spending some time discussing emotions. An early session generally includes the clinician providing some psychoeducation on the role of emotions, discussing what emotions are and how they work (i.e., to debunk overly strong beliefs in catharsis as a primary change strategy) as well determining the patient's ability to label and describe emotional experiences. It can be helpful for therapists new to working with older adults to be aware of cultural and generational differences in the labeling of emotions (Wuthrich et al., 2015). Older women, for example, are less likely to endorse feeling "anxious" and "angry" than younger patients, instead preferring other labels such as "tense" and "frustrated."

> Mrs. J. is able to describe her negative emotions; she uses "blah" more often than "sad" and commonly refers to feeling "tense" and "stressed" about getting worse and becoming more homebound. It was difficult for her to describe positive feelings – except when listening to music, which evokes positive memories, and as she describes "brings gladness to my heart." She strongly prefers "glad" and "pleased" over "happy" to describe positive emotional moments of her day.

All older patients, including those with a restricted range of emotional experiences and/ or vocabulary, will benefit from printed lists of feeling terms available to look at during the therapy session. Recognition memory is far easier than recall for all of us, and this phenomenon increases with age. A nice source of clinical information and practice suggestions related to working with emotions in CBT is provided by Hofmann (2015).

Behavioral Activation

Behavioral activation (BA) is an excellent starting point for most older adults as it is relatively straightforward to understand, addresses a common aspect of depression (reduced positive daily activities), improves mood, and decreases depressive symptomatology. BA has a very solid evidence base as a treatment for depression (Alexopoulos et al., 2016; Hawley et al., 2017), for use with depressed older adults in primary care, long-term care (Meeks, Looney, et al., 2008, Meeks et al., 2015, 2019), and prison nursing homes (Meeks, Sublett, et al., 2008), as well as with depressed caregivers of persons with cognitive impairment (Au et al., 2015; 2019; Bilbrey et al., 2020). Importantly, BA has shown to be effective for a diverse range of older individuals, including African-American older adults in the US (Szanton et al., 2014) and those experiencing cognitive loss, such as mild cognitive impairment or early-stage Alzheimer's disease (Bilbrey et al., in press). For these reasons, we strongly recommend that clinicians consider BA as a key change strategy and apply it in a coherent manner at the outset of treatment.

An early goal in therapy is to use self-monitoring and guided discovery to help older depressed patients appreciate that (1) their depressive symptoms vary in intensity across the day and from day to day and that (2) intentionally engaging in valued and rewarding activities can be a powerful way to reduce depression and increase positive emotional experiences. Some older adults already have that mindset, allowing therapy to progress rapidly toward implementing activity scheduling and then problem solving certain activities. Other patients may have only a vague sense of these relationships, and need a slower and more methodical approach. Clinicians can also expect to work with some depressed older adults who (1) have a firmly entrenched personal conceptualization of their depression as reactive to biological, environmental, or historical factors that are out of their control, as well as some (2) with mild cognitive impairments for whom any form of therapy is challenging For these patients, BA is just as valuable but needs more within- and between-session time to work on specific components of this process.

Because Mrs. J. was somewhat socially isolated, and one of her initial therapy goals was to increase her activity level, BA was initiated at the second session. A detailed description of how to modify standard BA for effective use with older adults is found in Bilbrey et al. (in press) and Bilbrey et al. (2020).

Many of the challenges faced by clinicians in implementing BA with older adults are the same as those with younger adult patients – with some notable exceptions. It can be difficult to figure out what activities patients still enjoy but are not doing at all, and activities they used to enjoy but now do much less often. These changes are usually for medical reasons (e.g., functional issues such as pain from arthritis that limits standing and walking which therefore limits related hobbies like gardening, golf, or bowling). Clinicians may want to employ the Older Persons Pleasant Events Schedule (COPPES; Rider et al., 2016) to help with identifying key activities. This questionnaire has 66 items that are rated for frequency of engagement in the past month, and for enjoyability (i.e., regardless of whether they occurred). This allows the clinician to see if there are activities that are rated high for enjoyability but are low in frequency. Discussing these activities is a fruitful way to develop options that the patient probably did not think of on their own. These specific activities often lead to further discussion about related things the person likes to do but thinks are no longer possible. This discussion, in turn, encourages behavioral experimentation to test out what is possible at this stage of life.

The worlds of many older adults will have shrunk due to limited ability to drive (or use other transportation) and lack of access to friends or family members for shared activities. These issues can be addressed by incorporating a problem-solving approach to connecting with others (Solomonov et al., 2019) from the outset. Example questions can include: Are there activities of interest that can be done close to home? Are there neighbors who may be in a similar situation who would also enjoy visiting with someone nearby? Can a ride service be used? What community resources might assist? Questions such as these can elicit a broad spectrum of responses that, in turn, lead to a list of potentially positive activities for the patient to incorporate into their daily life.

Many older adults lack regular routines in their day. Using the session time to explicitly schedule positive daily activities increases the likelihood that BA will succeed, because the therapist can help ensure consideration of details and potential barriers. A significant part of BA involves identifying and problem solving potential barriers. Scheduled activities can be written on a simple form to take home for practice. On this home practice sheet, the patient is asked to indicate which activities were completed, along with a rating of enjoyability. This information is reviewed at the next session, and adjustments are made based on home practice experience.

Because BA is commonly implemented relatively early in treatment, this becomes the context for managing many aspects of CBT. Clinicians are responsible for managing the pacing of sessions to allow enough time for developing and reviewing home practice assignments. Most older patients will benefit from consistent use of session summary forms completed toward the end of session (see Box 3.1) and session preparation forms (see Box 3.2). Tompkins (2004) is an excellent resource for therapists who wish to continue to build their skills in between-session assignments.

Box 3.1. Mrs. J.'s Session Number 4 Summary Form

My Session Summary Form

Date of Session: *Friday, June 5, 2020*

Name of My Therapist: *Dr. Dolores Gallagher-Thompson*

Today, we focused on:

- *Sometimes having a bad day is related to what I do that day (not the other way around).*
- *If I am busy, my brain has less time to focus on how much my back hurts.*

I'd like to especially remember:

- *I have some control over how I feel.*
- *There are specific things that help me feel better if I remember to do them.*

Before my next appointment, I am going to specifically work on:

1. *Check off what activities I did, and rate my mood, right before bed.*
2. *Reread over activities listed in COPPES to see if I get new ideas.*
3. *Write down any new/old things I am willing to try.*
4. *Ask Hannah if she is willing to set up weekly phone chat late Sunday afternoon (or another time that works better for her).*

This will involve these specific sheets (list here):

Activities and Mood Form

Older Persons Pleasant Events Schedule (COPPES) form

My next appointment is on *Friday, June 12th, 2020* at *11:00* am/pm.

Box 3.2. Mrs. J.'s Preparing for Session Number 5 Form

My Preparing for Session Form

Date of Session: *Friday, June 12th, 2020*

Name of My Therapist: *Dolores*

Instructions: Either at home or in the waiting room before my session, I should spend no more than 5–10 minutes to jot down a few words or phrases in each section below....

What did we talk about or work on in the most recent session?
- *Some things I could do to help with my depression.*
- *Even little positive things count.*
- *I am not alone.*

What was I trying to practice at home? Did I have a specific between-sessions assignment?
- *Check off activities and rate mood every day.*
- *Look over COPPES form and find some new things to do – walking? Art class?*

Did I have any difficulties with this? Learn anything new?
I'm not sure that I did this right; just circle numbers? Or was I supposed to make notes? Didn't know how much detail to put down.

Getting out of my apartment helps some – walking around the block — even though it feels like a lot of work.

What do I want my therapist to know about the past week? Have there been any major changes in my condition or life?
My eye doctor told me I have early signs of macular degeneration. I will need to start taking eye vitamins, and go in for more frequent appointments. I'm worried about whether I might go blind down the road.

What would I like to be sure to talk about in today's session?
This new problem with my eyes – I might go blind. Why do these things always happen to me?

Mrs. J.'s responses on the COPPES showed that she really enjoyed listening to music but was already doing that frequently. She also really enjoyed going for walks at a nearby park but had not done that in the past month. Similarly, her mood improved when she talked with her sons and granddaughter but that was "hit or miss" and did not occur on any type of schedule. She wanted to join an art class at the local senior center (had painted as a means of stress relief many times earlier in life) but did not know when the class was held, how to use the computer to find out, or whether her senior apartment coordinator could help her find transportation to get there. Discussion and questioning elicited a list of a dozen potentially enjoyable things Mrs. J. could do in the next week. Together, the therapist and patient recorded this list and tentatively scheduled which days the various things would be done. Her home practice was to monitor these activities and record pain level when she was (or was not) engaged in them. Subsequent sessions were spent reviewing and fine-tuning this information.

Middle and Later Phases of Therapy With Depressed Older Adults

BA Continued and Cognitive Reframing Added

Often the bulk of CBT with depressed older adults is focused on increasing rewarding and meaningful activities. In the middle and later phases of treatment, this includes refining choices for positive activities and problem solving barriers so that they can realistically be accomplished. For example, many older adults put walking on their list. In some climates, walking outside is difficult (if not impossible) during some months of the year. Rather than stop walking, alternatives such as mall walking or joining a gym and using a treadmill can be explored. It is also common to discover that activities thought to be enjoyable are so not in actuality (e.g., joining a book club is not much fun if the club reads only mysteries, and the patient prefers historical nonfiction). Again, it is the clinician's job to encourage development of options. The therapeutic goal by the middle of therapy – typically Session 6 or so in a 12-session treatment – is an increase in daily positive activities to a range associated with reduced symptoms of depression. Often, at least four rewarding activities per day are needed. This goal will take more sessions to reach if the patient is severely depressed – in which case establishing new patterns of one or two positive activities each day may be the starting point – gradually working up to more. Additional time is often required if the patient is experiencing significant memory problems and other symptoms of cognitive impairment. In these cases, involving an interested family member or friend as a coach can be very helpful. The coach can help keep the patient on track and can more accurately report back as to what is working and what is not successful.

> With her granddaughter Hannah's help in scheduling and transportation, Mrs. J. was able to regularly engage in four to six positive activities daily by Session 8 and experienced a concomitant decrease in depressive symptoms (as evidenced on her PHQ-9 result, which dropped to 10, from 24, and was stable there for several weeks). Mrs. J. reported decreased pain interference as she learned that she could engage in rewarding and meaningful daily activities despite her chronic pain; this combined with careful pacing of activities enabled her to do more than she thought she could. Throughout this process, however, Mrs. J. also expressed several persistent negative thoughts about how bad the future was going to be, how little control she had over her health, and how she was likely to get more depressed again when some new health problem emerged. By mutual agreement, it was decided to spend several sessions on discussing these negative thoughts systematically, and questioning them, so that more adaptive thoughts could (potentially) be generated.

The decision whether or not to proceed with the more *cognitive* components of CBT is a clinical one that will vary depending on a number of factors: (1) depth of depression that remains, (2) whether or not persistent negative thought patterns are present that interfere with having a good quality of life, and (3) the cognitive capacity of the patient to process this more intellectually demanding aspect of CBT. For many patients, BA is sufficient to improve mood; CBT can be ended at the point that BA has taken hold as a new habit the patient is able to practice regularly, with associated mood benefit. For some patients, however, persistent negative thinking prevents them from engaging in BA successfully. If the patient believes, for example, that "nothing I do will make me feel any better," then they are unlikely to make the effort required for BA. Therapy can help the patient question that thought and hopefully modify it into something more flexible and realistic, such as "I may not be able to get rid of this depression completely, but there are things I can do to feel better day by day." Recording these thoughts (and associated feelings) is usually done to highlight the problem, followed by use of specific reappraisal strategies (e.g., examining the evidence, asking, "is this thought helpful?" thinking about what a friend would say or do in the same situation, and learning to think along a continuum rather than in *all or none* terms). In all of these reappraisal strategies, the goal is for the clinician to help the patient develop more adaptive ways of viewing their situation, which then lead to more willingness to engage in positive daily activities and initiate other behavioral coping strategies. Thus, cognitive reappraisal is in the service of behavior change, or maintaining recent changes in the face of new challenges. Illustrations of these methods can be found in Gallagher-Thompson et al. (2020) and Laidlaw and Kishita (2015).

> Mrs. J. agreed to record these negative thoughts for a week and bring them to next session where a pattern of catastrophizing about her future was obvious – the "fortune telling" error – along with minimizing her strengths and coping abilities ("I can't deal with this at my age. When I was younger, I was stronger; now I am weak and frail"). The technique of Mrs. J. asking herself, "Is this thought helping me?" and "Is there another way of thinking about this that is more helpful?" was used to help Mrs. J. distrust these automatic thoughts and gradually develop a more adaptive view of her future situation. Over the next few sessions, Mrs. J. kept a diary of both positive and negative thoughts – she was asked to record thoughts every few hours and label them as helpful, unhelpful, or neutral, and bring in the information to review in-session. This exercise revealed that she often discounted her strengths and instead focused on her weaknesses. When the therapist and Mrs. J. discussed this together, it became easier for Mrs. J. to recognize certain patterns as self-defeating and contributing to depressed mood (and sometimes, also leading to increased pain perceptions). Mrs. J. was willing to try reframing the harshly negative thoughts and came up with statements such as, "At my age it will probably be harder to cope with change than when I was younger – but, I'm intelligent, I can still walk and talk to people and do many things that a lot of people my age cannot do." She also began a gratitude journal which she found very helpful, as it refocused her on what was good about her present life – clearly it was not all bad, and there was no reason to believe it would be all bad in the future.

As is true for BA, many of the challenges of implementing cognitive reappraisal as a change strategy for depressed older adults are the same as for patients across the lifespan. Solid training and supervision and consultation in cognitive therapy will ensure that providers facilitate the development of these skills in their patients. It is the responsibility of the therapist to help *the patient* learn to monitor, assess, and respond to unhelpful and depressogenic thoughts that are triggered in daily life. Although there is an important role for guided discovery and facilitative questions by the therapist, older adults' development of reappraisal skills is primarily achieved though *their asking themselves key questions*, rather than the therapist taking on this role. It is strongly recommended that therapists provide a printed list of questions, so that patients can ask themselves about their own thoughts. Behavioral health providers utilizing cognitive therapy as a change strategy need to embrace their role as an instructor, and then (most importantly) as coach during the time these skills are generalized across a range of life events and social environments.

Modifications for this work with older adults, especially those with mild cognitive impairment (Coon et al., 2007), can include breaking down the five-column thought record first into a three-column one (e.g., situation, thought, feeling). Rather than providing older patients with a list of all the unhelpful thought patterns used in CBT, we provide a shorter list of the most common that occur with this age group and cohort (e.g., personalizing, catastrophizing, all-or-nothing thinking). In the case of older adults with mild cognitive impairment, for example, it can be helpful to identify a pattern of key unhelpful thoughts, develop alternatives, and provide the alternative thoughts in written form so patients can read through them once each day as a reminder.

Readers will note that we have not mentioned schema work or therapy targeting core maladaptive schemas. It is our position, and one that is supported by the literature, that a focus on core schemas is often unnecessary and sometimes iatrogenic (harmful). For example, in a study with adults using *mind over mood* to treat depression (Hawley et al., 2017), attention to core beliefs led to an increase in depressive symptoms over the course of treatment. BA and cognitive reappraisal strategies, in contrast, reduced depressive symptoms. For these reasons, we recommend reserving work on core schemas for treatment failures or refractory patients. Clinicians who find themselves curious about their client's core negative schemas may decide to include these as part of their case conceptualization. Schema therapy should be implemented, however, only by a therapist formally trained and supervised in these change strategies. It is important to be aware that therapeutic strategies used to elicit negative schemas, such as the downward arrow technique (i.e., "If that was true, what would that mean about you? And if that was true, what would that mean about you?...") function as negative mood inductions when used with depressed patients. Inappropriately timed or poorly implemented, schema-related interventions can be harmful and exacerbate depression in older adults.

Later Phases of CBT With Older Adults

Therapy Termination

By Session 12, Mrs. J. said she did not feel she needed to come in weekly anymore because she was feeling much better (as supported by her PHQ-9 score of 8). Sessions were spaced out to every 2 weeks over 2 months, and then one monthly session for the next 6 months, for a total of 10 additional sessions. Because Mrs. J. maintained improvement over that time, a final follow-up session was scheduled for 3 months after that. At the final session, she remained stable with mild depression and mood fluctuations. Mrs. J. reported continuing to use BA and thought reframing (at times) and said BA had now become a "habit" – the importance of continuing this approach was reinforced by the clinician as well.

Termination can be difficult for older patients – particularly if a strong, trusting relationship was formed with the clinician. Many patients describe this relationship as "filling a void in my life" and are reluctant to give it up. This can be anticipated and dealt with by encouraging the patient to work on developing (or strengthening) a similar trusting relationship with another person in their lives, such as an existing friend (with whom friendship could be deepened) or a clergyperson or someone else they already trust but may not have opened up to much in the past. Discussing who this could be and how to work on that relationship so that it can be more satisfying are good topics for the final three to four sessions of CBT with older adults. A focus on relapse prevention is also encouraged; this includes developing a written review of what was successful for the patient, and what they tried that did not work so well, along with anticipation of future situations likely to result in depression again. Thinking through, and then writing down, what could be done when those situations occur can be a useful form of cognitive rehearsal – a technique often found to be helpful for relapse prevention. Recording this information (and giving it to the patient) is part of this process (Gallagher-Thompson & Thompson, 2010).

> Termination was difficult for Mrs. J., as she had developed a strong, trusting relationship with her therapist. To ease into the process, discussion focused on other meaningful relationships in her life and how she could enhance them so that she would have "someone to talk to" – such as using more self-disclosure and asking questions about the other person's struggles and how they are coping. Mrs. J. was willing to try this with another woman who lived down the hall in her senior apartment complex. Mrs. J. invited the resident over to her unit; over tea they were able to share more about their lives and struggles. Mrs. J. found this hopeful and felt encouraged that she could continue to build this relationship over time. When her granddaughter, Hannah, graduated and began a full-time job, Mrs. J. developed a stronger worry of "being a burden." One session near termination helped Mrs. J. identify some regular volunteers at her apartment complex who could both take her to medical appointments and function as friendly visitors. She then learned that one of these retired ladies shared her interest in art and music.

Two termination-related sessions were devoted to relapse prevention. A series of questions were explored: What signs or signals would alert Mrs. J. that depression was getting bad again? (e.g., in her case, it was difficulty sleeping, and more perceived pain and worry upon awakening). How could she cope? Could she apply anything she had learned in CBT at that time to reduce the depression? Or would she need to seek the services of a clinician again? A written *action plan* was developed, including relevant phone numbers, in case she felt she needed therapy. During the follow-up sessions, this information was reviewed and updated. Mrs. J. was asked what challenges she had faced since her last session and how she had dealt with them. The clinician provided feedback reinforcing Mrs. J.'s continued use of CBT practices and trusting her personal strengths.

Termination as such is not always able to be accomplished. Some patients do not have family or other trusted persons in their lives to provide support and feelings of social connectedness. In those cases, sessions may need to continue, spread out over many months, to maintain therapeutic gains and prevent relapse. The patient may also be referred to an ongoing CBT group (if available) or to other resources, such as peer counseling programs or *friendly visitor* programs, which exist in some communities. Effectively managing termination involves clinical decisions made in the patient's best interest and consistent with best practices in the region or agency for which the clinician works.

Treating Suicidality in Depressed Older Adults

Changes in functional abilities and onset of new disabilities are particularly strong risk factors for suicidality in older adults (Lutz & Fiske, 2018). In earlier years of CBT for depression, it was often assumed that targeting and reducing depressive symptoms would also successfully treat suicidality and reduce suicide risk. That is no longer consistent with current practice guidelines. Global suicide rates for older adults are high compared to those for other age groups (Sachs-Ericsson et al., 2016) and therapists have a responsibility to directly assess suicidal thoughts and behaviors in their depressed older patients using a validated screening tool; Chapter 2 of this book includes specific recommendations for this (Samarina et al, 2021). In the US, the Columbia Lighthouse Project provides free tools and online training for professionals in suicide risk assessment (https://cssrs.columbia.edu/).

If patients are evaluated as being at risk for suicide or self-harm, it is important to target the suicidal symptoms directly in therapy using an evidence-based treatment for suicidality. Within the US, the Joint Commission is responsible for accreditation of hospitals and acute care settings. In their National Patient Safety Goal 15.01.01, providers must conduct and document suicide risk assessment and the specific strategies implemented to manage risk. Three specific treatments are listed as effective and recommended: cognitive behavioral therapy for suicide prevention (CBT-SP; Brown et al., 2005; Kiosses et al., 2018), dialectical behavior therapy (Linehan, 2015), and collaborative assessment method for suicidality (CAMS; Jobes, 2016). These treatments appear to be appropriate for depressed older adults who are at elevated risk for suicide, yet the literature is still quite sparse in this area (Zeppegno et al., 2019). For readers who are especially interested in treatment for suicidality in depressed older adults, some case studies are available describing CBT-SP (Bhar & Brown, 2012) and problem-solving therapy (Lutz et al., 2019).

Exciting Developments in Geriatric Mental Health

There is a growing consensus on generalist (Hinrichsen et al., 2018) and specialist-level (Karel et al., 2010) attitudinal and knowledge-based competencies and skills that are vital to clinical practice with older adults. Interprofessional health care teams, for example, are important means of delivering behavioral health services to older adults with complex medical and psychosocial needs, and require a number of professional skills beyond those involved in psychotherapy (Decaporale-Ryan, et al., in press; Steffen & Zeiss, 2017). The Pikes Peak model for training in professional geropsychology (Knight et al., 2009) outlines the foundational and functional competencies required for behavioral health providers who work with older adults; these include general knowledge about adult development, aging, and the older adult population; and foundations of professional general practice, assessment, intervention, and consultation. The Pikes Peak Geropsychology Knowledge and Skills Assessment Tool (see Appendix 2; Karel et al., 2012) can be used as a way for licensed practitioners, trainees, and supervisors to consider their work in the context of these core Pikes Peak competencies. Behavioral anchors are provided across the continuum of novice, intermediate, advanced, proficient, and expert, allowing clinicians to evaluate their current status as well as target specific areas for future professional development.

In addition to those aging-specific domains, there are broader *best science* and *best practice* forces that are advancing behavioral health care of older adults, including depressed older adults. We discuss some of these in the final section of this chapter.

Intersectionality of Aging and Cultural Diversity

Gerontologists and geriatric specialists are very aware of the need to consider issues of diversity (Llorente & Valverde, 2019). Aging processes and health outcomes are characterized by significant intraindividual and interindividual differences that are shaped by cultural influences. CBT is very relevant for the mental health needs of diverse older adults (Lau & Kinoshita, 2019). Among other facets of diversity, gender and gender identity, sexual orientation, race and ethnicity, social class, and educational background are all relevant to how older individuals experience their health and interactions with health care. The conceptual framework of intersectionality was originally articulated by feminist scholars to acknowledge cultural influences in the experience of gender (Else-Quest & Hyde, 2016). This intersectionality lens has now been adopted by professional organizations to help behavioral health providers, researchers, and educators conceptualize what we mean by culture and how we work with diverse clients (Clauss-Ehlers et al., 2019; Ratts et al., 2016). This is an exciting development, because consideration of intersectionality places age and generational cohort firmly alongside other facets of diversity. The intersectionality model provides an increasingly familiar and powerful means of helping generalists or providers with culture-specific interests to consider the role of age and lifespan developmental processes. Specific examples of applications within behavioral health care can be seen in the ADDRESSING model articulated by Hays (2009) as well as the contextual adult lifespan theory for adapting psychotherapy (CALTAP) model (Pachana et al., 2015). An intersectional cultural lens can help providers consider psychotherapy adaptations that are firmly grounded in both cultural humility and evidence-based practice (Hays, 2009; Stirman et al., 2019).

Stepped-Care

Traditional individual psychotherapy is resource intensive and unavailable to many older adults who could benefit from some form of behavioral health care. A public health perspective involves considering the mental health needs of ALL older adults within a specific community and nation, and rethinking delivery strategies (Kazdin, 2018). The future of mental health care of older adults is expected to occur within the context of primary health care. Stepped-care approaches1 are developing rapidly (Maragakis & O'Donohue, 2018); in these models of mental health care, the recommended first-line treatment is the one that is least intensive and likely to provide significant benefit. Patients' outcomes are routinely monitored, with more intensive and costly *stepped-up* services provided only if the initial treatment does not lead to clinically significant gains. Mental health treatments for older adults (whether provided to individuals, couples, families, or within groups) can be offered across a continuum of needs and delivery mechanisms. Combined pharmacological and behavioral therapies, partial hospitalization, and inpatient care are all more intensive than individual psychotherapy. Self-help and clinician coaching via book (Moss et al., 2012), audio (Morthland et al., 2019), internet (Read et al., 2019), psychoeducational groups, telehealth (Lichstein et al., 2013; Scogin et al., 2018; Steffen & Gant, 2016), and assistance from behavioral technicians (Meeks et al., 2019) are all evidence-based interventions for depressed older adults on the lower end of the continuum of treatment. Stepped-care delivery models are one among many ways we can use the science of behavioral change to impact the health and well-being of older adults around the world. Because some of these less-intensive forms of behavioral health interventions are more amenable to being provided across distances, such approaches are important for older adults with limited transportation options or mobility problems, and/or who are living in rural communities.

This public health and stepped-care perspective of behavioral health supports contributions from a wide continuum of providers. Peer helpers and bachelor's degree–level behavioral technicians can be used to implement specific interventions under the supervision of licensed master's and doctoral degree–trained therapists (Kraus-Schuman et al., 2015). Doctoral degree–level professionals will be needed in the areas of training, program, and intervention development and evaluation. Across these levels of training, the goal is for each paraprofessional and professional to be working at the top of their own scope of practice. It has been demonstrated that, with adequate training and supervision, community peer-support specialists, behavioral technicians, and lower-level clinicians are effective front-line staff in some interventions for older adults (Stanley et al., 2016).

Process-Based Therapy: The Wave of the Future

The psychotherapy integration movement is now more than 3 decades old (a generation of clinicians!), and numerous conceptual models and therapeutic practices have been proposed for how mental health interventions help people. Moving beyond specific models of psychotherapy integration, some leaders in the development and evaluation of clinical interventions have predicted that traditional "schools" of psychotherapy (e.g., cognitive behavioral, family systems, interpersonal, psychodynamic, etc.) will disappear within the next 10 to 20 years (Hofmann & Barlow, 2014, Melchert, 2016). Instead, psychotherapies and other behavioral health interventions will be shaped by our growing knowledge of biopsychosocial processes that lead to functional impairments in daily life. In the same way that the growing fields of precision medicine and computational psychiatry aim to impact specific disease processes at the individual level, behavioral health clinicians will increasingly apply therapeutic strategies to target problems at the individual level. Within the US, this is articulated in the National Institute of Health's Science of Behavior Change program (described at https://commonfund.nih.gov/behaviorchange/ and at https://scienceofbehaviorchange.org/).

These efforts focus on key mechanisms that underlie a wide range of mental health problems, including self-regulation, stress reactivity and stress resilience, and interpersonal and social processes. Grounding interventions in a science of behavior change moves us away from categorical approaches of understanding psychopathology (i.e., the diagnostic categories in the *Diagnostic and Statistical Manual of Mental Disorders* [DSM]), instead using dimensional and transdiagnostic approaches to understand mental health problems and mechanisms of change. An excellent example of this in geropsychology and specific to BA is provided by Niu and Arean (2015); they demonstrate how applying *research domain criteria* (RDoC) to later-life depression can help clinicians identify and treat the specific processes at work. Instead of viewing BA as simply one component of CBT for depression, understanding how BA strategies target reward processes helps therapists make treatment decisions with their individual patients.

In this way, our field is moving beyond the use of set protocols for syndromes in both primary care and specialty behavioral health settings. This changed focus away from treatment manuals in delivery of CBTs will require providers to develop skills in precision therapy across all levels of care and care settings. This movement toward a *process-based* therapy (Hayes et al., 2019) has significant implications for dissemination and implementation. Helping clinicians identify problems and target areas of change for each individual client fits the preferences of most mental health clinicians, and is highly relevant for the subclinical symptoms that characterize many of the mental health conditions of older adults. Thus, language used to describe therapeutic approaches is expected to change, and move us away from labels such as "CBT" or "ACT" or "Interpersonal."

Conclusions and Implications

The research evidence on the therapeutic efficacy of CBT is very strong, including for depressed older adults. This chapter has described key facets of CBT with depressed older adults, focusing on elicitation of emotional experiences, BA, cognitive reappraisal, and positive psychotherapy as change strategies. Examples were provided to help clinicians think about and apply CBT to their depressed older patients. Considering the ongoing workforce shortage of professionals trained in aging (Hoge et al., 2015; Moye et al., 2019), it is our hope that this description inspires readers to join the community of professionals committed to evidence-based behavioral health for older adults.

Suggested Resources for CBT With Older Adults

Workbooks and Therapist Guides

Steffen, A. M., Thompson, L. W., & Gallagher-Thompson, D. (in press). *Treating later-life depression: A cognitive-behavioral therapy approach: Clinician guide* (2nd ed.). Treatments That Work Series, Oxford University Press.

Steffen, A. M., Dick-Siskin, L. P., Bilbrey, A. C., Powers, D. V., Gallagher-Thompson, D., & Thompson, L. W. (in press). *Treating later-life depression: A cognitive-behavioral therapy approach: Workbook* (2nd ed.). Treatments That Work Series, Oxford University Press.

Video Demonstrations of Behavioral Activation

Stanford Geriatric Education Center. (2011). Home [video] YouTube channel. https://www.youtube.com/user/StanfordGEC/ or https://sgec.stanford.edu/SGEC-Behavioral-Activation-Series.html

Cassidy-Eagle, E. (July 29, 2018) *Behavioral activation in a primary care setting* [video]. With Nancy Morioka-Douglas, MD, MPH. YouTube. https://www.youtube.com/watch?v=Vjq4Yap4gCo

Additional Recommended Works

Gallagher-Thompson, D., Steffen, A. M., & Thompson, L. W. (Eds.). (2008). *Handbook of behavioral and cognitive therapies with older adults.* Springer Science + Business Media. https://doi.org/10.1007/978-0-387-72007-4

Laidlaw, K. (2015). *CBT for older people: An introduction.*Sage. https://doi.org/10.4135/9781473910799.

Scogin, F., & Shah, A. (2012). *Making evidence-based psychological treatments work with older adults.* American Psychological Association. https://doi.org/10.1037/13753-000

Sorocco, K. H., & Lauderdale, S. (2011). *Cognitive behavior therapy with older adults: Innovations across care settings.* Springer.

Suggested Resources for General

Bennett-Levy, J., Thwaites, R., Haarhoff, B., & Perry, H. (2014). *Experiencing CBT from the inside out: A self-practice/self-reflection workbook for therapists.* Guilford Press.

Hayes, S. C., & Hofmann, S. G. (Eds.). (2018). *Process-based CBT: The science and core clinical competencies of cognitive behavioral therapy.* New Harbinger.

Hofmann, S. G., & Asmundson, G. J. G. (2017). *The science of cognitive behavioral therapy.* Elsevier.

Padesky, C. A. (2020). *Clinician's guide to CBT using mind over mood.* Guilford Press.

Tolin, D. F. (2016). *Doing CBT: A comprehensive guide to working with behaviors, thoughts, and emotions.* Guilford Press.

Asian Association for Cognitive Behaviour Therapy: https://asiancbt.weebly.com/
Australian Association for Cognitive and Behaviour Therapy: https://www.aacbt.org.au/
British Association for Behavioural and Cognitive Psychotherapies: https://www.babcp.com/
Association for Behavioral and Cognitive Therapies (USA): http://www.abct.org/
European Association for Behavioural and Cognitive Therapies: https://eabct.eu/
Indian Association for Cognitive Behaviour Therapy: http://iacbt.org/message.html

References

Alexopoulos, G. S., Raue, P. J., Gunning, F., Kiosses, D. N., Kanellopoulos, D., Pollari, C., ... Arean, P. A. (2016). "Engage" therapy: behavioral activation and improvement of late-life major depression. *American Journal of Geriatric Psychiatry, 24*(4), 320–326. https://doi.org/10.1016/j.jagp.2015.11.006

American Psychological Association. (2019). *Clinical practice guideline for the treatment of depression across three age cohorts.* https://www.apa.org/depression-guideline/guideline.pdf

Arnold, M. (2008). Polypharmacy and older adults: A role for psychology and psychologists. *Professional Psychology: Research and Practice, 39*(3), 283–289. https://doi.org/10.1037/0735-7028.39.3.283

Au, A., Gallagher Thompson, D., Wong, M., Leung, J., Chan, W. C., Chan, C. C., Lu, H. J., Lai, M. K., & Chan, K. (2015). Behavioral activation for dementia caregivers: Scheduling pleasant events and enhancing communications. *Clinical Interventions in Aging, 10,* 611–619. https://doi.org/10.2147/CIA.S72348

Au, A., Yip, H-M., Lai, S., Ngai, S., Cheng, S-T., Losada, A., Thompson, L. W., & Gallagher-Thompson, D. (2019). Telephone-based behavioral activation intervention for dementia family caregivers: Outcomes and mediation effect of a randomized controlled trial. *Patient Education and Counseling, 102,* 2049–2059. https://doi.org/10.1016/j.pec.2019.06.009

Beck, A. T., Steer, R. A., & Brown, G. K. (1996). *Manual for the Beck Depression Inventory-II.* Psychological Corporation.

Bhar, S. S., & Brown, G. K. (2012). Treatment of depression and suicide in older adults. *Cognitive and Behavioral Practice, 19*(1), 116–125. https://doi.org/10.1016/j.cbpra.2010.12.005

Bilbrey, A., Cassidy-Eagle, E., & Gallagher-Thompson, D. (2020). Working with depressed caregivers: Behavioral activation. In L. B. Dunn & E. L. Cassidy-Eagle (Eds.), *Practical strategies in geriatric mental health: Cases and approaches* (pp. 31–41). American Psychiatric Association.

Bilbrey, A., Laidlaw, K., Cassidy-Eagle, E. Thompson, L., & Gallagher-Thompson, D. (2020). Cognitive-behavioral therapy for late life depression: Evidence, issues, and recommendations. *Cognitive and Behavioral Practice.* https://doi.org/10.1016/j.cbpra.2020.02.003

Braun, M. M., Karlin, B. E., & Zeiss, A. (2016). Cognitive-behavioral therapies in older adult populations. In C. M. Nezu & A. M. Nezu (Eds.), *The Oxford handbook of cognitive and behavioral therapies* (pp. 349–362). Oxford University Press.

Brown, G. K., Ten Have, T., & Henriques, G. R. (2005). Cognitive therapy for the prevention of suicide attempts: A randomized controlled trial. *JAMA, 294*(5), 563–570. https://doi.org/10.1001/jama.294.5.563

Clauss-Ehlers, C. S., Chiriboga, D. A., Hunter, S. J., Roysircar, G., & Tummala-Narra, P. (2019). APA Multicultural Guidelines executive summary: Ecological approach to context, identity, and intersectionality. *American Psychologist, 74*(2), 232–244. https://doi.org/10.1037/amp0000382

Conti, E. C., Kraus-Schuman, C., & Stanley, M. A. (2017). Cognitive-behavioral therapy in older adults. In S. G. Hofmann & G. J. G. Asmundson (Eds.), *The science of cognitive behavioral therapy* (pp. 223–255). Academic Press. https://doi.org/10.1016/B978-0-12-803457-6.00010-6

Coon, D. W., Thompson, L. W., & Gallagher-Thompson, D. (2007). Adapting homework for an older adult client with cognitive impairment. *Cognitive and Behavioral Practice, 14*(3), 252–260. https://doi.org/10.1016/j.cbpra.2006.10.006

Cuijpers, P., Karyotaki, E., Pot, A. M., Park, M., & Reynolds, C. F., III. (2014). Managing depression in older age: Psychological interventions. *Maturitas, 79*(2), 160–169. https://doi.org/10.1016/j.maturitas.2014.05.027

Decaporale-Ryan, L., Warren, A. R., Steffen, A. M. (in press). Interprofessional health care teams. In G. Asmundson (Ed.), *Comprehensive clinical psychology* (2nd ed.). Elsevier.

Else-Quest, N. M., & Hyde, J. S. (2016). Intersectionality in quantitative psychological research: I. Theoretical and epistemological issues. *Psychology of Women Quarterly, 40*(2), 155–170. https://doi.org/10.1177/0361684316629797

Fiske, A., Wetherell, J. L., & Gatz, M. (2009). Depression in older adults. *Annual Review of Clinical Psychology, 5,* 363–389. https://doi.org/10.1146/annurev.clinpsy.032408.153621

Gallagher-Thompson, D., Bilbrey, A. C., Cassidy-Eagle, E. L., & Thompson, L. W. (2020). Late-life depression. In L. B. Dunn & E. L. Cassidy-Eagle (Eds.), *Practical strategies in geriatric mental health cases and approaches*. American Psychiatric Association.

Gallagher-Thompson, D., & Thompson, L. W. (2010). Effectively using cognitive/behavioral therapy with the oldest old: Case examples and issues for consideration. In N. A. Pachana, K. Laidlaw, & B. Knight (Eds.), *Casebook of clinical geropsychology: International perspectives on practice* (pp. 227–241). Oxford University Press. https://doi.org/10.1093/med/9780199583553.003.0014

Gallo, J. J., Hwang, S., Joo, J. H., Bogner, H. R., Morales, K. H., Bruce, M. L., & Reynolds, C. F., III. (2016). Multimorbidity, depression, and mortality in primary care: Randomized clinical trial of an evidence-based depression care management program on mortality risk. *Journal of General Internal Medicine, 31*(4), 380–386. https://doi.org/10.1007/s11606-015-3524-y

Gregg, J. J., Fiske, A., & Gatz, M. (2013). Physicians' detection of late-life depression: The roles of dysphoria and cognitive impairment. *Aging & Mental Health, 17*(8), 1030–1036. https://doi.org/10.1080/13607863.2013.805403

Gum, A. M., Areán, P. A., Hunkeler, E., Tang, L., Katon, W., Hitchcock, P., Steffens, D. C., Dickens, J., & Unützer, J. (2006). Depression treatment preferences in older primary care patients. *Gerontologist, 46*(1), 14–22. https://doi.org/10.1093/geront/46.1.14

Hawley, L. L., Padesky, C. A., Hollon, S. D., Mancuso, E., Laposa, J. M., Brozina, K., & Segal, Z. V. (2017). Cognitive-behavioral therapy for depression using mind over mood: CBT skill use and differential symptom alleviation. *Behavior Therapy, 48*(1), 29–44. https://doi.org/10.1016/j.beth.2016.09.003

Hayes, S. C., Hofmann, S. G., Stanton, C. E., Carpenter, J. K., Sanford, B. T., Curtiss, J. E., & Ciarrochi, J. (2019). The role of the individual in the coming era of process-based therapy. *Behaviour Research and Therapy, 117*, 40–53. https://doi.org/10.1016/j.brat.2018.10.005

Hays, P. A. (2009). Integrating evidence-based practice, cognitive–behavior therapy, and multicultural therapy: Ten steps for culturally competent practice. *Professional Psychology: Research and Practice, 40*(4), 354–360. https://doi.org/10.1037/a0016250

Hill, R. D. (2011). A positive aging framework for guiding geropsychology interventions. *Behavior Therapy, 42*(1), 66–77. https://doi.org/10.1016/j.beth.2010.04.006

Hinrichsen, G. A., Emery-Tiburcio, E. E., Gooblar, J., & Molinari, V. A. (2018). Building foundational knowledge competencies in professional geropsychology: Council of Professional Geropsychology Training Programs (Co PGTP) recommendations. *Clinical Psychology: Science and Practice, 25*(2), e12236. https://doi.org/10.1111/cpsp.12236

Hofmann, S. G. (2015). *Emotion in therapy: From science to practice*. Guilford Press.

Hofmann, S. G., & Barlow, D. H. (2014). Evidence-based psychological interventions and the common factors approach: The beginnings of a rapprochement? *Psychotherapy, 51*(4), 510–513. https://doi.org/10.1037/a0037045

Hoge, M. A., Karel, M. J., Zeiss, A. M., Alegria, M., & Moye, J. (2015). Strengthening psychology's workforce for older adults. *American Psychologist, 70*(3), 265–278. https://doi.org/10.1037/a0038927

James, I. A., Blackburn, I. M., & Reichelt, F. K. (2001). *Manual of the Revised Cognitive Therapy Scale (CTS-R)* [Unpublished manuscript]. https://doi.org/10.1037/t65807-000

Jobes, D. A. (2016). *Managing suicidal risk: A collaborative approach*. Guilford Press.

Kanfer, F. H., & Schefft, B. K. (1988). *Guiding the process of therapeutic change*. Research Press.

Karel, M. J., Holley, C. K., Whitbourne, S. K., Segal, D. L., Tazeau, Y. N., Emery, E. E., Molinari, V., Yang, J., & Zweig, R. A. (2012). Preliminary validation of a tool to assess competencies for professional geropsychology practice. *Professional Psychology: Research and Practice, 43*(2), 110–117. https://doi.org/10.1037/a0025788

Karel, M. J., Knight, B. G., Duffy, M., Hinrichsen, G. A., & Zeiss, A. M. (2010). Attitude, knowledge, and skill competencies for practice in professional geropsychology: Implications for training and building a geropsychology workforce. *Training and Education in Professional Psychology, 4*(2), 75–84. https://doi.org/10.1037/a0018372

Karpiak, C. P., Norcross, J. C., & Wedding, D. (2016). Evolution of theory in clinical psychology. In J. C. Norcross, G. R. VandenBos, D. K. Freedheim, & B. O. Olatunji (Eds.), *APA handbook of clinical psychology:*

Theory and research (Vol. 2; pp. 3–17). American Psychological Association. https://doi.org/10.1037/14773-001

Kazdin, A. E. (2018). *Innovations in psychosocial interventions and their delivery: Leveraging cutting-edge science to improve the world's mental health.* Oxford University Press. https://doi.org/10.1093/med-psych/9780190463281.001.0001

Kiosses, D. N., Alexopoulos, G. S., Hajcak, G., Apfeldorf, W., Duberstein, P. R., Putrino, D., & Gross, J. J. (2018). Cognitive Reappraisal Intervention for Suicide Prevention (CRISP) for middle-aged and older adults hospitalized for suicidality. *American Journal of Geriatric Psychiatry, 26*(4), 494–503. https://doi.org/10.1016/j.jagp.2017.11.009

Knight, B. G., Karel, M. J., Hinrichsen, G. A., Qualls, S. H., & Duffy, M. (2009). Pikes Peak model for training in professional geropsychology. *American Psychologist, 64*(3), 205–214. https://doi.org/10.1037/a0015059

Kraus-Schuman, C., Wilson, N. L., Amspoker, A. B., Wagener, P. D., Calleo, J. S., Diefenbach, G., Hopko, D., Cully, J. A., Teng, E., Rhoades, H. M., Kunik, M. E., & Stanley, M. A. (2015). Enabling lay providers to conduct CBT for older adults: Key steps for expanding treatment capacity. *Translational Behavioral Medicine, 5*(3), 247–253. https://doi.org/10.1007/s13142-015-0306-3

Kroenke, K., & Spitzer, R. L. (2002). The PHQ-9: A new depression diagnostic and severity measure. *Psychiatric Annals, 32*(9), 509–515. https://doi.org/10.3928/0048-5713-20020901-06

Laidlaw, K., & Kishita, N. (2015). Age-appropriate augmented cognitive behavior therapy to enhance treatment outcome for late-life depression and anxiety disorders. *GeroPsych: The Journal of Gerontopsychology and Geriatric Psychiatry, 28*(2), 57–66. https://doi.org/10.1024/1662-9647/a000128

Laidlaw, K., Thompson, L. W., & Gallagher-Thompson, D. (2004). Comprehensive conceptualization of cognitive behaviour therapy for late life depression. *Behavioural & Cognitive Psychotherapy, 32,* 389 – 399. https://doi.org/10.1017/S1352465804001584

Laidlaw, K., Thompson, L. W., Gallagher-Thompson, D., & Dick-Siskin, L. (2003). *Cognitive behaviour therapy with older people.* John Wiley & Sons. https://doi.org/10.1002/9780470713402

Lambert, M. J. (2012). Helping clinicians to use and learn from research-based systems: The OQ-analyst. *Psychotherapy (Chicago, Ill.), 49*(2), 109–114. https://doi.org/10.1037/a0027110

Lau, A. W., & Kinoshita, L. M. (2019). Cognitive behavior therapy with culturally diverse older adults. In G. Y. Iwamasa & P. A. Hays (Eds.), *Culturally responsive cognitive behavior therapy: Practice and supervision* (pp. 231–256). American Psychological Association. https://doi.org/10.1037/0000119-010

Levy, S. R. (2018). Toward reducing ageism: PEACE (positive education about aging and contact experiences) model. *Gerontologist, 58*(2), 226–232. https://doi.org/10.1093/geront/gnw116

Lichstein, K. L., Scogin, F., Thomas, S. J., DiNapoli, E. A., Dillon, H. R., & McFadden, A. (2013). Telehealth cognitive behavior therapy for co-occurring insomnia and depression symptoms in older adults. *Journal of Clinical Psychology, 69*(10), 1056–1065. https://doi.org/10.1002/jclp.22030

Linehan, M. M. (2015). *DBT skills training manual* (2nd ed.). Guilford Press.

Llorente, M. D., & Valverde, M. (2019). Mental health care of older adults: Does cultural competence matter? *Current Geriatrics Reports, 8*(3), 131–136. https://doi.org/10.1007/s13670-019-00284-8

Lutz, J., & Fiske, A. (2018). Functional disability and suicidal behavior in middle-aged and older adults: A systematic critical review. *Journal of Affective Disorders, 227,* 260–271. https://doi.org/10.1016/j.jad.2017.10.043

Lutz, J., Mashal, N., Kramer, A., Suresh, M., Gould, C., Jordan, J. T., Wetherell, J. L., & Beaudreau, S. A. (2019). A case report of problem solving therapy for reducing suicide risk in older adults with anxiety disorders. *Clinical Gerontologist: The Journal of Aging and Mental Health.* https://doi.org/10.1080/07317115.2019.1617378

Maragakis, A., & O'Donohue, W. T. (2018). *Principle-based stepped care and brief psychotherapy for integrated care settings.* Springer International. https://doi.org/10.1007/978-3-319-70539-2

McHugh, R. K., Whitton, S. W., Peckham, A. D., Welge, J. A., & Otto, M. W. (2012). Patient preference for psychological vs. pharmacological treatment of psychiatric disorders: A meta-analytic review. *Journal of Clinical Psychiatry, 74*(6), 595–602. https://doi.org/10.4088/JCP.12r07757

Meeks, S., Looney, S. W., Van Haitsma, K., & Teri, L. (2008). BE-ACTIV: A staff-assisted behavioral intervention for depression in nursing homes. *Gerontologist, 48*(1), 105–114. https://doi.org/10.1093/geront/48.1.105

Meeks, S., Sublett, R., Kostiwa, I., Rodgers, J. R., & Haddix, D. (2008). Treating depression in the prison nursing home: Demonstrating research-to-practice translation. *Clinical Case Studies, 7*(6), 555–574. https://doi.org/10.1177/1534650108321303

Meeks, S., Van Haitsma, K., Schoenbachler, B., & Looney, S. W. (2015). BE-ACTIV for depression in nursing homes: Primary outcomes of a randomized clinical trial. *Journals of Gerontology: Series B: Psychological Sciences and Social Sciences, 70*(1), 13–23. https://doi.org/10.1093/geronb/gbu026

Meeks, S., Van Haitsma, K., & Shryock, S. K. (2019). Treatment fidelity evidence for BE-ACTIV – A behavioral intervention for depression in nursing homes. *Aging & Mental Health, 23*(9), 1192–1202. https://doi.org/10.1080/13607863.2018.1484888

Melchert, T. P. (2016). Leaving behind our preparadigmatic past: Professional psychology as a unified clinical science. *American Psychologist, 71*(6), 486–496. https://doi.org/10.1037/a0040227

Morthland, M., Shah, A., Meadows, J. T., & Scogin, F. (2019). Development of an audio and computer cognitive behavioral therapy for depression in older adults. *Aging & Mental Health, 24*(8), 1207–1215. https://doi.org/10.1080/13607863.2019.1609901

Moss, K., Scogin, F., Di Napoli, E., & Presnell, A. (2012). A self-help behavioral activation treatment for geriatric depressive symptoms. *Aging & Mental Health, 16*(5), 625–635. https://doi.org/10.1080/13607863.2011.651435

Moye, J., Karel, M. J., Stamm, K. E., Qualls, S. H., Segal, D. L., Tazeau, Y. N., & DiGilio, D. A. (2019). Workforce analysis of psychological practice with older adults: Growing crisis requires urgent action. *Training and Education in Professional Psychology, 13*(1), 46–55. https://doi.org/10.1037/tep0000206

Niu, G., & Arean, P. (2015). Refining evidence-based treatments for late-life depression. *Geropsych: The Journal of Gerontopsychology and Geriatric Psychiatry, 28*(2), 67–76. https://doi.org/10.1024/1662-9647/a000127

Pachana, N. A., Mitchell, L. K., & Knight, B. G. (2015). Using the CALTAP lifespan developmental framework with older adults. *GeroPsych: The Journal of Gerontopsychology and Geriatric Psychiatry, 28*(2), 77–86. https://doi.org/10.1024/1662-9647/a000126

Padesky, C. A., & Mooney, K. A. (2012). Strengths-based cognitive–behavioral therapy: A four-step model to build resilience. *Clinical Psychology & Psychotherapy, 19*(4), 283–290. https://doi.org/10.1002/cpp.1795

Parks, A. C., & Layous, K. (2016). Positive psychological interventions. In J. C. Norcross, G. R. VandenBos, D. K. Freedheim, & R. Krishnamurthy (Eds.), *APA handbook of clinical psychology: Applications and methods* (Vol. 3; pp. 439–449). American Psychological Association. https://doi.org/10.1037/14861-023

Petkus, A. J., Lenze, E. J., & Wetherell, J. L. (2013). Anxious depression: Application of a unified model of emotional disorders to older adults. In H. Lavretsky, M. Sajatovic, & C. F. Reynolds III (Eds.), *Late-life mood disorders* (pp. 144–163). Oxford University Press.

Petrik, A. M., Kazantzis, N., & Hofmann, S. G. (2013). Distinguishing integrative from eclectic practice in cognitive behavioral therapies. *Psychotherapy (Chicago, Ill.), 50*(3), 392–397. https://doi.org/10.1037/a0032412

Ratts, M. J., Singh, A. A., Nassar-McMillan, S., Butler, S. K., & McCullough, J. R. (2016). Multicultural and social justice counseling competencies: Guidelines for the counseling profession. *Journal of Multicultural Counseling and Development, 44*(1), 28–48. https://doi.org/10.1002/jmcd.12035

Read, J., Sharpe, L., Burton, A. L., Arean, P. A., Raue, P. J., McDonald, S., Titov, N., Gandy, M., & Dear, B. F. (2019). A randomized controlled trial of internet-delivered cognitive behaviour therapy to prevent the development of depressive disorders in older adults with multimorbidity. *Journal of Affective Disorders, 264*, 464–473. https://doi.org/10.1016/j.jad.2019.11.077

Rider, K. L., Thompson, L. W., & Gallagher-Thompson, D. (2016). California Older Persons Pleasant Events Scale: A tool to help older adults increase positive experiences. *Clinical Gerontologist: The Journal of Aging and Mental Health, 39*(1), 64–83. https://doi.org/10.1080/07317115.2015.1101635

Sachs-Ericsson, N., Van Orden, K., & Zarit, S. (2016). Suicide and aging: Special issue of Aging & Mental Health. *Aging & Mental Health, 20*(2), 110–112. https://doi.org/10.1080/13607863.2015.1099037

Sales, C. M., & Alves, P. C. (2016). Patient-centered assessment in psychotherapy: A review of individualized tools. *Clinical Psychology: Science and Practice, 23*(3), 265–283. https://doi.org/10.1111/cpsp.12162

Samarina, V., Suresh, M., Picchiello, M., Lutz, J., Carpenter, B. & Beaudreau, S. A. (2021). Assessment approaches for psychiatric and cognitive syndromes. In N. Pachana, V. Molinari, L. Thompson & D. Gallagher-Thompson (Eds.), *Psychological Assessment and Treatment of Older Adults*. (pp. 15–44). Hogrefe Publishing.

Scogin, F., Lichstein, K., DiNapoli, E. A., Woosley, J., Thomas, S. J., LaRocca, M. A., ... Geyer, J. D. (2018). Effects of integrated telehealth-delivered cognitive-behavioral therapy for depression and insomnia in rural older adults. *Journal of Psychotherapy Integration, 28*(3), 292–309. https://doi.org/10.1037/int0000121

Solomonov, N., Bress, J. N., Sirey, J. A., Gunning, F. M., Flückiger, C., Raue, P. J., ... Alexopoulos, G. S. (2019). Engagement in socially and interpersonally rewarding activities as a predictor of outcome in "engage" behavioral activation therapy for late-life depression. *American Journal of Geriatric Psychiatry, 27*(6), 571–578. https://doi.org/10.1016/j.jagp.2018.12.033

Stanley, M. A., Wilson, N., Shrestha, S., Amspoker, A. B., Armento, M., Cummings, J. P., Evans-Hudnall, G., Wagener, P., & Kunik, M. E. (2016). Calmer life: A culturally tailored intervention for anxiety in underserved older adults. *American Journal of Geriatric Psychiatry, 24*(8), 648–658. https://doi.org/10.1016/j.jagp.2016.03.008

Steffen, A. M., & Gant, J. R. (2016). A telehealth behavioral coaching intervention for neurocognitive disorder family carers. *International Journal of Geriatric Psychiatry, 31*(2), 195–203. https://doi.org/10.1002/gps.4312

Steffen, A. M., & Zeiss, A. M. (2017). Interprofessional health care teams in geriatrics. In J. Stein (Ed.), *Reference module in neuroscience and biobehavioral psychology*. Elsevier. ISBN 9780128093245.

Stirman, S. W., Baumann, A. A., & Miller, C. J. (2019). The FRAME: An expanded framework for reporting adaptations and modifications to evidence-based interventions. *Implementation Science, 14*(1), 1–10. https://doi.org/10.1186/s13012-019-0898-y

Szanton, S. L., Thorpe Jr, R. J., & Gitlin, L. N. (2014). Beat the blues decreases depression in financially strained older African-American adults. *American Journal of Geriatric Psychiatry, 22*(7), 692–697. https://doi.org/10.1016/j.jagp.2013.05.008

Tompkins, M. A. (2004). *Using homework in psychotherapy: Strategies, guidelines, and forms.* Guilford Press.

Walsh, S., Cassidy, M., & Priebe, S. (2017). The application of positive psychotherapy in mental health care: A systematic review. *Journal of Clinical Psychology, 73*(6), 638–651. https://doi.org/10.1002/jclp.22368

Wuthrich, V. M., Johnco, C. J., & Wetherell, J. L. (2015). Differences in anxiety and depression symptoms: Comparison between older and younger clinical samples. *International Psychogeriatrics, 27*(9), 1523–1532. https://doi.org/10.1017/S1041610215000526

Yesavage, J. A., Brink, T. L., Rose, T. L., Lum, O., Huang, V., Adey, M., & Leirer, V. O. (1982). Development and validation of a geriatric depression screening scale: A preliminary report. *Journal of Psychiatric Research, 17*(1), 37–49. https://doi.org/10.1016/0022-3956(82)90033-4

Zeiss, A. (2016). Cognitive Behavioral Therapy as an integral component of interprofessional care. *Cognitive and Behavioral Practice, 23,* 441–445. https://doi.org/10.1016/j.cbpra.2016.01.004

Zeppegno, P., Gattoni, E., Mastrangelo, M., Gramaglia, C., & Sarchiapone, M. (2019). Psychosocial suicide prevention interventions in the elderly: A mini-review of the literature. *Frontiers in Psychology,* 9, 1–7. https://doi.org/10.3389/fpsyg.2018.02713

Chapter 4

Case-Based Approaches With Older Adults: ACT, IPT, and DBT

Laura Gallego-Alberto
María S. Pedroso-Chaparro
Andrés Losada
María Márquez-González
Lindsey Jacobs
Gregory A. Hinrichsen

Introduction

Although cognitive behavior therapy (CBT) currently enjoys the greatest amount of support in terms of empirical studies and meta-analyses regarding its efficacy with older adult populations, many other forms of psychotherapy have a solid empirical basis for use with this age cohort. This chapter describes three well-established therapeutic approaches for use with older persons: *acceptance and commitment therapy* (ACT), *interpersonal psychotherapy* (IPT), and *dialectical behavior therapy* (DBT). In treating older adults, part of the competencies of the clinician (as referenced in the Pikes Peak competencies; see the Appendix 1; and Knight et al., 2009) involve knowledge about various methods of intervention, including current research evidence about their efficacy and effectiveness as applied to diverse groups within the older adult population (Pikes Peak competencies G13 and G14). In the sections below, ACT, IPT, and DBT are each briefly described, and their main therapeutic emphases are explained. In each section, the psychotherapy processes are illustrated with a case example. (Acknowledgement: This work was in part supported by grants from the Spanish Ministry of Economy and Competitiveness: PSI2015-65152-C2-1-R & PSI2015-65152-C2-2-R.)

Acceptance and Commitment Therapy

Introduction

ACT (Hayes et al., 2011) is one of the most popular third-generation behavior therapies, and it has shown efficacy for emotional disorders such as depression, mixed anxiety, obsessive-compulsive disorder, psychosis, and distress related to chronic pain (American Psychological Association, 2016). ACT involves a subtle but essential change in the treatment focus, as compared with classic cognitive behavioral interventions. Specifically, ACT interventions do not try to produce direct changes in the frequency or topography of unpleasant internal experiences of the person (thoughts, emotions, or feelings), but instead aim to modify their function by altering the context in which they appear – that is, the relationship established between the person and those private events (Hayes et al., 2011). In this regard, ACT promotes the acceptance of aversive experiences that inevitably and naturally happen in the "walk of life" toward important personal values. ACT proposes the concept of *psychological inflexibility* as a transdiagnostic mechanism underlying psychological problems such as anxious or depressive problems (Hayes et al., 2006). Psychological inflexibility can be conceptualized as the person's unwillingness to stay in touch with private experiences (e.g., emotions, thoughts, or feelings) and their actions to alter the form or frequency of these events and the contexts that cause them (Hayes, 2004).

With this in mind, "the goal of ACT is to produce more psychological flexibility" (Hayes, 2004, p. 15). For achieving this objective, ACT interventions include different experiential techniques (such as metaphors and experiential exercises) that are aimed at increasing the person's ability to accept annoying internal experiences, and the situations involved in their origin, while at the same time helping the person to clarify and reorient their actions according to the most important values in their life (Hayes et al., 2011).

Previous research supports the use of ACT in older adults. Regarding chronic pain in older adults, ACT interventions have shown good results for this population. For example, studies by McCracken and Jones (2012) or Scott and colleagues (2017) have shown that ACT interventions for adults aged 60 and over obtained significant changes in functioning and mental health in posttreatment, showing improvements in the levels of pain intensity and pain acceptance, and decreasing the disability derived from the pain as well as depressive levels. Similarly, the results of an intervention that combined ACT with the model of *selective optimization with compensation* (Baltes & Baltes, 1990) for older adults with chronic pain residing in nursing homes suggested improvements in the satisfaction with the time and effort dedicated to living according to their own values (Alonso et al., 2013; Alonso-Fernández et al., 2016). Positive results have also been obtained for ACT with older people with heart disease–related distress (Kakavan et al., 2015).

In addition, ACT interventions in older adults have shown good results for anxiety disorders. In adults aged 60 and over with generalized anxiety disorder (GAD) the results of an ACT intervention showed reduction in worries and depressive symptoms after the intervention (Wetherell et al., 2011). In fact, ACT has been suggested as an intervention that may be particularly suited for older adults with treatment-resistant GAD (Lawrence et al., 2019). Furthermore, an ACT intervention showed an improvement of death anxiety and obsession in older adults with anxiety (Bayati et al., 2017). In addition, an ACT intervention in older men afflicted by heart disease increased positive perceived stress and reduced negative perceived stress (Kakavan et al., 2015).

ACT interventions have also been supported for the treatment of depression in older adults (Davison et al., 2017). Consistently, different studies have shown improvements in depression in people 55 years or older (Jacobs et al., 2018; Karlin et al., 2013). Finally, positive and significant effects of ACT on anxious and depressive symptoms have been also reported for the family caregivers of patients with dementia, suggesting that ACT may be useful for people exposed to significant and chronic levels of stress (Losada et al., 2015; Márquez-González et al., in press). In summary, the reviewed studies analyzing the effects of ACT interventions with older adults provide support for the use of this therapeutic approach with older adults.

When to Use ACT With Older Adults?

Several authors have argued that ACT may be a particularly helpful approach for working with older adults experiencing different forms of distress or suffering. Following Petkus and Wetherell's (2013) seminal work on ACT in older adults, there are many reasons underlying this suggestion of a particular suitability. Its transdiagnostic nature, which involves targeting the core dysfunctional dimensions (experiential and behavioral avoidance, cognitive fusion, clarity and commitment, together with personal values), makes it particularly suitable for emotional problems involving comorbidity, which is close to being ubiquitous in older adults (e.g., comorbidity between depression and anxiety in GAD or in chronic stress situations). Also, as compared with other approaches such as CBT, ACT is a more holistic therapy, in the sense that it more explicitly involves the whole life of the person: It deals with thoughts, emotions, and behaviors, but also with values, meaning, affective bonds, spirituality, etc. These characteristics may facilitate a higher "resonance" with this approach, for older adults. They also highlight the consistency between ACT and one of the main gerontological theoretical frameworks – namely, selective optimization with compensation (Baltes & Baltes, 1990), which places flexibility in the management of gains and losses (compensation for losses and optimization of maintained skills and activities) occurring across the lifespan, and in the selection of personal goals, at the core of well-being and adaptation in old age (Alonso-Fernández et al., 2016).

The use of an ACT approach is recommended when the psychological problem presented by the older adult involve patterns of experiential avoidance in which the person is "trapped" and which keep them from developing actions consistent with their values. As ACT frames psychological intervention in the context of the whole landscape of personal values, this makes it very helpful when people show distress conditions involving an excessive focalization on one facet or problem generating suffering, while neglecting or ignoring other aspects of their life.

The case of Mr. P. may be an example of this:

> His life is focused, almost exclusively, in his "bad performance" as a caregiver and he invests all of his energy and efforts in trying (unsuccessfully) not to behave in those "bad ways." Mr. P. is fused with a self-concept of "bad caregiver," and he lives his life from this label, trying hard to eradicate this "bad plant" from his "life garden" (e.g., avoiding guilt by not doing leisure activities), but eventually neglecting other important plants (other values: self-care, relationships with other persons, etc.), and finding the bad plant even stronger, despite his strong fight against it. Older adults may be more vulnerable to become fused with rigid ageist self-stereotypes (e.g., "At my age, I cannot...start new relationships...learn anything new," etc.), from which they perceive life and based on which they act in the world, and these can be serious barriers for the development of courses of action committed to their personal values. ACT facilitates acknowledging these barriers, and, in contrast to the CBT strategy of replacing these thoughts by more functional ones to change behavior, it fosters the ability of the person to act in the desired or valued directions, even in the presence of thoughts saying "You cannot do that!"

ACT's emphasis on "acceptance" of uncomfortable experiences makes it very useful for helping older adults facing irreversible and unchangeable losses or situations (e.g., chronic diseases, death of loved ones, caregiving of ill relatives, etc.). In these situations, change or problem-focused coping strategies may be not only ineffective but even maladaptive, with acceptance being more functional. Indeed Butler and Ciarrochi (2007) found acceptance to be positively associated with quality of life in older adults living in retirement communities to be positively associated with quality of life in older adults living in retirement communities. ACT fosters work on meaning and making sense of the hassles and obstacles in daily life, and hence it is particularly useful to help people who do not necessarily show clinical distress, but that present with normal suffering associated with the facing of normal life problems or situations. In this regard, we identify two additional reasons to use ACT with older adults: (1) age brings with it many unchangeable situations such as just described; and (2) research has shown that older adults present with a higher prevalence of subclinical presentations of psychological symptoms, such as depression (American Psychiatric Association, 2013).

Intervention Based on ACT: Working With the Anxious, Depressive, and Guilt Feelings of a Caregiver of an Older Adult

In this section, we describe the ACT intervention in which Mr. P. participated. As we mentioned in the Introduction to this section, ACT interventions have two main objectives: (a) to increase awareness and acceptance of unpleasant internal events (e.g., negative emotions or thoughts) and the factors involved in their origin (e.g., the behaviors of the care recipient) and (b) to increase the person's commitment to personal values. Table 4.1 summarizes the principal objectives for each intervention objective or module.

Table 4.1. Objectives of the main therapeutic modules in ACT-based interventions

Acceptance module	Commitment to personal values module
Increase emotional awareness Understand experiential avoidance and its costs	Clarify the most important values (e.g., caregiving, parenting, friendship, etc.) for the person
Learn the adaptive alternative to avoidance: acceptance (e.g., of unchangeable conditions such as dementia diagnosis, negative emotions...)	Increase awareness of the level of commitment to those values. Behavioral activation toward the chosen values; performance of committed actions
Increase acceptance skills: mindfulness techniques, metaphors, and experiential exercises	Learn to cope with barriers to committed actions (e.g., feeling guilty for involvement in activities different from caregiving duties)

Note. ACT = acceptance and commitment therapy.

Case Study

> Mr. P. is 70 years old. For the last 3 years, he has been caring for his 68 years old wife, who has frontotemporal dementia. Mr. P. comes to therapy because he feels anxious and depressed when he interacts with his wife. He does not understand why he "loses his nerves" when his wife forgets things (e.g., the cutlery place). Frequently, when he reminds her of the correct word or place that she has forgotten, she yells at him, and he usually behaves in either of two different ways: (a) shouting at her, starting a big argument, or (b) leaving home, with his wife being left alone. Irrespective of the performed behavior, he feels anxious, sad, and guilty. During the past months, the frequency of arguments with his wife has increased, and he feels very anxious about it. He says, "I shouldn´t act this way...I must be patient with her...." On some occasions, he inhibits the expression of his feelings (mostly, anger and sadness), so as not to worry his wife and other relatives. Before becoming a caregiver, Mr. P. was a very active man (e.g., travelling with friends, visiting museums, etc.); however, since his caregiving started 3 years ago, he has not met his friends or had any leisure activity since. "I would feel terribly guilty if I left her just to have fun." Also, he confesses that he has severe difficulties accepting the dementia-related changes in his wife, and their relationship ("I married another person...."), and now he reports high levels of hopelessness, saying, "I don't know what can I do. I do not see any good chance. I face a bleak future."

In the case of Mr. P., the ACT-based intervention was focused mainly on his feelings of guilt. Guilt is a frequent emotion reported by family caregivers of patients with dementia (Gonyea et al., 2008), and it has been suggested as a dimension that significantly contributes to the appearance of depressive symptoms (Losada et al., 2018). Guilt may appear due to self-judgment of one's own actions as insufficient (e.g., being angry with the cared relative, forgetting important care-related dates or tasks, etc.) or be an assessment of the experience of negative feelings or thoughts derived from caregiving (e.g., sadness, thinking about the death of the relative, etc.) as inappropriate. In addition, based on the authors' clinical experience, guilt feelings usually function as barriers for performing actions committed actions based on personal values. Hence, guilt frequently appears when caregivers plan to do or perform some committed activity different from caregiving (e.g., leaving the relative for some time to go out with friends). This way, guilt may facilitate the caregiver's avoidance of non-caregiving valued-based behaviors, prompting them to stay at home with the relative being cared for. With this in mind, ACT interventions with a special focus on guilt may be a useful alternative for caregivers, as they may help them to increase their acceptance of this guilt, understand the function (consequences) of this feeling in their behavior, and reorient their life toward chosen values.

In the case example of Mr. P., the assessment and functional analysis suggested the important role of guilt in the maintenance of his distress (anxious and depressive symptoms). Mr. P. commented on feeling guilty about his anger or anxious reactions directed at his wife, something that increases his stress and sadness. In addition, his baseline score of 40 on the Caregiver Guilt Questionnaire (CGQ; Losada et al., 2010) suggested the presence of elevated levels of guilt feelings in his daily life. Furthermore, the prevention or avoidance of feelings of guilt for "abandoning" his wife explained the lack of realization of potentially rewarding activities. For all of these reasons, Mr. P. participated in an ACT-based intervention with a special focus on guilt – namely, the Guilt-Focused Intervention (Gallego-Alberto et al., 2019), a specific and structured intervention consisting of eight weekly 2-hr sessions, which are outlined in Table 4.2.

Table 4.2. Content of sessions of the ACT-based Guilt-Focused Intervention

Session	Main objective	Content of the session
1	Identifying and understanding guilt feelings	• Experiential exercise: activating and observing my guilt feelings (OC) • Debate: definition of guilt. Unhealthy versus healthy guilt; consequences of unhealthy guilt • Work with personal values: identifying my values (Valued Living Questionnaire Adapted to Dementia Caregiving; Romero-Moreno et al., 2017)
2	Working with perfectionist beliefs	• Experiential exercise: experiencing guilt about doing wrong with my relative with dementia (OC) • Focus on perfectionism and the consequences of acting fused with this belief • Working with personal values: garden metaphor (Hayes et al., 1999) • Mindfulness exercise: breathing exercise (Hayes et al., 1999)

Table 4.2. continued

Session	Main objective	Content of the session
3	Working with "selfishness" beliefs	• Case exercise: the case of Maria (Part 1). Analyzing Maria's garden, non-self-caring behavior and its consequences (OC) • Garden metaphor (Hayes et al., 1999), illustrated in the case example of Mr. P. on the next page • Mindfulness exercise: working with uncomfortable emotions (Márquez-González et al., 2010) • Working with personal values: schedule for committed actions
4	Increasing the new strategy of acceptance	• Exercise: guilt as a sign of change in my life. Working with guilt as a barrier for committed actions (OC) • Bus metaphor (Hayes et al., 1999) • Working with personal values: scheduling new committed actions
5	Acceptance of negative emotions	• Case exercise: the case example of Maria (Part 2; based on the exercise of Isabel the supercaregiver in Márquez-González et al., 2010) • Exercises for accepting guilt and negative thoughts: mindfulness exercises for negative and uncomfortable thoughts (Márquez-González et al., 2010) • Working with personal values: scheduling new committed actions
6	Reviewing the concept of good caregiver	• Exercise: Analyzing my caregiver role and my dysfunctional beliefs about caregiving (OC) • Mindfulness exercise: working with uncomfortable emotions (Márquez-González et al., 2010) • Working with personal values: scheduling new committed actions
7	Reviewing my guilt sources and my own limitations	• Assertive rights: the right of making mistakes • Self-compassion experiential exercise: self-compassion as a strategy to accept my limitations and my mistakes (OC; based on Gilbert, 2010) • Working with personal values: scheduling new committed actions
8	Final	• Closing, summarizing, and reinforcement of the advances obtained through the intervention

Note. ACT = acceptance and commitment therapy; OC= techniques originally created for this program. Based on Gallego-Alberto et al. (2019)

During the first three sessions, the therapeutic work was aimed at increasing Mr. P.'s willingness to observe and get in contact with his emotions, such as guilt or anger. Moreover, the therapist helped him to identify the consequences of some rigid beliefs (e.g., perfectionism) that might be leading him to carry out behaviors that increased the chances of feeling guilty, that were acting as barriers to performing committed activities, and that also were serving as a factor in increasing his distress derived from negative and rigid self-judgments. In addition to that, the work on values focused on clarifying the most important values for Mr. P.. He chose caregiving, friendship, and grandparenting, and new committed actions in those life areas were scheduled.

In the fourth and fifth sessions, the work focused on Mr. P.'s ability to accept negative emotions and thoughts, and on normalizing the occurrence of these experiences in the context of dementia caregiving. Simultaneously, the work on commitment to personal values was maintained. The guilt feelings that emerged during his committed actions were addressed with the exercise of Guilt as a Sign of Change in My Life. The main goal of this exercise was to increase Mr. P.'s acknowledgement of the interference of guilt or another uncomfortable thoughts (e.g. "If I go out with friends, I am a bad caregiver") on the performance of valued, oriented actions and the consequences of not performing committed actions based on personal values due to guilt and other negative emotions. Also, the exercise supports and promotes the use of the skill of acceptance, encouraging the caregiver to experience and explore those feelings, avoiding attempts to stop or control them.

Finally, the last three sessions were directed to reinforcing the acceptance of guilt and other negative emotions, as well as promoting more flexible and compassionate self-judgments.

The delivery of treatment with Mr. P. was fluid, and adherence was successful. During the sessions, Mr. P. worked on his ability to accept those negative thoughts and emotions derived from the caregiving situation. At the beginning of treatment, he presented high levels of anger and frustration, derived from the changes in the relationship with his wife, and worsened by his attempts to avoid their expression. Over the sessions, his willingness to observe and express those feelings increased, even allowing him to find some functionality in some of them. This can be seen in the following statement during the seventh session:

> I am learning to live with those sad feelings.... It is hard, but when I let them ... although I feel sad and melancholic, they remind me of how much I love my wife, and how important is to me the task of taking care of her.... (Mr. P., ACT patient)

> The work on acceptance was conducted simultaneously with work on clarifying Mr. P.'s values and reorienting his actions to the most important ones. The garden metaphor (Hayes et al., 1999) was used to clarify and represent the current state of his commitment to his values. In that exercise, Mr. P. had to draw his life as a garden, composed by different plants. In his first garden, Mr. P. drew a cactus representing his wife, cypresses as his children, some tulips as his friends, and two lamppost as his granddaughters. Finally, at the end of the treatment, Mr. P. drew the same garden, but he introduced two new areas: He included himself in the middle of the garden, representing the need for self-care, and in one corner, he added a lighthouse representing those abilities learned at the intervention, which may help him to cope with the caregiving situation. In fact, at the last session, Mr. P. said, "We have removed the component of guilt and added letting me get pampered.... Although it's hard and hard, I see light at the end of the tunnel."

After completing the intervention, Mr. P. reported lower levels of psychological distress; indeed, his scores for the outcome variables assessed (depressive and anxious symptomatology) decreased significantly (to under the clinical cutoff scores). These significant reductions were accompanied by improvements in the abilities promoted by the ACT intervention: acceptance skills, cognitive defusion strategies, and frequency of committed actions. These results provide additional support for implementing ACT interventions focused on guilt feelings with family caregivers of patients with dementia (Losada et al., 2015; Márquez-González et al., in press), a population mainly composed of older adults.

Treatment Considerations for Older Adults

ACT is a particularly suitable therapeutic approach for older adults for the reasons discussed above. However, some of its components may involve important challenges for some older cohorts, not because of chronological age, but more probably due to variables related to context (e.g., lack of socialization on psychological constructs, introspection skills, etc.) that may shape their experiences with their emotions.

Cognitive defusion techniques may be difficult to apprehend for some older adults, as they involve metacognitive strategies aimed at "distancing" from one's thoughts and emotions, analyzing them from a certain "distance." In our clinical work, we have found some older adults, particularly those with a low educational level, to have a hard time understanding and performing these exercises. As Petkus and Wetherell (2013) note, older adults may present difficulties with introspecting, identifying, and acknowledging thoughts and other internal experiences. Hence, it seems reasonable to be sensitive to the possible presence of these difficulties, to lower the complexity of defusion techniques or reduce their importance or centrality in the therapy.

Although framed in the context of CBT therapies, Laidlaw's (2015) suggestion that older adults' larger number of experiences – and larger experience in facing problems and regulating associated emotions – may be of help to reframe narratives in a way that promotes resilience, growth, and wisdom, something that can foster self-forgiveness and acceptance, promoting new ways of coping with adversities, is apt here. In the context of difficulties, in addition to acknowledging older adults' experiences and reducing the impact of negative aging stereotypes, behavioral activation may be initiated through the use of selection, optimization, and compensation strategies, with the work on their personal values being essential for this purpose (Kishita et al., 2016).

Interpersonal Psychotherapy

Introduction

IPT was developed as an individual treatment for depression by Gerald Klerman, Myrna Weissman, and their colleagues in the 1970s. Along with CBT, IPT is one of the most researched psychotherapeutic interventions which has consistently demonstrated efficacy in the treatment of depression (Cuijpers et al., 2011). Professional clinical treatment guidelines in the US and other nations recommend IPT as a treatment for depression (e.g., American Psychiatric Association, 2010; American Psychological Association, 2019). IPT has been adapted from its original individual format to marital or dyadic and group versions, and a maintenance form of IPT exists. IPT has been found efficacious in different populations, including adolescent, adults, older adults, and medical patients, and military service veterans. In addition to depression, IPT has been found useful in the treatment of bipolar disorder, eating disorder, personality disorder, and posttraumatic stress disorder (Weissman et al., 2018). International studies have found that IPT is efficacious in the treatment of depression in non-Western cultures (e.g., Bolton et al., 2003).

In the early history of IPT, it was observed that it might be a useful treatment for late-life depression, and two pilot studies provided promising evidence (Rothblum et al., 1982; Sloane et al., 1985). Other studies found IPT useful in the treatment of depressive symptoms in medically ill older adults with depression and those with moderate to severe depression (Mossey et al., 1996; Van Schaik et al., 2006). One of two studies found IPT reduced the likelihood of depressive relapse (Reynolds et al., 1999). A recent report found IPT efficacious in the treatment of depressed military service members, many of whom were older adults (Stewart et al., 2014).

The four IPT problem areas that are a focus of this psychotherapy seem especially useful for the life problems often seen among older depressed adults in outpatient practice (see Table 4.3). The problem areas include interpersonal role disputes (conflict with another), role transitions (life change), grief (death of an important person), and social isolation and/or loneliness (problems establishing and sustaining relationship, also referred to as "interpersonal deficits"). In clinical practice, the IPT problem area most commonly seen in older adults treated with IPT is role transitions, examples of which include residential move, financial problems, change in work status, care for a family member, and onset or exacerbation of health problems (Hinrichsen, 2008; Hinrichsen & Clougherty, 2006). The second most common IPT problem area among older adults is interpersonal role disputes which includes problems with spouse or partner, sibling, adult child, and sometimes institutions. The IPT problem area grief is usually in relationship to death of spouse or partner, adult child, or sibling. Social isolation and/or loneliness is the least commonly treated problem area with older adults but has been found to be much more common among older military service veterans (Stewart et al., 2014).

IPT is a time-limited psychotherapy. As originally developed, it involved 16 sessions. It is frequently delivered in three phases of treatment: initial sessions, intermediate sessions, and termination. The initial sessions are the evaluation and goal-setting stage. The lion's share of treatment is in the intermediate sessions, where one, or at most two, of the four IPT problem areas are addressed. Termination is a review of the course of treatment, progress made in treatment, and a look to the future. Goals and strategies exist for each of the four problem areas.

Various treatment techniques are used, the most common of which are noted in Table 4.3. These techniques are implemented in the service of the therapeutic strategies and goals of the respective problem area. An example of the use of these techniques is given in the following case example of an *interpersonal role dispute*.

Table 4.3. Overview of interpersonal psychotherapy for depression

Therapeutic stance	Phases of treatment	Problem areas and associated goals	Commonly used techniques
Collaborative Hopeful Encouraging Educational	Initial sessions (weeks 1–3): (1) Assess and educate about depression, (2) Identify life event(s) tied to depression, (3) Conduct interpersonal inventory, and (4) Provide formulation and plan	Role transitions: (1) Come to emotional terms with changed life, (2) Build new skills to better manage new life situation	Communications analysis: In-depth review of a recent interpersonal interaction
	Intermediate sessions (weeks 4–14): Implement goals associated with identified problem area(s)	Grief: (1) Facilitate the grieving progress, (2) Reestablish a more satisfying and meaningful life without the deceased	Decision analysis: Identification of options to address issues tied to depression
	Termination (weeks 15–16): (1) Elicit feelings about ending, (2) Assess current status of depression and problem area, (3) Identify possible future life problems and warning signs of depression onset, and (4) Explore if further treatment needed	Interpersonal role disputes: (1) Clarify issues and expectations in the dispute, (2) Change expectations as needed, and/or (3) Acquire skills to better manage the dispute	Interpersonal skills building: Learn ways to more productively communicate
		Social isolation and/or loneliness: (1) Reduce isolation, (2) Encourage formation of new relationships	Role play: Enactment of a planned conversation
			Work-at-home: Between-session efforts to address some aspect of a problem area

Case Example: IPT in an Interpersonal Role Dispute

Mrs. C., a 77-year-old married women with three children, was told by a friend that her husband had had an affair with a mutual acquaintance several years earlier. When she confronted her husband with this information, he denied it but then later said it was true. He avowed that the affair had ended. What followed were frequent arguments between them including long periods in which she refused to speak to him. She grew increasingly depressed and sought psychological services. At first, the therapist asked her to describe, in detail, incidents in which they fought (a "communications analysis"), which revealed that she would accuse him of being "selfish," "a bad person," and "heartless," to which he would respond with his own allegations of her moral failings. These arguments left her feeling more depressed and hopeless. The therapist engaged Mrs. C. in a review of options to address her marital problem. She came up with a variety of options (a "decision analysis"), including listing the advantages and disadvantages of each option (e.g., leave him, live together but lead separate lives, continue to argue, find a way to have a different kind of conversation about the infidelity with him). She chose the last option. Working with the therapist, she learned skills in how to have a more productive conversation with her husband (interpersonal skills building), practiced a planned conversation with him (role play), and then had the conversation (work-at-home), followed by a review of how the conversation went.

Most IPT intermediate sessions focus on current life issues in the identified problem area(s) with a focus on events from the prior week. Depression symptoms are monitored throughout IPT using a structured assessment measure (e.g., the Patient Health Questionnaire [PHQ-9]) or general standardized inquiry about the status of the patient's depression (e.g., subjective rating of depression severity on a scale from 1 to 10). IPT is less structured than most CBTs, yet treatment is guided by the goals and strategies associated with the identified IPT problem area(s), issues relevant to the problem area that developed in the past week, and the impact of those issues on the patient's depression. The therapist is collaborative, hopeful, encouraging, and psychoeducational. Treatment gains are attributed to efforts made by the patient to address problems to further enhance the individual's sense of mastery.

Case Example: IPT for Depression and Grief

Initial Sessions

Mrs. J. was an 82-year-old White woman with an adult daughter who was referred for IPT by her primary care physician because of concerns about how she was contending with the loss of her husband who had died a year and a half earlier. In addition to grieving, Mrs. J. evidenced symptoms consistent with a major depressive episode. The apparent trigger to her depression was not only the death of her husband but a move across country from her home in the Midwest to the East Coast where her daughter lived. Mrs. J. found it difficult to establish a new life in this eastern city where she lived in assisted living. She had few friends, little interest in social or recreational activities, and regretted that she had moved. The patient was educated about grief and depression by the therapist, including the fact that major depression impairs people's ability to function. Grief and role transitions (i.e., move to a new city) were identified as the IPT problem areas. The goal of treatment was further resolution of grief, improved ability to adapt to her new living environment, and reduced depressive symptoms.

Intermediate Sessions

Mrs. J.'s depressive symptoms were monitored throughout treatment. Change in depressive symptoms was often associated with an issue in the prior week tied to either grief or role transitions. The therapist facilitated the grieving process by engaging the patient in a discussion of both positive and negative aspects of her relationship with her husband and the circumstances surrounding his illness and death. The difficulties with which she was contending in her new life on the East Coast were elicited, as well as feelings about her prior life that included her husband, friends, and community involvements. Both positive and negative aspects of her life in the Midwest were identified. Clarification of discontent with her current living circumstances was made, including the fact that she did not want to live in assisted living. She found that most of the residents of the assisted living residence had health and functional problems greater than her own. Originally, she had resisted her daughter's suggestion that she move to assisted living but then acquiesced. Other living options were explored by Mrs. J., including the possibility of moving to her own independent apartment for which she weighed the advantages and disadvantages. During the course of therapy, she identified an apartment building in a neighborhood that appealed to her; and by the end of therapy, she was making plans for a move to it. Her depressive symptoms slowly improved during the course of treatment.

Termination

> Feelings about ending IPT were elicited by the therapist. Mrs. J. said that she had found therapy more helpful than she had anticipated and, in fact, felt sad about ending it. The therapist reviewed change in her depressive symptoms from the beginning of treatment and said that they had significantly improved. Mrs. J. felt that it had been helpful to talk further about her relationship with her husband – a topic which she felt her friends and family no longer wanted to discuss. The plan to move to an apartment made her feel more in control of her life, and she was more hopeful about establishing a new network of friends and meaningful activities. The therapist reviewed with her, the future stressors that might increase depressive symptoms and the options for addressing them.

As noted, the fourth IPT problem area, social isolation and/or loneliness (also known as interpersonal deficits), is less commonly seen in older adults than the other problem areas. One explanation is that older adults often seek mental health services at the behest of a family member or friend, and socially isolated individuals are less likely to have such persons in their lives. Two clinical examples of older individuals with social isolation and/or loneliness are those of Ms. Greenberg and Mr. Holden – cases that are discussed in detail elsewhere (Hinrichsen & Clougherty, 2006). Ms. Greenberg was a 62-year-old woman, never married and with no children, who became depressed following the death of her mother. After an evaluation, it appeared that the depression was less tied to the death of her mother than to longstanding social isolation: "I now have nobody except my brother." The goal of treatment was to reduce her social isolation by slowly helping to her find avenues for engagement with others and to build fundamental social skills as part of that engagement.

Mr. Holden was a 78-year-old divorced man with no children who lived in a nursing home. He had only one friend, who visited him on a regular basis. After his friend moved out of state and the visits stopped, he became increasingly depressed. Further, he had increasing conflicts with the nursing home staff, which included making racially offensive remarks to them. The focus of IPT was acquiring skills to better negotiate differences with nursing staff, as well as make efforts to engage other residents for some measure of companionship. For both Ms. Greenberg and Mr. Holden, reduction of social isolation was tied to an improvement in depression.

Treatment Considerations for Older Adults

IPT requires little adaptation when provided to older adults (Hinrichsen, 2008; Hinrichsen & Clougherty, 2006). As with any psychotherapeutic intervention with older adults, treatment is informed by a solid familiarity with attitudes toward aging, facts about aging, the lifespan developmental perspective, how the presentation of mental disorders may be different in older versus younger adults, skillful assessment, and knowledge of how to optimize psychological interventions with this population (Hinrichsen et al., 2018).

IPT is a highly researched and widely recommended treatment for depression. It seems especially well-suited to the life problems often evident in older adults with depression seen in outpatient clinical practice. It is a flexibly applied psychotherapy guided by goals and strategies associated with one, or at most two, of the four IPT problem areas. Clinical research studies and clinical practice with older adults indicate that it is helpful for most older patients, as evidenced by improved depression and capacity to contend with life problems associated with their depression.

Dialectical Behavior Therapy

Introduction

DBT is a multicomponent, cognitive behavioral intervention developed by Marsha Linehan to treat individuals with borderline personality disorder (BPD), persistent suicidal ideation, and self-harming behaviors (Linehan, 1993a, 1993b). Though relatively little research has investigated the use of DBT in older adults compared with CBT, IPT, and ACT, it may be the best treatment choice for individuals with treatment-resistant depression and/or chronic moderate to severe depression with chronic suicidal ideation and/or self-harming behaviors, especially when there is a suspected or diagnosed comorbid personality disorder. DBT includes one or more components of all three psychotherapies mentioned in this chapter to promote a "life worth living" (Linehan & Wilks, 2015). Like IPT, DBT teaches skills to improve interpersonal functioning. Similar to CBT, DBT encourages "checking the facts" to challenge unhelpful appraisals and interpretations. Like ACT, DBT uses mindfulness as a core process to notice and accept internal experiences. Finally, as in both CBT and ACT, DBT uses exposure by challenging the client to notice distressing emotions and urges (i.e., often characterized by intense feelings, impulsive desires, and avoidance behaviors) and behave in a way that is the opposite of their lifelong patterns of behavior.

The dialectical framework, which differentiates DBT from other CBTs, supports the notion that reality consists of opposing forces, such as feelings of intense anger and yet also a desire to have meaningful connections with others, and both can exist simultaneously. The process of DBT, with its focus on validation and problem solving, promotes a balance between acceptance and change (Linehan, 1993a). Acceptance is rooted in Zen and contemplative practices, and is facilitated through the use of mindfulness and other skills to improve a person's tolerance to distress (Linehan & Wilks, 2015). DBT was the first psychotherapy to use mindfulness practice, which is a core skill that is central to the treatment. Based on behavioral theory, change is promoted through use of effective problem-solving strategies and acquisition of skills to improve interpersonal functioning and emotion regulation.

DBT is an evidence-based, empirically supported intervention that has been endorsed by the Society of Clinical Psychology for the treatment of BPD (https://www.div12.org/treatments/). Standard DBT has four components: group skills training, individual therapy, telephone coaching, and therapist consultation. Treatment is delivered over a minimum of 28 weeks and typically lasts 12 months (Rizvi et al., 2013). Linehan separated skills training from individual therapy for several reasons. For individuals with BPD, skills training alone may be perceived as invalidating and is not effective as a stand-alone treatment in reducing distress (Linehan, 1993b; Linehan & Wilks, 2015). Group skills training is used as the vehicle to provide psychoeducation about specific skills, and individual therapy is meant to reinforce the use of the skills in a flexible and effective manner. Telephone coaching is provided between sessions primarily to reinforce the use of skills in different contexts and environments. It should not be used in isolation during acute suicidal ideation, due to the potential impact this behavior can have in reinforcing suicidality (Linehan & Wilks, 2015). Lastly, therapist consultations occur weekly in a DBT team and model the same validation and problem-solving process as the therapy. Consultation is included as a core component of standard DBT due to the high potential for burnout among therapists working with individuals with BPD.

Research has shown promising benefits of DBT across a range of clinical populations (Robins & Chapman, 2004). Randomized controlled trials using standard DBT for individuals with BPD have demonstrated its efficacy in reducing suicide attempts, self-harm behaviors, depression, anxiety, and attrition (Linehan et al., 2015; Panos et al., 2014). It has been effective at reducing anger and aggression in BPD and other clinical populations (Frazier & Vela, 2014). When applied to other populations, researchers and clinicians have modified DBT to fit their specific setting and client needs with success (Robins & Chapman, 2004). Modifications have included, but are not limited to, reducing the number of treatment sessions for individual therapy and group skills training, using only the individual therapy component and applying skills training during individual sessions, and using only group skills training. DBT skills training is a popular treatment component among clinicians and has been effectively used and written about in the literature (Valentine et al., 2014). More research is needed to understand the incremental clinical value of each treatment component of standard DBT, but it is clear that skills training is a key component attributed to improved clinical outcomes (Linehan et al., 2015).

Less attention has been paid to the investigation of DBT in older adults. To date, only two randomized studies in this population have been published. Lynch and colleagues (2003) conducted a randomized pilot study to assess the feasibility, acceptability, and benefits of augmenting pharmacotherapy with a DBT skills training group and DBT-consistent telephone coaching in older adults with depression. The study group received medication and participated in both the skills training group and scheduled telephone coaching (DBT+MED), while the control group received medication only (MED). While interviewer-rated depression scores significantly decreased in participants in both groups, only the participants in DBT+MED demonstrated significant decreases in self-rated depression. In addition, only one participant dropped out DBT+MED, indicating overall feasibility and acceptability of the treatment (described in Lynch, Cheavens, Cukrowicz et al., 2007). Finally, more participants in DBT+MED met the cutoff for depression remission at posttreatment, compared to controls (MED) (71% vs. 47%) and 6-month follow-up (75% vs. 31%).

A second randomized study investigated the benefit of DBT individual therapy and group skills training for older adults with major depressive disorder and personality disorders, who did not benefit from an 8-week medication trial (Lynch, Cheavens, Cukrowicz et al., 2007). Of note, only 14% of participants experienced at least a 50% reduction in symptoms after the initial medication trial, resulting in over two thirds of participants being randomized in the DBT+MED and MED groups. While participants in both groups eventually reached remission, remittance of symptoms occurred more quickly for participants in the DBT+MED group. Moreover, the DBT+MED group was associated with improvements in interpersonal sensitivity and aggression, while the MED-only group was not.

Other research has been conducted with older caregivers. Drossel et al. (2011) used the DBT skills training group component in a small sample of caregivers for persons with dementia who had one or more risk factors for elder abuse. The group was modified in language content (focused on caregiving situations instead of self-harm behaviors) and duration (reduced to 8 weeks). The 16 caregivers who completed the group experienced improvements in problem-focused coping, emotional well-being, and fatigue, and they participated in separate individual therapy at a higher rate while in the group, which was interpreted as improved help-seeking behavior.

Patient Selection

Because DBT was developed to treat individuals with BPD, Linehan needed a theoretical model of BPD on which to base the treatment (Linehan & Wilks, 2015). The *biosocial theory* was developed to explain the factors that lead to and maintain BPD. The theory posits that a biological predisposition for emotional vulnerability, coupled with an invalidating environment, produces emotional dysregulation that is continuously reinforced. As such, DBT was developed to target these factors.

Based on clinical expertise and research in DBT with older adults with comorbid depression and personality disorder, Lynch and Cheavens (2007) expanded the biosocial theory to include heightened negative affect as a biological precursor and reinforcement of maladaptive coping characterized by avoidance. They proposed that these elements lead to disruptions in interpersonal relationships as well as excessive rigidity and guardedness against new experiences. Difficulty regulating emotions and impulses is also a consequence of the aforementioned predisposing factors, but it is less pronounced in older adults compared with younger adults (Lynch & Cheavens, 2007).

When considering DBT as a potential treatment option for a patient, clinicians should consider three factors: suicidality and/or high-risk behaviors, chronicity of depression, and presence of maladaptive personality characteristics, such as rigidity or paranoia. Suicide is of significant concern in the older population since rates of suicide are highest for men aged 75 and older (Hedegaard et al., 2018).

DBT Treatment Elements

As previously mentioned, standard DBT comprises four components (i.e., individual therapy, group skills training, telephone coaching, and therapist consultation). Skills training, which is a vital component of DBT, is focused on psychoeducation and skill acquisition, whereas the individual therapy and telephone coaching components further reinforce the skills and facilitate flexibility in skill application. For the purpose of this chapter, we will focus on the skills training component for four reasons: (1) it requires less therapist training compared with what is needed for the provision of standard DBT, (2) it is the most studied component of DBT, (3) it can be delivered in individual or group therapy, and (4) preliminary research supports its use as a stand-alone treatment. Acceptance skills are taught in the mindfulness and distress tolerance modules, while change skills are taught in the interpersonal effectiveness and emotion regulation modules (Linehan & Wilks, 2015). For detailed descriptions of skills, exercises, and session outlines, see Linehan's (1993b) *Skills Training Manual for Treating Borderline Personality Disorder,* and McKay, Wood, and Brantley's (2007) *The Dialectical Behavior Therapy Skills Workbook.*

Mindfulness

Mindfulness comprises one module and is also incorporated in the other skills modules because it is a core skill. Simply put, mindfulness is intentionally being aware of internal and external experiences in the present moment without judgment of self, others, or experiences. It is a practice that facilitates awareness and exploration of the self in a curious yet gentle manner.

In DBT, mindfulness is initially presented as a way to "take control of the mind" rather than "letting the mind take control of you" (Linehan, 1993b). Note that the purpose of mindfulness, as presented in DBT, is slightly different from mindfulness and acceptance in ACT, which purports that suffering is perpetuated by the control agenda (i.e., attempting to control the mind). States of mind reflect the dialectic of *reasonable mind* versus *emotion mind.* Reasonable mind is the rational, logical, and planful state of mind, whereas emotion mind is characterized by thinking and behavior that is controlled by emotions. The balanced state is *wise mind,* which is only achieved by way of mindfulness.

Mindfulness skills are separated into the "what" skills (i.e., focused and specific) and the "how" skills (i.e., principles for the application). "What" skills consist of (a) noticing and (b) describing what is observed, while fully attending to and participating in the activity. An exercise to highlight noticing would be to simply pay undivided attention to a single component of one's internal experience, be it thoughts, emotions, physical sensations, sounds, sights, etc. Describing can begin with the simple practice of describing an object, moving to more complex exercises, such as describing one's emotions. Similar to in ACT, in DBT it is important to highlight that thoughts are not facts, and they primarily consist of judgments or evaluations rather than pure descriptions. Finally, the "how" skills are (a) practicing mindfulness with a nonjudgmental attitude, (b) focusing on one thing at a time, and (c) doing what is workable and effective.

Distress Tolerance

Individuals in DBT typically have intense emotions or, rather, extreme sensitivity to emotions, and thus have difficulty accepting their internal experiences without acting on them. Skills taught in the distress tolerance module facilitate radical acceptance, which is defined as complete willingness and acceptance of internal experiences, one's ability to tolerate and survive crises.

Four methods of distress tolerance taught in this module are (a) identifying the pros and cons of tolerating distress, (b) distracting oneself from distress, (c) soothing oneself by focusing on the five senses, and (d) improving the moment by replacing negatives with positives. Distracting (b) and improving (d) skills use acronyms for easy recall and are shown in Table 4.4.

Table 4.4. Distress tolerance skills

Distracting (ACCEPTS)	Improving (IMPROVE)
Activities: engage in pleasurable activities	**I**magery: imagine a pleasant and safe situation, or imagine effective coping
Contributing: do something to help others	**M**eaning: find meaning in the distressing situation
Comparison: compare self with others who are less well-off	**P**rayer: use prayer to open up to the moment
Emotions: generate opposing emotions (half smile when feeling distressed)	**R**elax: relax the body
Push away: leave a distressing situation either physically or mentally	**O**ne thing in the moment: use the "how" skills of mindfulness
Thoughts: distract with other thoughts	**V**acation from adulthood: take a brief retreat and allow oneself to be taken care of
Sensations: create a benign but intense sensation (e.g., hold ice cubes)	**E**ncouragement: Be your own cheerleader

Note. Based on Linehan, 1993b, pp. 166, 168.

Interpersonal Effectiveness

Interpersonal effectiveness skills are based largely on assertiveness training and focus on managing conflict and initiating and maintaining healthy relationships. Psychoeducation on the characteristics of interpersonal styles (i.e., passive, assertive, and aggressive) is an ideal starting point. From there, the client can begin to apply mindfulness skills in interactions with others to develop an understanding of their own interpersonal style. The clinician highlights the importance of balancing the client's priorities and the demands of others, linking it to an assertive communication style. Several acronyms are used to highlight the key skills of interpersonal effectiveness, as shown in Box 4.1.

Box 4.1. Interpersonal effectiveness skills

Core strategy – DEAR MAN
Describe: describe the situation using facts and avoiding judgments
Express: describe how you feel using "I" statements and avoid blaming
Assert: clearly state your wish, and avoid telling the person what he or she should do
Reinforce: reward the person for a positive response, or describe how achieving your request would positively impact the situation
Mindful: keep your focus on the objective and do not get distracted by negative responses from the other person
Appear confident: appear confident in your tone of voice, posture, and eye contact
Negotiate: be willing to compromise

Improve relationship – GIVE
Gentle: be courteous and gentle in your approach
Interested: be interested in the other person's opinions and point of view
Validate: acknowledge the other person's feelings, opinions, and struggles
Easy manner: be light-hearted and use a soft approach

Maintain respect – FAST
Fair: be fair to yourself and the other person
Apologies: apologize when warranted, but do not apologize for having an opinion or disagreeing with the other person
Stick to values: know your values and stick to them
Truthful: be true to yourself and others

Note. Based on Linehan 1993b, pp. 125, 127, 128.

Emotion Regulation

The emotion regulation module uses cognitive and behavioral strategies to decrease distressing emotions and increase positive emotions. Skills focus on identifying and labeling emotions, identifying and problem solving personal obstacles to changing emotions, reducing vulnerability to difficult emotions (i.e., emotion mind), and managing difficult emotions when they arise. A useful starting point in this module is providing psychoeducation on the cognitive behavioral framework and impact of cognitive appraisals on emotions. Then, the therapist can begin to facilitate exploration and understanding of the client's emotions, as well as of additional factors that contribute to emotional vulnerability, such as physical well-being, diet and exercise, sleep, alcohol, and drugs. Time should be taken to identify and intervene in self-destructive behaviors.

Similar to traditional CBT, the emotion regulation module utilizes cognitive restructuring by "checking the facts" of cognitive appraisals. Behavioral activation to increase pleasurable activities is a method used to increase positive emotions. It is common to use tracking logs for thoughts, emotions, behaviors, and consequences, to facilitate learning and use of skills. Exposure is used via "taking the opposite action," which encourages clients to do the opposite of what their emotions or urges dictate. Finally, imaginal rehearsal can be used to facilitate visualization of effectively using emotion regulation skills in an anticipated distressing situation.

Case Example: Individual Therapy for Depression

Mr. S. was 71-year-old, divorced, African-American, noncombat Vietnam War era veteran who was referred by his psychiatrist for individual therapy. His psychiatrist had been treating him for recurrent and severe major depressive disorder for 7 years, and he had not experienced much benefit from pharmacotherapy except for a slight improvement in sleep. He had had individual therapy with two therapists in the past but terminated both abruptly because he felt those were not helpful.

Upon intake with his new therapist in a small private practice, Mr. S. reported a long history of depressed and irritable mood, anhedonia, sense of hopelessness and emptiness, fatigue, poor concentration, and suicidal ideation that began before his military service. In his 30s and 40s, he coped with his depression by using alcohol and other substances, which resulted in the end of his marriage, a rupture in his relationship with his two daughters, and 4 years of homelessness. Mr. S. was treated for alcohol and substance misuse in an inpatient program 25 years ago and has generally maintained sobriety without the use of support, which he cited as a source of pride. However, he has had three suicide attempts in the past 3 decades, all in the context of drinking that was precipitated by feelings of rejection and the thought, "What is the point of living?"

Since completing the inpatient program years ago, Mr. S. had reconnected with his daughters but spoke to them infrequently and visited them only during holidays. He reported having no support network and has difficulty maintaining relationships because either he ends relationships with people who do not meet his expectations, or others end the relationship when they are offended by his irritability and his critiques of them. Mr. S. has isolated himself from others for years, and his current activities are limited to doing chores around his home, shopping for groceries, going to medical appointments, and occasionally going to a local coffee shop. He actively avoids being around others, especially when he feels irritable and angry, which occurs often.

The therapist spent the initial sessions gathering additional information about Mr. S.'s background and current functioning, taking care to validate his emotions in an effort to develop rapport and ease his initial guardedness, and collaboratively developing a safety plan. Mr. S. was frank about his nihilistic perception of therapy and his belief that he will likely die by suicide in the future. Though he did not readily report experiencing feelings of sadness, guilt, and rejection, it appeared that his anger functioned to protect him from these vulnerable emotions. Moreover, his rigid thought patterns, unrealistic expectations and negative judgment of others, isolation, and suicide attempts served as avoidance patterns and behaviors. The combination of these factors negatively impacted his ability to initiate and maintain respectful and meaningful relationships with others. Given Mr. S.'s presentation, current functioning, suicide attempts, chronic suicidal ideation, and lack of success with past mental health treatment, the therapist chose to use DBT.

Mr. S. identified his anger as a primary target for treatment and acknowledged that it negatively impacted all aspects of his life. Therefore, the therapist began with introducing the concept of wise mind and mindfulness skills. Because of past failed therapy attempts and

Mr. S.'s nihilistic view of therapy, the therapist helped Mr. S. identify distressing emotions that came up in his past therapy sessions and linked them to the abrupt termination of therapy. Mr. S. began learning to use his senses to ground himself in the present moment and to self-soothe when feeling distressed, both inside and outside the therapy room. In addition, Mr. S. weighed the pros and cons of tolerating distress in the therapy room, which positively impacted his commitment to the treatment.

Using emotion regulation skills, Mr. S. identified two emotions underlying his anger – guilt at causing emotional harm to his family and fear of their rejection. Recognizing these emotions allowed him to acknowledge his desire to have a closer relationship with his daughters. Using DEAR MAN, GIVE, and "taking the opposite action," Mr. S. reached out to his daughters and began visiting them almost every week. Initially, he had strong reactions of feeling rejected when one of his daughters was not available to visit him for a month. However, he was open to "checking the facts" of his initial cognitive appraisal in session and was able to identify that his daughter's work obligations limited her availability.

Mr. S. engaged in other behavioral experiments throughout therapy. Using DEAR MAN and GIVE skills in his interactions with others ultimately improved his interpersonal interactions, leading to less negative judgments of others. Using ACCEPTS and going out in public when feeling distressed (i.e., "taking the opposite action") decreased his isolation and improved his ability to tolerate frustration with minor stressors, such as encountering an annoyed or slow customer representative in the checkout line at a grocery store.

Treatment Considerations for Older Adults

When using DBT with older adults, clinicians are encouraged to consider several factors. Compared with younger adults, older adults with life-long depression, especially with comorbid personality disorders, are more likely to have difficulty making cognitive and behavioral changes, due to the chronicity of symptoms and years of reinforcement of maladaptive behaviors (Lynch & Cheavens, 2007). However, on a positive note, emotion regulation tends to improve with age. Therefore, rigidity and steady negative emotionality, as opposed to emotional lability, are more likely to be primary treatment targets when using DBT with older adults.

Related to this, years of negative emotionality and rigidity can have long-lasting impacts on relationships, resulting in desired or undesired isolation. It can be difficult for older adults to reestablish damaged relationships and tolerate the distress of attempting to mend relationships. Distress tolerance and emotional regulation skills are vital in helping older clients choose, and act on, reestablishing past relationships.

Lynch and Cheavens (2007) identified additional concepts to include in DBT for older adults. Their proposed framework for reducing rigidity, titled "path to a fluid mind," involves decreasing bitterness (e.g., resentment and distrust), emotional inhibition (i.e., thought and emotion suppression), rigid thinking (e.g., assumptions), and unimportant behaviors (e.g., downplaying importance of relationships). They encourage challenging the myths of a fixed mind, such as, "You can't teach an old dog new tricks" "These techniques are for stupid young people" and "Even if I did try something different, it wouldn't help, because I've tried everything" (Lynch & Cheavens, 2007, p. 279). Finally, forgiveness is likely to be a key element, as forgiveness of self and others may be needed to move forward and create a life worth living.

Conclusions and Implications

As discussed in the introductory part, although CBT interventions have stronger empirical support, the ACT, IPT and DBT approaches have also been shown efficacious options for addressing the distress and the management of the uncontrollable interpersonal events which usually occur in late life (e.g., loss of a family member, role transitions, isolation).

Summarizing, ACT interventions are aimed at fostering the acceptance of these events and promoting the performance of committed actions with the personal values (e.g., family relationships, etc.). IPT is aimed at improving the interpersonal skills of the individual in order to cope effectively with these problematics. And, finally, DBT seems to be a potential option for severe depression cases (including cases with high risk of suicide), including acceptance techniques, exposure and training in interpersonal abilities.

Keeping in mind the therapeutic objectives, ACT interventions may be a potential option for older adults facing uncontrollable situations (e.g., diagnosis of a chronic disease, change in abilities), and for patients with high rates of distress avoidance patterns of behavior. The IPT would be a potential treatment for those patients who may present dysfunctional interpersonal abilities and are facing situations which need some reformulation (e.g., reformulation and adjustment to new roles after retirement). Finally, DBT has been shown an efficacious treatment option for patients presenting severe psychopathologies (e.g. as severe depression and bipolar personality disorder).

Despite the different techniques and objectives raised, all of them are aimed at improving the adjustment of the older adults to the changes and events that aging may entail, such as, loss and grief, role transitions and loneliness.

Suggested Resources for Case-Based Approaches

Frazer, D. W., Hinrichsen, G. A., & Jongsma, A. E. (2015). *The older adult psychotherapy treatment planner, with DSM-5 updates* (2nd ed.). Wiley.

Hayes, S. C., Strosahl, K. D., & Wilson, K. G. (2011). *Acceptance and Commitment Therapy, second edition: The process and practice of mindful change.* Guilford Press.

Hinrichsen, G. A. (2019). *Assessment and treatment of older adults: A guide for mental health professionals.* American Psychological Association.

Hinrichsen, G. A., & Clougherty, K. F. (2006). *Interpersonal psychotherapy for depressed older adults.* American Psychological Association. https://doi.org/10.1037/11429-000

Knight, B. G., & Pachana, N. A. (2015). *Psychological assessment and therapy with older adults.* Oxford University Press. https://doi.org/10.1093/med:psych/9780199652532.001.0001

Linehan, M. M. (1993a). *Cognitive behavioral therapy of borderline personality disorder.* Guilford Press.

Linehan, M. M. (1993b). *Skills training manual for treating borderline personality disorder.* Guilford Press.

McKay, M., Wood, J. C., & Brantley, J. (2007). *The dialectical behavior therapy skills workbook: Practical DBT exercises for learning mindfulness, interpersonal effectiveness, emotion regulation, & distress tolerance.* New Harbinger.

References

Alonso, M., López, A., Losada, A., & González, J. L. (2013). Acceptance and commitment therapy and selective optimization with compensation for older people with chronic pain. *Behavioral Psychology, 21,* 59–79. https://doi.org/10.1111/pme.12885

Alonso-Fernández, M., López-López, A., Losada, A., González, J. L., & Wetherell, J. L. (2016). Acceptance and commitment therapy and selective optimization with compensation for institutionalized older people with chronic pain. *Pain Medicine, 17*(2), 264–277. https://doi.org/10.1111/pme.12885

American Psychiatric Association. (2010). *Practice guidelines for patients with major depressive disorder* (3rd ed.). http://psychiatryonline.org/pb/assets/raw/sitewide/practice_guidelines/guidelines/mdd.pdf

American Psychiatric Association. (2013). *Diagnostic and statistical manual of mental disorders* (5th ed.). https://doi.org/10.1176/appi.books.9780890425596

American Psychological Association. (2019). *Clinical practice guideline for the treatment of depression across three age cohorts.* American Psychological Association Guideline Development Panel for the Treatment of Depressive Disorders. https://www.apa.org/depression-guideline/

American Psychological Association, Division 12. (2016). *Psychological treatments.* https://www.div12.org/treatments/-

Baltes, P. B., & Baltes, M. M. (1990). Psychological perspectives on successful aging: The model of selective optimization with compensation. In P. B. Baltes, & M. M. Baltes (Eds.), *Successful aging: Perspectives from the behavioral sciences* (pp. 1–34). Cambridge University Press. https://doi.org/10.1017/CBO9780511665684.003

Bayati, A., Parvin, A., & Arash, Z. (2017). Effectiveness of acceptance and commitment therapy on death anxiety and death obsession in the elderly. *Journal of Family Medicine, 15*(10), 122–128. https://doi.org/10.5742/MEWFM.2017.93148

Bolton, P., Bass, J., Neugebauer, R., Verdeli, H., Clougherty, K. F., Wickramaratne, P., Speelman, L., Ndogoni, L., & Weissman, M. (2003). Group interpersonal psychotherapy for depression in rural Uganda: a randomized controlled trial. *JAMA, 289,* 3117–3124. https://doi.org/10.1001/jama.289.23.3117

Butler, J., & Ciarrochi, J. (2007). Psychological acceptance and quality of life in the elderly. *Quality of Life Research, 16*(4), 607–615. https://doi.org/10.1007/s11136-006-9149-1

Cuijpers, P., Geraedts, A. S., van Oppen, P., Andersson, G., Markowitz, J. C., & van Straten, A. (2011). Interpersonal psychotherapy for depression: a meta-analysis. *American Journal of Psychiatry, 168*(6), 581–592. https://doi.org/10.1176/appi.ajp.2010.10101411

Davison, T. E., Eppingstall, B., Runci, S., & O'Connor, D. W. (2017). A pilot trial of acceptance and commitment therapy for symptoms of depression and anxiety in older adults residing in long-term care facilities. *Aging & Mental Health, 21*(7), 766–773. https://doi.org/10.1080/13607863.2016.1156051

Drossel, C., Fisher, J. E., & Mercer, V. (2011). A DBT skills training group for family caregivers of persons with dementia. *Behavior Therapy, 42*(1), 109–119. https://doi.org/10.1016/j.beth.2010.06.001

Frazier, S. N., & Vela, J. (2014). Dialectical behavior therapy for the treatment of anger and aggressive behavior: A review. *Aggression and Violent Behavior, 19*(2), 156–163. https://doi.org/10.1016/j.avb.2014.02.001

Gallego-Alberto, L., Márquez-González, M., Romero-Moreno, R., Cabrera, I., & Losada, A. (2019). Pilot study of a psychotherapeutic intervention for reducing guilt feelings in highly distressed dementia family caregivers (innovative practice). *Dementia.* Advance online publication. https://doi.org/10.1177/1471301219886761

Gilbert, P. (2010). *Compassion focused therapy: Distinctive features.* Routledge. https://doi.org/10.4324/9780203851197

Gonyea, J. G., Paris, R., & de Saxe Zerden, L. (2008). Adult daughters and aging mothers: The role of guilt in the experience of caregiver burden. *Aging & Mental Health, 12*(5), 559–567. https://doi.org/10.1080/13607860802343027

Hayes, S. C. (2004). Acceptance and commitment therapy and the new behavior therapies: Mindfulness, acceptance, and relationship. In S. C. Hayes, V. M. Follette, & M. M. Linehan (Eds.), *Mindfulness and acceptance: Expanding the cognitive-behavioral tradition* (pp. 1–29). Guilford Press.

Hayes, S. C., Luoma, J. B., Bond, F. W., Masuda, A., & Lillis, J. (2006). Acceptance and commitment therapy: Model, processes and outcomes. *Behaviour Research and Therapy, 44*(1), 1–25. https://doi.org/10.1016/j.brat.2005.06.006

Hayes, S. C., Strosahl, K. D., & Wilson, K. G. (1999). *Acceptance and commitment therapy: An experiential approach to behaviour change.* Guilford Press.

Hayes, S. C., Strosahl, K., & Wilson, K. G. (2011). *Acceptance and commitment therapy: The process and practice of mindful change* (2nd ed.). Guilford Press.

Hedegaard, H., Curtin, S. C., & Warner, M. (2018). *Suicide mortality in the United States,* 1999–2017. https://www.cdc.gov/nchs/data/databriefs/db330-h.pdf

Hinrichsen, G. A., & Clougherty, K. F. (2006). *Interpersonal psychotherapy for depressed older adults.* American Psychological Association. https://doi.org/10.1037/11429-000

Hinrichsen, G. A., Emery-Tiburcio, E. E., Gooblar, J., & Molinari, V. A. (2018). Building foundational knowledge competencies in professional geropsychology: Council of Professional Geropsychology Training Programs (CoPGTP) recommendations. *Clinical Psychology: Science and Practice, 25*(2), 1–8. https://doi.org/10.1111/cpsp.12236

Hinrichsen, G. A. (2008). Interpersonal psychotherapy as a treatment for depression in late life. *Professional Psychology: Research and Practice, 39,* 306–312. https://doi.org/10.1037/0735-7028.39.3.306

Jacobs, M. L., Luci, K., & Hagemann, L. (2018). Group-based Acceptance and Commitment Therapy (ACT) for older veterans: Findings from a quality improvement project. *Clinical Gerontologist, 41*(5), 458–467. https://doi.org/10.1080/07317115.2017.1391917

Kakavan, A., Reza, B. M., & Farhad, S. (2015). The effectiveness of Acceptance and Commitment therapy on stress reduction in afflicted elderly men to heart diseases. *Journal of Aging Psychology, 1*(3), 169–178. https://doi.org/10.21859/jgn.3.2.89

Karlin, B. E., Walser, R. D., Yesavage, J., Zhang, A., Trockel, M., & Taylor, C. B. (2013). Effectiveness of acceptance and commitment therapy for depression: Comparison among older and younger veterans. *Aging & Mental Health, 17,* 555–563. https://doi.org/10.1080/13607863.2013.789002

Kishita, N., Laidlaw, K., Wuthrich, V. M., Egan, S. J., & Chellingsworth, M. (2016). Evidence-based developments of CBT for late life anxiety. In R. G. Menzies, M. Kyrios, & N. Kazantzis (Eds.), *Innovations and future directions in the behavioural and cognitive therapies* (pp. 56–60). Australian Academic Press.

Knight, B. G., Karel, M. J., Hinrichsen, G. A., Qualls, S. H., & Duffy, M. (2009). Pikes Peak model for training in professional geropsychology. *American Psychologist, 64*(3), 205–214. https://doi.org/10.1037/a0015059

Laidlaw, K. (2015). *Cognitive behaviour therapy for older people: An introduction.* Sage.

Lawrence, V., Kimona, K., Howard, R., Serfaty, M., Wetherell, J. L., Livingston, G., Wilkinson, P., Walters, K., Jones, R., Wuthrich, V. M., & Gould, R. (2019). Optimising the acceptability and feasibility of acceptance and commitment therapy for treatment-resistant generalised anxiety disorder in older adults. *Age and Aging, 48*(5), 741–750. https://doi.org/10.1093/ageing/afz082

Linehan, M. M. (1993a). *Cognitive behavioral therapy of borderline personality disorder.* Guilford Press.

Linehan, M. M. (1993b). *Skills training manual for treatment borderline personality disorder.* Guilford Press.

Linehan, M. M., & Wilks, C. R. (2015). The course and evolution of dialectical behavior therapy. *American Journal of Psychotherapy, 69*(2), 97–110. https://doi.org/10.1176/appi.psychotherapy.2015.69.2.97

Linehan, M. M., Korslund, K. E., Harned, M. S., Gallop, R. J., Lungu, A., Neacsiu, A. D., McDavid, J., Comtois, K. A., & Murray-Gregory, A. M. (2015). Dialectical behavior therapy for high suicide risk in individuals with borderline personality disorder: A randomized clinical trial and component analysis. *JAMA, 72*(5), 475–482. https://doi.org/10.1001/jamapsychiatry.2014.3039

Losada, A., Márquez, G. M., Vara, G. C., Gallego, A. L., Romero, M. R., & Pillemer, K. (2018). Ambivalence and guilt feelings: Two relevant variables for understanding caregivers' depressive symptomatology. *Clinical Psychology & Psychotherapy, 25*(1), 59–64. https://doi.org/10.1002/cpp.2116

Losada, A., Márquez-González, M., Peñacoba, C., & Romero-Moreno, R. (2010). Development and validation of the Caregiver Guilt Questionnaire. *International Psychogeriatrics, 22*(4), 650–660. https://doi.org/10.1017/S1041610210000074

Losada, A., Márquez-González, M., Romero-Moreno, R., Mausbach, B. T., López, J., Fernández-Fernández, V., & Nogales-González, C. (2015). Cognitive behavioral therapy (CBT) versus acceptance and commitment therapy (ACT) for dementia family caregivers with significant depressive symptoms: Results of a randomized clinical trial. *Journal of Consulting and Clinical Psychology, 83,* 760–772. https://doi.org/10.1016/S1878-7649(14)70088-9

Lynch, T. R., & Cheavens, J. S. (2007). Dialectical behavior therapy for depression with comorbid personality disorder: An extension of standard dialectical behavior therapy with a special emphasis on the treatment of older adults. In L. A. Dimeff & K. Koerner (Eds.), *Dialectical behavior therapy in clinical practice: Applications across disorders and settings.* Guilford Press.

Lynch, T. R., Cheavens, J. S., Cukrowicz, K. C., Thorp, S. R., Bronner, L., & Beyer, J. (2007). Treatment of older adults with co-morbid personality disorder and depression: A dialectical behavior therapy approach. *International Journal of Geriatric Psychiatry, 22*(2), 131–143. https://doi.org/10.1002/gps.1703

Lynch, T. R., Morse, J. Q., Mendelson, T., & Robins, C. J. (2003). Dialectical behavior therapy for depressed older adults. *American Journal of Geriatric Psychiatry, 11*(1), 33–45. https://doi.org/10.1097/00019442-200301000-00006

Márquez-González, M., Romero-Moreno, R., & Losada, A. (2010). Caregiving issues in a therapeutic context: New insights from the acceptance and commitment therapy approach. In N. A. Pachana, K. Laidlaw, & B. Knight (Eds.), *Casebook of clinical geropsychology: International perspectives on practice* (pp. 33–53). Oxford University Press. https://doi.org/10.1093/med/9780199583553.003.0003

Márquez-González, M., Romero-Moreno, R., Cabrera, I., Olmos, R., Pérez-Miguel, A., & Losada, A. (2020). Tailored versus manualized interventions for dementia caregivers: The functional analysis-guided modular intervention. *Psychology and Aging, 35*(1), 41–54. https://doi.org/10.1037/pag0000412

McCracken, L. M., & Jones, R. (2012). Treatment for chronic pain for adults in the seventh and eighth decades of life: A preliminary study of Acceptance and Commitment Therapy (ACT). *Pain Medicine, 13,* 860–867. https://doi.org/10.1111/j.1526-4637.2012.01407.x

McKay, M., Wood, J. C., & Brantley, J. (2007). *The dialectical behavior therapy skills workbook: Practical DBT exercises for learning mindfulness, interpersonal effectiveness, emotion regulation, & distress tolerance.* New Harbinger.

Mossey, J. M., Knott, K. A., Higgins, M., & Talerico, K. (1996). Effectiveness of a psychosocial intervention, interpersonal counseling, for subdysthymic depression in medically ill elderly. *Journals of Gerontology Series A: Biological Sciences and Medical Sciences, 51*(4), 172–178. https://doi.org/10.1093/gerona/51A.4.M172

Panos, P. T., Jackson, J. W., Hasan, O., & Panos, A. (2014). Meta-analysis and systematic review assessing the efficacy of dialectical behavior therapy (DBT). *Research on Social Work Practice, 24*(2), 213–223. https://doi.org/10.1177/1049731513503047

Petkus, A. J., & Wetherell, J. L. (2013). Acceptance and commitment therapy with older adults: Rationale and considerations. *Cognitive and Behavioral Practice, 20,* 47–56. https://doi.org/10.1016/j.cbpra.2011.07.004

Reynolds, C. F., III, Frank, E., Perel, J. M., Imber, S. D., Cornes, C., Miller, M. D., Mazumdar, S., Houck, P. R., Dew, M. A., Stack, J. A., Pollock, B. G., & Kupfer, D. J. (1999). Nortriptyline and interpersonal psychotherapy as maintenance therapies for recurrent major depression: a randomized controlled trial in patients older than 59 years. *JAMA, 281*(1), 39–45. https://doi.org/10.1001/jama.281.1.39

Rizvi, S. L., Steffel, L. M., & Carson-Wong, A. (2013). An overview of dialectical behavior therapy for professional psychologists. *Professional Psychology: Research and Practice, 44*(2), 73–80. https://doi.org/10.1037/a0029808

Robins, C. J., & Chapman, A. L. (2004). Dialectical behavior therapy: Current status, recent developments, and future directions. *Journal of Personality Disorders, 18*(1), 73–89. https://doi.org/10.1521/pedi.18.1.73.32771

Romero-Moreno, R., Gallego-Alberto, L., Márquez-González, M., & Losada, A. (2017). Psychometric properties of the Valued Living Questionnaire Adapted to Dementia Caregiving. *Aging and Mental Health, 21*(9), 983–990. https://doi.org/10.1080/13607863.2016.1191055

Rothblum, E. D., Sholomskas, A. J., Berry, C., & Prusoff, B. A. (1982). Issues in clinical trials with the depressed elderly. *Journal of the American Geriatrics Society, 30,* 694–699. https://doi.org/10.1111/j.1532-5415.1982.tb01982.x

Scott, W., Daly, A., Yu, L., & McCracken, L. M. (2017). Treatment of chronic pain for adults 65 and over: Analyses of outcomes and changes in psychological flexibility following interdisciplinary Acceptance and Commitment Therapy (ACT). *Pain Medicine, 18*(2), 252–264. https://doi.org/10.1093/pm/pnw073

Sloane, R. B., Staples, F. R., & Schneider, L. S. (1985). Interpersonal therapy versus nortriptyline for depression in the elderly. In G. D. Burrows, T. R. Norman, & L. Dennerstein (Eds.), *Clinical and pharmacological studies in psychiatric disorders. Biographical psychiatry: New prospects* (pp. 344–346). John Libbey.

Stewart, M. O., Raffa, S. D., Steele, J. L., Miller, S. A., Clougherty, K. F., Hinrichsen, G. A., & Karlin, B. E., (2014). National dissemination of interpersonal psychotherapy for depression in veterans: Therapist and patient-level outcomes. *Journal of Consulting and Clinical Psychology, 82,* 1201–1206. https://doi.org/10.1037/a0037410

Valentine, S. E., Bankoff, S. M., Poulin, R. M., Reidler, E. B., & Pantalone, D. W. (2014). The use of dialectical behavior therapy skills training as stand-alone treatment: A systematic review of the treatment outcome literature. *Journal of Clinical Psychology, 71*(1), 1–20. https://doi.org/10.1002/jclp.22114

Van Schaik, A., Van Marwijk, H., Adèr, H., Van Dyck, R., De Haan, M., Penninx, B., Van der Kooij, K., Van Hout, H., & Beekman, A. (2006). Interpersonal psychotherapy for elderly patients in primary care. *American Journal of Geriatric Psychiatry, 14*(9), 777–786. https://doi.org/10.1097/01.JGP.0000199341.25431.4b

Weissman, M. M., Markowitz, J. C., & Klerman, G. L. (2018). *The guide to interpersonal psychotherapy: Updated and expanded edition.* Oxford University Press.

Wetherell, J. L., Afari, N., Ayers, C. R., Stoddard, J. A., Ruberg, J., Sorrell, J. T., Liu, L., Petkus, A. J., Thorp, S. R., Kraft, A., & Patterson, T. L. (2011). Acceptance and commitment therapy for generalized anxiety disorder in older adults: A preliminary report. *Behaviour Therapy, 42,* 127–134. https://doi.org/10.1016/j.beth.2010.07.002

Chapter 5
Therapeutic Approaches for Anxiety and PTSD in Late Life

Alisa O'Riley Hannum
Danielle N. Berkel
Rachael Spalding
Nancy A. Pachana

Introduction

This chapter combines discussions of anxiety in later life and posttraumatic stress disorder (PTSD) in later life (in the *Diagnostic and Statistical Manual of Mental Disorders*, 5th edition [DSM-5], PTSD is no longer considered an anxiety disorder but classified under trauma- and stressor-related disorders), in terms of diagnostic criteria, assessment issues, and intervention strategies. Cultural considerations regarding both anxiety and PTSD are discussed where appropriate. These disorders often have presentations which can cause confusion in older patients, given a range of comorbidities, and they are also disorders receiving increasing research attention in terms of diagnoses, assessment, and treatment in later life. Given this, both assessment and interventions for anxiety disorders and PTSD require competencies mentioned among the Pikes Peak geropsychology competencies (see Appendix 1; Knight et al., 2009), particularly with respect having a good knowledge of differential presentations of anxiety, and being sensitive to cohort-related expressions of anxiety and its manifestations in everyday life. Anxiety which causes distress and lowered functioning is not a part of normal aging and often requires appropriate assessment and intervention to restore well-being.

As defined in the DSM-5, anxiety disorders encompass a group of mental disorders characterized by symptoms related to excessive worry, hyperarousal, and fear. Anxiety disorders include generalized anxiety disorder (GAD), panic disorder (PD), social anxiety disorder (SAD), agoraphobia, and specific phobias. Global estimated prevalence rates of anxiety disorders among individuals in later life (over age 60) range from 4.4% to 14.2% (Wolitzky-Taylor et al., 2010). In the US, lifetime prevalence and 1-year prevalence rates for anxiety disorders among older adults have been reported to be as high as 15.1% and 11.6%, respectively (Reynolds et al., 2015; Kessler et al., 2005).

Prevalence estimates among older adults, of anxiety symptoms occurring in the absence of depressive symptoms, are on average around 15% (Mehta et al., 2003)is the most frequently diagnosed anxiety disorder among this age group (lifetime prevalence as high as 11%; Zhang et al., 2015) and is particularly common among individuals suffering from chronic illnesses (19%; Kunik et al., 2005), many of whom tend to be older. GAD is likely underdiagnosed and undertreated among older adults, since anxiety symptoms as reported by older adults often overlap with physiological symptoms associated with the aging process (Calleo et al., 2009; Ramos & Stanley, 2018). Older people with cognitive dysfunction also tend to experience anxiety disorders at a higher rate than cognitively intact older adults (Monastero et al., 2009), with prevalence rates of anxiety among older adults with mild cognitive impairment ranging from 11% to 75% (Monastero et al., 2009; Yates et al., 2013).

Anxiety prevalence rates vary across sociodemographic groups. Globally, women are nearly twice as likely as men to experience an anxiety disorder at some point in their lives (Remes et al., 2016). Moreover, individuals with lower educational backgrounds are at greater risk for developing an anxiety disorder, while being married or cohabitating with a partner is considered a protective factor (Byers et al., 2010). In terms of racial and ethnic differences, non-Hispanic Whites and Latinos exhibit the highest rates of anxiety disorders (Jimenez et al., 2010). Lifetime prevalence of GAD diagnoses were about the same for Hispanics (4.9%, 0.9 standard error [s.e.]) and non-Hispanic Blacks (5.1%, 0.9 s.e.) as opposed to non-Hispanic Whites (8.6%, 0.5 s.e.) in a large study by Breslau et al. (2006). In the same study, the presence of any anxiety disorder, across the same three groups, was (24.9%, 2.2 s.e.) for Hispanics, (23.8%, 1.9 s.e.) for non-Hispanic Blacks, and (29.4%, 1.0 s.e.) for non-Hispanic Whites. Recent work teasing out variations within larger ethnic groups have found that, for example, US-born Caribbean Black men are more likely to meet criteria for lifetime psychiatric disorders, including anxiety disorders, than African-American and non-US-born Caribbean men (Mays et al., 2018). It is worth noting that these cultural and ethnic prevalence data are likely not giving a true picture, due to lack of research, but also because of biases and barriers in this area; see Williams et al. (2013) for a discussion of such issues with respect to anxiety surveys in African-American populations.

Cross-cultural differences in older adults' presentation and experience of anxiety disorders are vital to consider, particularly in the US. According to recent US census data, by 2030, one in five Americans will be 65 or older; by 2045, less than half of all Americans are projected to be non-Hispanic Whites; and by 2060, almost one in five of the total US population will have been born outside the US (Colby & Ortman, 2015). In general, research in the US suggests that ethnic minority immigrants of ethnic minorities are at less risk for developing mental disorders than those born in the US (e.g., Ortega et al., 2000; Vega et al., 1998). However, notions of the protective effects of ethnicity or immigration status must be regarded with caution, particularly when considering older samples and anxiety disorders. For instance, a more recent investigation of prevalence rates for specific disorders among older adults in the US found that older immigrant Asians and Latinos presented higher lifetime prevalence rates for GAD than those born in the US (Jimenez et al., 2010). Mental health treatment disparities are particularly salient among older adults in the US, as minority older adults are significantly more likely than non-Hispanic Whites to drop out of treatment (Vega, 2005).

Assessing Anxiety in Later Life

The clinical interview is one of the most important parts of the assessment of older persons presenting with anxiety in later life (Mohlman et al., 2012). A good interview yields detailed data on the nature and circumstances surrounding the presentation of anxiety symptoms, and puts these in their medical and historical context. It is important, particularly for novice clinicians, not to fall prey to stereotypes regarding aging in older persons that might cloud diagnostic judgments. For example, it is not normal for older adults to be more socially isolated or to visit people less often. Current behavior also must be viewed alongside immediate past behavior, so that acute or more gradual changes may become apparent, along with behavior changes coinciding with health, interpersonal, or medication events and changes.

Older adults are less likely to describe their anxiety symptoms as excessive or uncontrollable, and tend to use words such as "concerns" or "issues" when describing their worries (Mohlman et al., 2012). The older adult's conceptualization of anxiety, in addition to age-specific symptom presentations, can contribute to the presentation of anxiety symptoms that fail to meet diagnostic criteria (i.e., are subthreshold), but still result in significant social and functional impairment (i.e., anxiety disorder, other specified or unspecified). Furthermore, there is mounting evidence that older adults experience anxiety differently from younger adults and may present with a different constellation of symptoms. Lawton and colleagues (1993), in a seminal study, were the first to show that older adults report fewer negative emotions than young and middle-aged adults, and lower levels of depression, hostility, shyness, anxiety, and guilt. More recent work has examined the positivity effect and older adults' tendency to direct less attention to negative stimuli and presentations of negative emotions (Carstensen et al., 2000).

The nature of worries also varies across the lifespan, with older adults worrying more than young adults about health, world issues, and family concerns (Hunt et al., 2003). The nature of fears differs across age groups. Kogan and Edelstein (2004) identified several fears that were frequently endorsed by older adults but not by young adults (e.g., mental decline, poor well-being, inability to care for oneself, being a burden to others). Also, it is easier for older adults to avoid social situations that evoke anxiety compared with young adults (Bryant et al., 2008). Older adults also experience panic attacks less frequently compared with younger adults (Depp et al., 2005). Correlates of panic attack frequency also differ for the two age groups such that cognitive symptoms are associated with greater panic attack frequency for older adults, and somatic symptoms are associated with greater panic attack frequency for young adults (Depp et al., 2005). Clinically, the concerns of older adults about cognitive decline and the possibility of having a diagnosis of dementia is a topic that deserves the attention of all health care professionals, including, of course, psychologists. Concerns in this regard should be taken seriously, and psychoeducation about age-related cognitive changes, and clinical referrals if appropriate, should be carried out.

Use of a structured interview, such as the Semi-Structured Clinical Interview for DSM-IV (SCID), may help enormously with arriving at diagnoses of specific anxiety disorders (Spitzer et al., 1992). Such structured clinical interview instruments may be useful to guide initial clinical hypotheses and prompt the use of additional measures to assess for more specific anxiety disorders. Careful attention to such issues as anxiety symptoms confounded by comorbidities, and issues regarding biases in thinking that such behaviors as social avoidance are more common in later life, often lead to misdiagnosis or lack of a diagnosis of anxiety disorders in later life; excellent reviews of particular usefulness for novice clinicians include those by Bryant et al. (2013) and Mohlman et al. (2012).

Given the relative paucity of research regarding anxiety disorders among older adults in general, little guidance exists regarding best-practice means of assessing anxiety among this population. Systematic reviews of this literature have found that self-report tends to be the dominant means of assessment (Therrien & Hunsley, 2012). To be considered valid, clinical diagnoses formed from self-reported symptoms must also take into account comorbid physical health problems and medication side effects, given the prevalence of chronic illness and polypharmacy among this population. Physiological anxiety symptoms (e.g., muscle rigidity, chest discomfort) reported by older adults may be wrongly attributed to a medical condition, and some anxiety symptoms can appear as side effects of medications or symptoms of physical disorders such as cardiovascular disease or hyperthyroidism (Therrien & Hunsley, 2012). Many self-report measures of anxiety originally designed for use with young adults weigh these somatic symptoms heavily. Thus, ascertaining whether the anxiety symptoms reported by older adults on these measures arise from psychological or medical underpinnings is more difficult.

To date, few self-report measures of anxiety have been developed for use specifically with adults over age 65. Of those that do exist, the Anxiety in Cognitive Impairment and Dementia Scales (ACIDS; Gerolimatos et al., 2015), the Adult Manifest Anxiety Scale–Elderly Version (AMAS-E; Reynolds, 2003), the Geriatric Anxiety Inventory (GAI; Pachana et al., 2007), and the Geriatric Anxiety Scale (GAS; Segal et al., 2010) have demonstrated good psychometric properties among diverse samples of older adults. Among these, the GAI and the GAS have been the subjects of the most empirical research on their psychometric properties (e.g., Gould et al., 2014; Johnco et al., 2015) as well as their use in various clinical populations (e.g., Matheson et al., 2012) and across a variety of cultures (e.g., Karahan et al., 2018). The GAI has a short 5-item form useful for either brief screening or epidemiological work (Byrne & Pachana, 2011); a similar 10-item form of the GAS has also been published (Mueller et al., 2015).

In assessing anxiety in older adults with comorbid cognitive declines, the Rating Scale of Anxiety in Dementia (RAID; Shankar et al., 1999) is a useful instrument. The RAID demonstrates satisfactory psychometric properties (Shankar et al., 1999) and provides a comprehensive evaluation of a patient's anxiety symptoms based on self-reports, caregiver reports, clinical observations, and medical records.

Comorbidities With Anxiety Symptoms and Disorders

Among older adults, anxiety disorders, cognitive decline, and dementia diagnoses are often comorbid (Seignourel et al., 2008). Cognitive deficits and memory impairments may also affect an older adult's ability to self-report their symptoms. Collateral information from close family members, partners, and caregivers can therefore be helpful in developing a full clinical picture.

When working with older patients, clinicians must be sensitive to how anxiety symptoms manifest among this population, with unique features and patterns. Older adults most often report worry content related to issues specific to later life, such as health, retirement planning, financial security, loss of loved ones, and caregiving (Ramos & Stanley, 2018). Several topics that older adults report as being a strong source of anxiety, such as mental and physical decline and being a burden to others, are endorsed very rarely, if at all, by younger adults (Kogan & Edelstein, 2004). With regard to phobias, the most common specific fear reported by older adults, other than agoraphobia, is fear of falling (Ramos & Stanley, 2018). Fear of falling has its own literature and set of assessment and intervention approaches; the interested reader is referred to reviews by Greenberg (2012) and El-Khoury et al. (2013). Prevalence rates of fear of falling range from 12% to 65%, with higher rates reported by individuals with a history of falls (Grenier et al., 2011).

Relative to younger adults, older adults are less likely to report experiencing panic attacks (Depp et al., 2005) and endorse less uncontrollable worry (Gould & Edelstein, 2010) and lower levels of negative emotions, including depressive and anxiety symptoms (Lawton et al., 1993). Related to social anxiety, the types of social situations that are found distressing by socially anxious older adults may differ from those of their younger counterparts. Asking others for help or appearing incompetent or forgetful in public, for example, are concerns more frequently reported by older adults (Ciliberti et al., 2011). Finally, when describing their symptoms, the language used by older adults may also differ from that of younger adults. A common misconception exists that older adults are less likely to report anxiety symptoms or seek mental health treatment; however, research suggests this may be a cohort effect, as the current cohort of older adults appears particularly less comfortable than those of later generations with discussing emotional problems and mental health (Pachana, 2008). Clinicians should be mindful that terms such as "anxiety" may not be familiar to their clients, and should be alert to other descriptions of worry, anxiety, and distress that they may be discounting.

Anxiety and depression are highly comorbid in young adults (e.g., Kessler et al., 2005), and a similar pattern holds among older adults (see Chapter 3 for a discussion of the conceptualization of depression in later life). One study evaluating a large population-based sample of Canadian adults over age 55 found that comorbidity between anxiety and depressive disorders was common, with the most common pattern being a primary diagnosis of depression with one or more concurrent anxiety disorders (Cairney et al., 2008). This is consistent with earlier findings that roughly half of older adults with major depressive disorder also meet criteria for an anxiety disorder (Beekman et al., 1998). Across studies specifically assessing prevalence rates among adults over age 55, the prevalence of anxiety, mood, and comorbid disorders appears to decline with age (Byers et al., 2010). In general, more research is needed regarding anxiety symptomatology among the oldest-old (85+) demographic. According to the United Nations (2015), this is the fastest-growing demographic group globally. Recently, research has begun to more specifically target the relation between anxiety symptoms and cognitive decline among the oldest-old. For example, in one of the first of such studies, Kassem et al. (2018) found among a sample of oldest-old women that mild anxiety symptoms tended to predict future dementia risk.

Treatment of Anxiety in Late Life

In general, psychological interventions that are efficacious with younger adults are often efficacious with older clients. The evidence base for the effectiveness of psychotherapy with anxious older adults is also strong. In a meta-analysis, strong effects of cognitive behavior therapy (CBT) for anxiety with older adults were reported by Cuijpers et al. (2014), with similar effect sizes for the relief of both depressive and anxious symptoms in older adults. Comorbid presentations of anxiety with depression can be particularly challenging, especially when one or more medical illnesses are present (Lecrubier, 2001).

Many concerns in later life involving anxiety (health, caregiving responsibilities, etc.) may have more similarities than differences across cultural groups, thus, while cultural considerations in both assessment and treatment are important, they do not necessarily make treatment more complex (Knight & Pachana, 2015). Degrees of acculturation, language skills shared between therapist and client, and social support structures are all important for the therapist to consider. Issues among migrants, particularly in recent times, have implications for anxiety treatment, whether it is adjustment to a new country (recent immigrant) or adjustments to the acculturation of children (if a less recent immigrant). Underreporting of affective disorders in Asian cultural groups has been noted in the literature (Woodward et al., 2012), and this has implications for diagnosis, assessment, and treatment in this population.

While progressive muscle relaxation and other relaxation methods often work quite well with older adults, problems with arthritis can mean imaginal relaxation techniques are better tolerated. Similarly, deep breathing exercises for relaxation should be tailored around any illnesses that affect breathing, or previous surgeries that may make deep breathing distressing. Finally, while some older adults are lifelong practitioners of yoga, meditation, and deep breathing, others may need more time and guided practice to master the techniques.

A number of types of therapies have been shown to be effective in treating anxiety in later life, most prominently CBT and relaxation training (e.g., Ayers et al., 2007) as well as CBT in combination with pharmacological approaches (Goncalves & Byrne, 2012). CBT has also been proven effective with older persons living with both anxiety and dementia (Spector et al., 2015). Other therapeutic approaches require more substantial empirical study in older populations, despite some promising preliminary data, including Acceptance and Commitment Therapy (ACT; Wetherell et al., 2011; Petkus & Wetherell, 2013) and mindfulness-based stress reduction techniques (Lenze et al., 2014).

Effective treatment of anxiety disorders in later life is important for improved quality of life and well-being, particularly in light of the fact that we have many modes of treatment that might be effective for an individual. Effective treatment is often stymied by the belief on the part of both the health professional and the older adult themselves that anxiety in later life is something that must be tolerated – this is very far from true, and anxiety symptoms are not a part of normal aging. Anxiety is less-often assessed and treated than depression, often for the simple reason of beliefs about the heightened consequences of depression as opposed to anxiety. Again, this myth or stereotype is untrue and also potentially damaging. For example, one often neglected topic in anxiety is its relation to suicide. Suicide has been shown to be related to anxiety in later life (Oude Voshaar et al., 2015), but often anxiety is overlooked in favor of depression being more closely linked with suicide.

Both anxiety and depression are important factors that may influence risk of suicide in later life. With an increased understanding of the importance of anxiety as it relates to suicide in later life, researchers are turning their attention to this area, and developing interventions for those with late-life anxiety at risk for suicide. For example, Van Orden et al. (2012) describe the adaptation of interpersonal psychotherapy (IPT), discussed in Chapter 4 of this book, as informed by the interpersonal theory of suicide, to assist in guiding the IPT process with a suicidal client. For example, this approach helps the therapist in selecting which problem to focus on during treatment. Such research is just beginning, and more focused research on such interventions with older adults is required.

Similarly, anxiety in persons with dementia has a growing empirical database, although the types of interventions that have been examined are more numerous than in the previous example of anxiety and suicide. For example, Spector et al. (2015) report promising effects of a pilot randomized controlled trial (RCT) of a 10-session CBT approach to anxiety in persons living with dementia, although in their trial only depressive, and not anxiety, symptoms were significantly reduced. Stanley and colleagues (2013) reported significant decreases in anxiety symptoms and improvements in quality of life following a 12-week CBT-based intervention called Peaceful Mind, which included self-monitoring for anxiety and deep breathing. Mindfulness-based interventions, which are growing in popularity for use in people living with dementia, were found in a meta-analysis to not significantly reduce anxiety in this group (Wang et al., 2020). The interested reader is referred to an excellent review by Kishita et al. (2020) for an overview of systematic reviews of the treatments for both anxiety and depression in those living with dementia.

PTSD Diagnostic Criteria and Prevalence Rates

PTSD is a mental health condition triggered by exposure to a traumatic event, in which an individual experiences a maladaptive pathological response to stress. To be diagnosed with PTSD, the DSM-5 (American Psychiatric Association, 2013) requires that an individual be exposed to real or threatened serious injury or death through direct exposure to the trauma, witnessing the trauma, learning that a close friend or relative was exposed to trauma, or indirect exposure to aversive details of the trauma (known as a Criterion A event). PTSD is characterized by four thematically organized clusters of symptoms, including intrusion symptoms (e.g., distressing memories or nightmares), avoidance of trauma reminders (e.g., avoiding situations or thoughts), negative alterations in cognitions and mood (e.g., feeling detached from others or negative beliefs), and alterations in arousal and reactivity (e.g., hypervigilance or irritability). Lastly, to achieve a PTSD diagnosis, the patient's symptoms must begin or worsen following the trauma, last longer than 1 month, cause distress or functional impact, and not be due to medication, substance use, or other illness.

The estimated lifetime and current prevalence rates of PTSD among adults in the US are 6.1% and 4.7%, respectively (Goldstein et al., 2016). Women are more than twice as likely to be diagnosed with PTSD during their lifetime compared with men, with lifetime prevalence rates of 9.7% and 3.6%, respectively (National Comorbidity Survey, 2005). Studies of trauma exposure indicate women with PTSD were significantly more likely to report sexual assault in adulthood and before the age of 18, interpersonal violence (IPV) victimization, physical abuse before the age of 18, and being stalked. Meanwhile, men with PTSD were more likely to report trauma exposure such as combat, serious or life-threatening injury, or non-IPV physical assault (Goldstein et al., 2016).

For older adults in the US, lifetime prevalence rates range from 4.5% for PTSD and 5.5% for partial PTSD (Pietrzak et al., 2012). Past-year PTSD prevalence of 2.6% has been reported among older adults (Reynolds et al., 2016). It is estimated that between 50% and 90% of older adults in the US have been exposed to at least one potentially traumatic event in their lifetime (Forman-Hoffman et al., 2012; Monson et al., 2016). Combat experience is a relevant traumatic event endorsed by a large number of older adult men, with a PTSD prevalence rate in older adult veterans of 8.4% (Williamson et al., 2018). In older women, lifetime physical or emotional IPV and sexual assault are commonly reported traumatic events, with reports of current PTSD prevalence as high as 22.5% (Gibson et al., 2019).

PTSD Symptoms Across the Lifespan

Generally, rates of PTSD among older adults tend to be slightly lower compared with their young and middle-age adult counterparts despite high prevalence of trauma exposure (Frans et al., 2005; Kessler et al., 2005; Spitzer et al., 2008). In the face of acute traumatic stressors, older adults display lower rates of PTSD and lower symptom severity when compared with younger individuals (Böttche et al., 2012), potentially suggesting decreased susceptibility to the effects of trauma exposure. Lower rates may also be attributable to reporting biases. Older adults with PTSD tend to endorse symptom severity in the mild or moderate range as opposed to the extreme range (Yehuda et al., 1997). Some researchers have suggested older adults, particularly older men, are hesitant to report psychological symptoms due to traditional gender role expectations and fear of stigma, thus leading to underestimated prevalence of PTSD among older generations (Fontana & Rosenheck, 1994; Lipton & Schaffer, 1988). This is supported by evidence that elderly veterans' PTSD symptoms tend to present more somatically (Petkus et al., 2009). The presence of comorbidities that may complicate assessment (i.e., depression, substance use, cognitive deficits) leading to misdiagnosis, and selective mortality may serve as a barrier to obtaining accurate prevalence rates in older adults (Averill & Beck, 2000; Liptzin, 2004; Owens et al., 2005). Despite potential methodological limitations, the majority of studies indicate PTSD symptom severity declines with age (Norris et al., 2002; Reynolds et al., 2016). Longitudinal research has confirmed similar trends across time (Yehuda et al., 2009).

Fluctuations in PTSD symptoms have been observed throughout the lifespan. Symptoms are often highest in the acute phase, declining or remitting during middle age, and then increasing in late life (Port et al., 2001; den Velde et al., 1993). Over time, PTSD symptom profiles indicate decreased re-experiencing and intrusive symptoms, and increased avoidance symptoms (Böttche et al., 2012; Yehuda & Bierer, 2009). The course of hyperarousal symptoms is less understood, as reports regarding symptom worsening or improvement are inconsistent (Böttche et al., 2012; Yehuda & Bierer, 2009). Despite findings of improvement in PTSD across the lifespan, not all trauma-exposed individuals follow this pattern over time.

Specific subgroups of older adults exposed to severe traumas (e.g., survivors of natural disasters, combat veterans, prisoners of war, or Holocaust survivors) report significantly higher PTSD symptoms compared with the general population (Böttche et al., 2012; Jia et al., 2010; Landau & Litwin, 2000; Solomon et al., 2012).

Additionally, some researchers report groups that show a gradual increase of symptoms over time or a delayed onset of symptoms, despite being asymptomatic for years, with some as late as 50 years after the event (Port et al., 2001; Solomon & Ginzburg, 1998; Spiro et al., 1994). Several explanations have been offered to explain this phenomenon. The first is a failure to repress trauma memories and subsequent symptoms (Horowitz, 1974). Researchers point to the effects of cognitive aging, speculating that age-related decreases in attention increase the likelihood of intrusive trauma-related memories (Floyd et al., 2002), while other decreases across domains impair the ability to adequately employ coping strategies, create disorganized trauma narratives, and generally increase distress (Floyd et al., 2002).

Future vulnerability or *sensitization* from past trauma exposure has been theorized to increase the likelihood of PTSD symptoms reemergence in later life (Resnick et al., 1995; Solomon & Ginzburg, 1998; Dannefer, 2003). This explanation is supported by evidence that individuals with multiple traumas report higher PTSD symptom severity compared with those with single traumas (Schnurr et al., 2002). The reemergence of PTSD symptoms later in life may be triggered by more recent stressors and changes such as loss of social support (Barlow, 1988), retirement (Busuttil, 2004), and institutionalization (i.e., in nursing homes or assisted living facilities; Cook et al., 2005). Health concerns may also trigger reemergence or worsening of PTSD symptoms (Port et al., 2001). Various illnesses have been shown to worsen PTSD symptomology later in life, such as neurological illness (Grossman et al., 2004), cancer (Wachen et al., 2014), terminal illnesses (Feldman, 2017), or more general ill health (Macleod, 1994). Together these findings illustrate the nuances involved in conceptualizing PTSD course across the lifespan and special considerations for managing PTSD in aging populations.

Assessment of PTSD in Late Life

PTSD researchers have provided significant guidance on assessing PTSD in late life (Cook et al., 2014; Thorp et al., 2011). They point out that there may be cohort differences in the expression of PTSD symptoms (especially given that social desirability may be more pronounced in certain cohorts), that it may be helpful to take into account sensory issues that may interfere with assessment (e.g., it may be helpful to print measures in larger font), and that it might be helpful to use multiple assessment methods (especially if the older adult being assessed has some cognitive impairment).

In terms of specific measures, the gold standard diagnostic instrument for PTSD in the US is the Clinician-Administered PTSD Scale for DSM-5 (CAPS-5; Weathers et al., 2018). The CAPS-5 is a structured interview that provides a categorical diagnosis of PTSD and information about PTSD symptom severity based on the DSM-5 (American Psychiatric Association, 2013) PTSD diagnostic criteria. The CAPS-5 requires some training and 30–60 minutes to administer. In psychometric evaluations, the CAPS-5 has demonstrated strong interrater reliability, test-retest reliability, and correspondence to previous versions of the measure (i.e., the CAPS-IV; Weathers et al, 2018); however, it is important to note that very few older adults were included in psychometric evaluations of this measure.

For screening and measurement based care, the Posttraumatic Stress Disorder Checklist for DSM-5 (Blevins et al., 2015) is the most commonly used instrument in the US. In research, this measure has been found to have strong reliability and convergent validity; however, older adults were not included in psychometric evaluations of this measure. The International Trauma Questionnaire (ITQ; Cloitre et al., 2018) is another self-report measure with strong validity and reliability data. The original psychometric studies for this measure included adults up to age 90. As of yet, we are not aware of any studies that have compared younger and older adult responses on the Posttraumatic Stress Disorder Checklist for DSM-5 (PCL-5) or the ITQ.

Treatment of PTSD in Late Life

In 2019, the International Society for Traumatic Stress Studies released their latest PTSD Prevention and Treatment Guidelines (Berliner et al., 2019). In these guidelines, three psychotherapy treatments: cognitive processing therapy (CPT; Resick et al., 2017), eye movement desensitization and reprocessing (EMDR) therapy (Shapiro, 2018), and prolonged exposure (PE) therapy (Foa et al., 2019) were given "strong recommendations" (Berliner et al., 2019). In addition to these psychotherapy treatments, four selective serotonin reuptake inhibitors (SSRIs; i.e., fluoxetine, paroxetine, sertraline, and venlafaxine) were considered treatments with "low effects" (Berliner et al., 2019). We will briefly discuss what is known about the use of these treatments in older adults, below.

Most pharmacotherapy treatment studies for PTSD have not included older adults in their participants (Cook et al., 2014). In addition, other authors (Cook et al., 2014) have noted that many of the pharmaceutical treatments for PTSD are listed on the American Geriatrics Society (AGS) Beers Criteria as medications that might result in problematic side effects in older adults (AGS, 2019). In terms of psychotherapy treatments for PTSD, Dinnen et al. (2014) published a comprehensive review of psychotherapy treatment literature for PTSD in older adults. Overall, they determined that evidence-based PTSD interventions that have been validated in younger and middle aged adults are likely also to be acceptable and efficacious in older adults (Dinnen et al., 2014).

In terms of specific literature for CPT, at this time we are not aware of any studies examining the use of CPT in specifically older adults that have been published; however, in the CPT manual (Resick et al., 2017), the authors note that older adults (primarily older US veterans seeking treatment within the Department of Veterans Affairs) have been participants in many CPT research studies and clinical programs. Conversely, Resick et al. (2002) found that some evidence suggests older adults respond better to exposure-based therapies. Specifically, research on older and younger women who survived sexual assault indicates that older women who received PE had better treatment responses than older women who received CPT (Resick et al., 2002); however, it is worth noting that the sample size of older women in this study was small, and additional research is needed to confirm this finding. In RCTs of CPT, analyses have been done indicating that CPT can be used effectively for individuals with organic brain disorders (e.g., traumatic brain injury or dementia; Resick et al., 2017) and that significant changes to the CPT worksheet format are not necessary in this population.

Several case studies have been published on the use of EMDR with older adults, demonstrating that at least some older adults can tolerate and benefit from EMDR treatment (e.g., Burgmer & Heuft, 2004; Thomas & Gafner, 1993). One case study has also been published describing the successful use of EMDR treatment with an older adult diagnosed with dementia (Hyer, 1995).

Of the three gold standard evidence-based PTSD treatments, PE has been examined the most extensively in terms of use with older adults. Several case studies have been published describing the effective use of PE with older adults with PTSD (see, e.g., Yoder et al., 2010), including one study with an older veteran diagnosed with PTSD and early-stage dementia (Duax et al., 2013). In addition, Yoder and colleagues (2013) published a post hoc effectiveness study examining the effectiveness of PE in 65 older US veterans. This study resulted in large *d*-type effect sizes (1.13–1.90) and high retention rates (85%). Also of note, none of the 65 participants in this study experienced adverse medical or psychiatric events as a result of participating in this exposure-based treatment. Finally, Thorp and colleagues (2012) published a pre-post design comparing PE treatment versus a nonrandomized treatment-as-usual comparison group in older US veterans. This study demonstrated that PE was feasible and efficacious in the treatment of PTSD in older adults.

In addition to research examining the use of CPT, EMDR, and PE in older adults with PTSD, two RCTs have examined alternative treatments for PTSD in older adults. The first study examined the effectiveness of narrative therapy (vs. a psychoeducational treatment) for the treatment of PTSD in older adults ($n = 9$ in each group) who had been political detainees in communist Romania (Bichescu et al., 2007). The results of this study indicated that narrative therapy was more effective for this very small sample than psychoeducation.

A second study examined the effectiveness of a group "spiritually focused" intervention (vs. control group) in 22 older, Christian women who had experienced interpersonal trauma (Bowland et al., 2012). The results of this study showed improvements in depressive symptoms, anxiety, physical symptoms, and PTSD symptoms in the treatment group versus the control group.

Overall, while it is the case that more research examining the treatment of PTSD in older adults is certainly warranted (especially of CPT, EMDR, and PE), taken together, the existing research suggests that there is reason to be optimistic that older adults with PTSD can tolerate and benefit from PTSD treatments validated in younger and middle-aged adults. At the current time, the use of one of the gold standard evidence-based PTSD treatments with older adults can likely be considered a good standard of care.

Case Example of PTSD Treatment in an Older Adult

Within the US Veterans Health Administration (VHA), treatment of PTSD is a prominent priority for all veterans, including for veterans older than 65. In this system, CPT, EMDR, and PE are regularly provided to older adults. This case example illustrates some of the prominent treatment issues related to PTSD in late life discussed above.

Mr. N., a cisgender male, 67-year-old US Army veteran was referred to a PTSD Clinical Team (PCT; a specialized team that focuses solely on PTSD treatment) in an outpatient VHA clinic by his psychiatrist. In the referral, Mr. N.'s psychiatrist noted that Mr. N. was a veteran of the Vietnam War who had first been diagnosed with traumatic stress–related issues shortly after his return from Vietnam in 1972. At that time, he had a psychiatric hospitalization related to severe hypervigilance (bordering on paranoia), nightmares, dissociative flash backs, and comorbid substance abuse. He received significant treatment for several years after his return from Vietnam and eventually experienced a significant reduction in PTSD symptoms and stabilization that allowed Mr. N. to maintain employment and start a family. Mr. N. was able to maintain this stability without mental health treatment for over 30 years. Eighteen months prior to his referral to the PCT, Mr. N. was diagnosed with stage III liver cancer and told that his condition was life threatening. As Mr. N. progressed through cancer treatment, he started to experience a marked exacerbation of PTSD symptoms that eventually led him to be referred for mental health treatment. At the time of his referral to the PCT, Mr. N.'s cancer was considered in remission; however, he was told that he was at risk for having the cancer return again in the future. Despite this relatively positive news about his cancer, Mr. N. found that his PTSD symptoms continued to increase and expressed a desire for more intensive PTSD psychotherapy treatment.

Mr. N. was initially seen in the PCT for a clinical interview, a CAPS-5 interview, and several self-report measures. At his initial visit, Mr. N.'s total severity CAPS-5 score was 33, and his PCL-5 score was 64 (both of which are above recommended cutoff scores). He was diagnosed with PTSD. Mr. N. presented as very motivated for treatment (he stated multiple times that he wished intensive treatment had been available when he had initially sought assistance with trauma-related symptoms after his return from Vietnam) with goals very consistent with PTSD evidence-based treatment. At the end of this visit, the treating psychologist used a shared decision-making model to help Mr. N. choose an appropriate PTSD evidence-based treatment. Together, the decision was made to try PE treatment.

PE treatment is a time-limited exposure-based CBT that focuses on addressing both the internal and external avoidance common in individuals with PTSD (Foa et al., 2019) using both exercises in-session and significant homework. Much of the in-session exposure work focuses on processing a specific index trauma, and the work outside of session focuses on tapes created in-session and engaging in exposure in vivo exercises (Foa et al., 2019).

Overall, Mr. N. was a very active participant in both components of PE treatment and successfully completed treatment in 11 sessions of PE. For his in vivo exposure exercises, Mr. N. focused on engaging in previously avoided activities related to crowds, activities that he found frustrating, and triggers that specifically reminded him of traumatic events. A challenge for some older adults centers on choosing one appropriate index trauma (this is a particularly salient challenge for war veterans who have often experienced multiple events that meet Criterion A for PTSD). In Mr. N.'s case, although he had had several traumatic experiences during his service in Vietnam, he was able to identify a specific index trauma that was more distressing than any of his other traumatic memories, involving watching one of his fellow soldiers step on a mine.

Over the course of treatment, Mr. N. required very little modification of treatment protocol to effectively participate in treatment. Many VHA patients that complete PE use a VA/DOD app to make recordings of sessions; however, Mr. N. did not have a smart phone to download the app, so he made use of a simple digital recorder instead. In addition, Mr. N.'s wife attended some sessions so that she could be oriented to his homework assignments and could remind him to complete homework. Finally, aging-related topics, including Mr. N.'s recent experience with life-threatening cancer, were discussed in debriefings about Mr. N.'s experience in exposure sessions. Other than these small modifications, the treating psychologist adhered strictly to the PE manual.

By the end of PE treatment, Mr. N. had experienced a clinically significant decline in PTSD symptoms as measured by the PCL-5 (his final PCL-5 score was 14). Mr. N. also experienced a significant improvement in depressive symptoms and in social functioning as a result of treatment. Mr. N. was seen for a follow-up session 2 months posttreatment and reported he had maintained treatment gains despite another (milder) health scare.

Conclusions and Implications

Despite anxiety disorders in later life receiving much more recent attention in the empirical literature, anxiety is less likely to be diagnosed or treated in older persons, and treatment options, including long-term treatment outcomes, still require more research, particularly for those over age 75. Both burden of disease and health care service utilization are significant for late-life anxiety (Schuurmans & van Balkom, 2011). Research suggests that, while PTSD symptoms may decline over the course of the lifespan, many individuals experience PTSD symptoms as they age, and these symptoms are associated with a host of emotional and physical problems. Although more research is needed examining treatment of PTSD in late life, there is good reason to be optimistic that treatments validated in younger and middle aged adults can be used effectively with other adults as well.

Suggested Psychotherapy Resources for Anxiety and PTSD in Late Life

Ayers, C. R., Sorrell, J. T., Thorp, S. R., & Wetherell, J. L. (2007). Evidence-based psychological treatments for late-life anxiety. *Psychology and Aging, 22*(1), 8. https://doi.org/10.1037/0882-7974.22.1.8

Böttche, M., Kuwert, P., & Knaevelsrud, C. (2012). Posttraumatic stress disorder in older adults: An overview of characteristics and treatment approaches. *International Journal of Geriatric Psychiatry, 27*(3), 230–239. https://doi.org/10.1002/gps.2725

Byrne, G. J. A., & Pachana, N. A. (Eds.). (in press). *Anxiety in older people: Clinical and research perspectives.* Cambridge University Press.

Dinnen, S., Simiola, V., & Cook, J. M. (2014). Posttraumatic stress disorder in older adults: A systematic review of the psychotherapy treatment literature. *Aging and Mental Health, 19*(2), 144–150. https://doi.org/10.1080/13607863.2014.920299

Pachana, N. A., Laidlaw, K., & Knight, B. G. (Eds.). (2010). *Casebook of clinical geropsychology: International perspectives on practice.* Oxford University Press. https://doi.org/10.1093/med/9780199583553.001.0001

References

American Geriatrics Society. (2019). American Geriatrics Society 2019 updated AGS Beers Criteria for potentially inappropriate medication use in older adults. *Journal of the American Geriatrics Society, 67*(4), 674–694. https://doi.org/10.1111/jgs.15767

American Psychiatric Association. (2013). *Diagnostic and statistical manual of mental disorders* (5th ed.). https://doi.org/10.1176/appi.books.9780890425596

Averill, P. M., & Beck, J. G. (2000). Posttraumatic stress disorder in older adults: A conceptual review. *Journal of Anxiety Disorders, 14*(2), 133–156. https://doi.org/10.1016/S0887-6185(99)00045-6

Ayers, C. R., Sorrell, J. T., Thorp, S. R., & Wetherell, J. L. (2007). Evidence-based psychological treatments for late-life anxiety. *Psychology and Aging, 22*(1), 8. https://doi.org/10.1037/0882-7974.22.1.8

Barlow, D. H. (1988). *Anxiety and its disorders.* Guilford Press.

Beekman, A. T., Bremmer, M. A., Deeg, D. J., van Balkom, A. J., Smit, J. H., DeBeurs, E., van Dyck, R., & van Tilburg, W. (1998). Anxiety disorders in later life: A report from the longitudinal aging study Amsterdam. *International Journal of Geriatric Psychiatry, 13,* 717–726. https://doi.org/10.1002/(SICI)1099-1166(1998100)13:10<717::AID-GPS857>3.0.CO;2-M

Berliner, L., Bisson, J., Cloitre, M., Forbes, D., Goldbeck, L., Jensen, T., Lewis, C., Monson, C., Olff, M., Pilling, S., Riggs, D., Roberts, N., Shapiro, F. (2019). *ISTSS PTSD prevention and treatment guidelines methodology and recommendations.* https://www.istss.org/treating-trauma/new-istss-prevention-and-treatment-guidelines

Bichescu, D., Neuner, F., Schauer, M., & Elbert, T. (2007). Narrative exposure therapy for political imprisonment-related chronic posttraumatic stress disorder and depression. *Behaviour Research and Therapy, 45*(9), 2212–2220. https://doi.org/10.1016/j.brat.2006. 12.006

Blevins, C. A., Weathers, F. W., Davis, M. T., Witte, T. K., & Domino, J. L. (2015). The Posttraumatic Stress Disorder Checklist for DSM-5 (PCL-5): Development and initial psychometric evaluation. *Journal of Traumatic Stress, 28,* 489–498. https://doi.org/10.1002/jts.22059

Böttche, M., Kuwert, P., & Knaevelsrud, C. (2012). Posttraumatic stress disorder in older adults: An overview of characteristics and treatment approaches. *International Journal of Geriatric Psychiatry, 27*(3), 230–239. https://doi.org/10.1002/gps.2725

Bowland, S., Edmond, T., & Fallot, R. D. (2012). Evaluation of a spiritually focused intervention with older trauma survivors. *Social Work, 57,* 73–82. https://doi.org/10.1093/sw/swr001

Breslau, J., Aguilar-Gaxiola, S., Kendler, K. S., Su, M., Williams, D., & Kessler, R. C. (2006). Specifying race-ethnic differences in risk for psychiatric disorder in a USA national sample. *Psychological Medicine, 36*(1), 57–68. https://doi.org/10.1017/S0033291705006161

Bryant, C., Jackson, H., & Ames, D. (2008). The prevalence of anxiety in older adults: methodological issues and a review of the literature. *Journal of affective disorders, 109*(3), 233–250.

Bryant, C., Mohlman, J., Gum, A., Stanley, M., Beekman, A. T., Wetherell, J. L., Thorp, S. R., Flint, A. J., & Lenze, E. J. (2013). Anxiety disorders in older adults: Looking to DSM5 and beyond.... *American Journal of Geriatric Psychiatry, 21*(9), 872–876. https://doi.org/10.1016/j.jagp.2013.01.011

Burgmer, M., & Heuft, G. (2004). Occurrence and treatment of post-traumatic stress disorder in elderly patient after a traffic accident. *International Journal of Geriatric Psychiatry, 19*(2), 185–188. https://doi.org/10.1002/gps.1047

Busuttil, W. (2004). Presentations and management of post traumatic stress disorder and the elderly: A need for investigation. *International Journal of Geriatric Psychiatry, 19*(5), 429–439. https://doi.org/10.1002/gps.1099

Byers, A. L., Yaffe, K., Covinsky, K. E., Friedman, M. B., & Bruce, M. L. (2010). High occurrence of mood and anxiety disorders among older adults: The National Comorbidity Survey Replication. *Archives of General Psychiatry, 67*(5), 489–496. https://doi.org/10.1001/archgenpsychiatry.2010.35

Byrne, G. J. A., & Pachana, N. A. (2011). Development and validation of a short form of the Geriatric Anxiety Inventory – the GAI-SF. *International Psychogeriatrics, 23*(1), 125–131. https://doi.org/10.1017/S1041610210001237

Cairney, J., Corna, L. M., Veldhuizen, S., Herrmann, N., & Streiner, D. L. (2008). Comorbid depression and anxiety in later life: Patterns of association, subjective well-being, and impairment. *American Journal of Geriatric Psychiatry, 16*(3), 201–208. https://doi.org/10.1097/01.JGP.0000300627.93523.c8

Calleo, J., Stanley, M. A., Greisinger, A., Wehmanen, O., Johnson, M., Novy, D., Wilson, N., & Kunik, M. (2009). Generalized anxiety disorder in older medical patients: diagnostic recognition, mental health management and service utilization. *Journal of clinical psychology in medical settings, 16*(2), 178–185.

Carstensen, L. L., Pasupathi, M., Ulrich, M., & Nesselroade, J. R. (2000). Emotional experience in everyday life across the adult life span. *Journal of Personality and Social Psychology, 79,* 644–655. https://doi.org/10.1037/0022-3514.79.4.644

Ciliberti, C., Gould, C., Smith, M., Chorney, D., & Edelstein, B. (2011). A preliminary investigation of developmentally sensitive items for the assessment of social anxiety in late life. *Journal of Anxiety Disorders, 25*(5), 686–689. https://doi.org/10.1016/j.janxdis.2011.03.003

Cloitre, M., Shevlin, M., Brewin, C. R., Bisson, J. I., Roberts, N. P., Maercker, A., Karatzias, T., & Hyland, P. (2018). The International Trauma Questionnaire: Development of a self-report measure of ICD-11 PTSD and complex PTSD. *Acta Psychiatrica Scandinavica, 138*(6), 536–546. https://doi.org/10.1037/t73478-000

Colby, S. L., & Ortman, J. M. (2015). Projections of the size and composition of the U.S. population: 2014 to 2060. *Current Population Reports,* P25-1143, U.S. Census Bureau.

Cook, J. M., Elhai, J. D., Cassidy, E. L., Ruzek, J. I., Ram, G. D., & Sheikh, J. I. (2005). Assessment of trauma exposure and post-traumatic stress in long-term care veterans: Preliminary data on psychometrics and post-traumatic stress disorder prevalence. *Military Medicine, 170*(10), 862–866. https://doi.org/10.7205/MILMED.170.10.862

Cook, J. M., Spiro, A., & Kaloupek, D. G. (2014). Trauma in older adults. In M. J. Friedman, T. M. Keane, & P. A. Resick (Eds.), *Handbook of PTSD: Science and practice* (pp. 351–366). Guilford Press.

Cuijpers, P., Sijbrandij, M., Koole, S., Huibers, M., Berking, M., & Andersson, G. (2014). Psychological treatment of generalized anxiety disorder: a meta-analysis. *Clinical psychology review, 34*(2), 130-140.

Dannefer, D. (2003). Cumulative advantage/disadvantage and the life course: Cross-fertilizing age and social science theory. *Journals of Gerontology Series B: Psychological Sciences and Social Sciences, 58*(6), S327–S337. https://doi.org/10.1093/geronb/58.6.S327

den Velde, W. O., Falger, P. R., Hovens, J. E., de Groen, J. H., Lasschuit, L. J., Van Duijn, H., & Schouten, E. G. (1993). Posttraumatic stress disorder in Dutch resistance veterans from World War II. In J. P. Wilson & B. Raphael (Eds.), *International handbook of traumatic stress syndromes* (pp. 219–230). Springer. https://doi.org/10.1007/978-1-4615-2820-3_18

Depp, C., Woodruff-Borden, J., Meeks, S., Gretarsdottir, E., & DeKryger, N. (2005). The phenomenology of non-clinical panic in older adults in comparison to younger adults. *Journal of Anxiety Disorders, 19*(5), 503–519. https://doi.org/10.1016/j.janxdis.2004.04.007

Dinnen, S., Simiola, V., & Cook, J. M. (2014). Posttraumatic stress disorder in older adults: A systematic review of the psychotherapy treatment literature. *Aging and Mental Health, 19*(2), 144–150. https://doi.org/10.1080/13607863.2014.920299

Duax, J. M., Waldron-Perrine, B., Rauch, S. A., & Adams, K. M. (2013). Prolonged exposure therapy for a Vietnam veteran with PTSD and early-stage dementia. *Cognitive and Behavioral Practice, 20,* 64–73. https://doi.org/10.1016/j.cbpra.2012.02.001

El-Khoury, F., Cassou, B., Charles, M. A., & Dargent-Molina, P. (2013). The effect of fall prevention exercise programmes on fall induced injuries in community dwelling older adults: Systematic review and meta-analysis of randomised controlled trials. *BMJ, 347,* f6234. https://doi.org/10.1136/bmj.f6234

Feldman, D. B. (2017). Stepwise psychosocial palliative care: A new approach to the treatment of posttraumatic stress disorder at the end of life. *Journal of Social Work in End-of-Life & Palliative Care, 13*(2–3), 113–133. https://doi.org/10.1080/15524256.2017.1346543

Floyd, M., Rice, J., & Black, S. R. (2002). Recurrence of posttraumatic stress disorder in late life: A cognitive aging perspective. *Journal of Clinical Geropsychology, 8*(4), 303–311. https://doi.org/10.1023/A:1019679307628

Foa, E. B., Henbree, E. A., Rothbaum, B. O., & Rauch, S. A. M. (2019). *Prolonged exposure therapy for PTSD* (2nd ed.). Oxford University Press.

Fontana, A., & Rosenheck, R. (1994). Traumatic war stressors and psychiatric symptoms among World War II, Korean, and Vietnam War veterans. *Psychology and Aging, 9*(1), 27. https://doi.org/10.1037/0882-7974.9.1.27

Forman-Hoffman, V. L., Mengeling, M., Booth, B. M., Torner, J., & Sadler, A. G. (2012). Eating disorders, post-traumatic stress, and sexual trauma in women veterans. *Military Medicine, 177*(10), 1161–1168. https://doi.org/10.7205/MILMED-D-12-00041

Frans, Ö., Rimmö, P. A., Åberg, L., & Fredrikson, M. (2005). Trauma exposure and post-traumatic stress disorder in the general population. *Acta Psychiatrica Scandinavica, 111*(4), 291–290. https://doi.org/10.1111/j.1600-0447.2004.00463.x

Gerolimatos, L. A., Ciliberti, C. M., Gregg, J. J., Nazem, S., Bamonti, P. M., Cavanagh, C. E., & Edelstein, B. A. (2015). Development and preliminary evaluation of the anxiety in cognitive impairment and dementia (ACID) scales. *International psychogeriatrics, 27*(11), 1825.

Gibson, C. J., Huang, A. J., McCaw, B., Subak, L. L., Thom, D. H., & Van Den Eeden, S. K. (2019). Associations of intimate partner violence, sexual assault, and posttraumatic stress disorder with menopause symptoms among midlife and older women. *JAMA Internal Medicine, 179*(1), 80–87. https://doi.org/10.1001/jamainternmed.2018.5233

Goldstein, R. B., Smith, S. M., Chou, S. P., Saha, T. D., Jung, J., Zhang, H., Pickering, R. P., Ruan, W. J., Huang, B., & Grant, B. F. (2016). The epidemiology of DSM-5 posttraumatic stress disorder in the United States: results from the National Epidemiologic Survey on Alcohol and Related Conditions-III. *Social Psychiatry and Psychiatric Epidemiology, 51*(8), 1137–1148. https://doi.org/10.1007/s00127-016-1208-5

Gould, C. E., & Edelstein, B. A. (2010). Worry, emotion control, and anxiety control in older and young adults. *Journal of anxiety disorders, 24*(7), 759–766.

Goncalves, D. C., & Byrne, G. J. (2012). Interventions for generalized anxiety disorder in older adults: systematic review and meta-analysis. *Journal of Anxiety Disorders, 26*(1), 1–11. https://doi.org/10.1016/j.janxdis.2011.08.010

Gould, C. E., Segal, D. L., Yochim, B. P., Pachana, N. A., Byrne, G. J., & Beaudreau, S. A. (2014). Measuring anxiety in late life: a psychometric examination of the geriatric anxiety inventory and geriatric anxiety scale. *Journal of Anxiety Disorders, 28*(8), 804–811. https://doi.org/10.1016/j.janxdis.2014.08.001

Greenberg, S. A. (2012). Analysis of measurement tools of fear of falling for high-risk, community-dwelling older adults. *Clinical Nursing Research, 21*(1), 113–130. https://doi.org/10.1177/1054773811433824

Grenier, S., Préville, M., Boyer, R., O'Connor, K., Béland, S. G., Potvin, O., Hudon, C., & Brassard, J. (2011). The impact of DSM-IV symptom and clinical significance criteria on the prevalence estimates of subthreshold and threshold anxiety in the older adult population. *The American Journal of Geriatric Psychiatry*, 19(4), 316–326. https://doi.org/10.1097/JGP.0b013e3181ff416c

Grossman, A. B., Levin, B. E., Katzen, H. L., & Lechner, S. (2004). PTSD symptoms and onset of neurologic disease in elderly trauma survivors. *Journal of Clinical and Experimental Neuropsychology, 26*(5), 698–705. https://doi.org/10.1080/13803390409609793

Horowitz, M. (1974). Stress response syndromes: Character style and dynamic psychotherapy. *Archives of General Psychiatry, 31*(6), 768–781. https://doi.org/10.1001/archpsyc.1974.01760180012002

Hunt, S., Wisocki, P., & Yanko, J. (2003). Worry and use of coping strategies among older and younger adults. *Journal of anxiety disorders, 17*(5), 547-560. https://doi.org/10.1016/s0887-6185(02)00229-3

Hyer, L. (1995). Use of EMDR in a "dementing" PTSD survivor. *Clinical Gerontologist, 16*(1), 70–73.

Jia, Z., Tian, W., Liu, W., Cao, Y., Yan, J., & Shun, Z. (2010). Are the elderly more vulnerable to psychological impact of natural disaster? A population-based survey of adult survivors of the 2008 Sichuan earthquake. *BMC Public Health, 10*(1), 172. https://doi.org/10.1186/1471-2458-10-172

Jimenez, D. E., Alegría, M., Chen, C. N., Chan, D., & Laderman, M. (2010). Prevalence of psychiatric illnesses in older ethnic minority adults. *Journal of the American Geriatrics Society, 58*(2), 256–264. https://doi.org/10.1111/j.1532-5415.2009.02685.x

Johnco, C., Knight, A., Tadic, D., & Wuthrich, V. M. (2015). Psychometric properties of the Geriatric Anxiety Inventory (GAI) and its short-form (GAI-SF) in a clinical and non-clinical sample of older adults. *International Psychogeriatrics, 27*(7), 1089–1097. https://doi.org/10.1017/S1041610214001586

Karahan, F. S., Hamarta, E., & Karahan, A. Y. (2018). The Turkish adaptation and psychometric properties of the Geriatric Anxiety Scale. *Mental Illness, 10*(1):7580. https://doi.org/10.4081/mi.2018.7580

Kassem, A. M., Ganguli, M., Yaffe, K., Hanlon, J. T., Lopez, O. L., Wilson, J. W., Ensrud, K., Cauley, J. A., & Study of Osteoporotic Fractures (SOF) Research Group. (2018). Anxiety symptoms and risk of dementia and mild cognitive impairment in the oldest old women. *Aging & Mental Health, 22*(4), 474–482. https://doi.org/10.1080/13607863.2016.1274370

Kessler, R. C., Berglund, P., Demler, O., Jin, R., Merikangas, K. R., & Walters, E. E. (2005). Lifetime prevalence age-of-onset distributions of DSM-IV disorders in the National Comorbidity Survey replication: Erratum. *Archives of General Psychiatry, 62*(6), 768. https://doi.org/10.1001/archpsyc.62.6.593

Kishita, N., Backhouse, T., & Mioshi, E. (2020). Nonpharmacological interventions to improve depression, anxiety, and quality of life (QoL) in people with dementia: An overview of systematic reviews. *Journal of Geriatric Psychiatry and Neurology, 33*(1), 28–41. https://doi.org/10.1177/0891988719856690

Kogan, J. N., & Edelstein, B. A. (2004). Modification and psychometric examination of a self-report measure of fear in older adults. *Journal of Anxiety Disorders, 18*(3), 397–409. https://doi.org/10.1016/S0887-6185(02)00260-8

Knight, B. G., Karel, M. J., Hinrichsen, G. A., Qualls, S. H., & Duffy, M. (2009). Pikes Peak model for training in professional geropsychology. *American Psychologist, 64*(3), 205–214. https://doi.org/10.1037/a0015059

Knight, B. G., & Pachana, N. A. (2015). *Psychological assessment and therapy with older adults.* Oxford University Press, USA.

Kunik, M. E, Roundy, K., Veazey, C., Souchek, J., Peter, R., Wray, N., Stanley, M. A. (2005). Surprisingly high prevalence of anxiety and depression in chronic breathing disorders. *Chest, 127*(4), 1205–1211. https://doi.org/10.1016/S0012-3692(15)34468-8

Landau, R., & Litwin, H. (2000). The effects of extreme early stress in very old age. *Journal of Traumatic Stress, 13*(3), 473–487. https://doi.org/10.1023/A:1007737425260

Lawton, M. P., Kleban, M. H., & Dean, J. (1993). Affect and age: Cross-sectional comparisons of structure and prevalence. *Psychology and aging, 8*(2), 165.

Lecrubier, Y. (2001). The burden of depression and anxiety in general medicine. *Journal of clinical psychiatry, 62*, 4-11.

Lenze, E. J., Hickman, S., Hershey, T., Wendleton, L., Ly, K., Dixon, D., Doré, P., & Wetherell, J. L. (2014). Mindfulness-based stress reduction for older adults with worry symptoms and co-occurring cognitive dysfunction. *International Journal of Geriatric Psychiatry, 29*(10), 991–1000. https://doi.org/10.1002/gps.4086

Lipton, M. I., & Schaffer, W. R. (1988). Physical symptoms related to post-traumatic stress disorder (PTSD) in an aging population. *Military Medicine, 153*(6), 316–318. https://doi.org/10.1093/milmed/153.6.316

Liptzin, B. (2004). Delirium. In J. Sadavoy, L. F. Jarvik, G. T. Grossberg, & B. S. Myers (Eds.), *Comprehensive textbook of geriatric psychiatry* (3rd ed., pp. 525–544). W. W. Norton.

Macleod, A. D. (1994). The reactivation of post-traumatic stress disorder in later life. *Australian and New Zealand Journal of Psychiatry, 28*(4), 625–634. https://doi.org/10.1080/00048679409080786

Matheson, S. F., Byrne, G. J., Dissanayaka, N. N. W., Pachana, N. A., Mellick, G. D., O'Sullivan, J. D., Silburn, P. A., Sellbach, A., & Marsh, R. (2012). Validity and reliability of the Geriatric Anxiety Inventory in Parkinson's disease patients. *Australasian Journal on Ageing, 31*(1), 13–16. https://doi.org/10.1111/j.1741-6612.2010.00487.x

Mays, V. M., Jones, A. L., Cochran, S. D., Taylor, R. J., Rafferty, J., & Jackson, J. S. (2018, June). Chronicity and mental health service utilization for anxiety, mood, and substance use disorders among black men in the United States: Ethnicity and nativity differences. *Healthcare, 6*(2), 53. https://doi.org/10.3390/healthcare6020053

Mehta, K. M., Simonsick, E. M., Penninx, B. W., Schulz, R., Rubin, S. M., Satterfield, S., & Yaffe, K. (2003). Prevalence and correlates of anxiety symptoms in well-functioning older adults: findings from the health aging and body composition study. *Journal of the American Geriatrics Society, 51*(4), 499-504.

Mohlman, J., Bryant, C., Lenze, E. J., Stanley, M. A., Gum, A., Flint, A., Beekman, A. T. F., Wetherell, J. L., Thorp, S. R., & Craske, M. G. (2012). Improving recognition of late life anxiety disorders in Diagnostic and Statistical Manual of Mental Disorders: Observations and recommendations of the Advisory Committee to the Lifespan Disorders Work Group. *International Journal of Geriatric Psychiatry, 27*(6), 549–556. https://doi.org/10.1002/gps.2752

Monastero, R., Mangialasche, F., Camarda, C., Ercolani, S., & Camarda, R. (2009). A systematic review of neuropsychiatric symptoms in mild cognitive impairment. *Journal of Alzheimer's Disease, 18*(1), 11–30. https://doi.org/10.3233/JAD-2009-1120

Monson, E., Lonergan, M., Caron, J., & Brunet, A. (2016). Assessing trauma and posttraumatic stress disorder: Single, open-ended question versus list-based inventory. *Psychological Assessment, 28*(8), 1001. https://doi.org/10.1037/pas0000223

Mueller, A. E., Segal, D. L., Gavett, B., Marty, M. A., Yochim, B., June, A., & Coolidge, F. L. (2015). Geriatric Anxiety Scale: Item response theory analysis, differential item functioning, and creation of a ten-item short form (GAS-10). *International Psychogeriatrics, 27*(7), 1099–1111. https://doi.org/10.1017/S1041610214000210

National Comorbidity Survey. (2005). *NCS-R appendix tables: Table 1. Lifetime prevalence of DSM-IV/WMH-CIDI disorders by sex and cohort. Table 2. Twelve-month prevalence of DSM-IV/WMH-CIDI disorders by sex and cohort.* http://www.hcp.med.harvard.edu/ncs/publications.php

Norris, F. H., Kaniasty, K., Conrad, M. L., Inman, G. L., & Murphy, A. D. (2002). Placing age differences in cultural context: A comparison of the effects of age on PTSD after disasters in the United States, Mexico, and Poland. *Journal of Clinical Geropsychology, 8*(3), 153–173. https://doi.org/10.1023/A:1015940126474

Ortega, A. N., Rosenheck, R., Alegria, M., & Desai, R. A. (2000). Acculturation and the lifetime risk of psychiatric and substance use disorders among Hispanics. *Journal of Nervous and Mental Disease, 188*(11), 728–735. https://doi.org/10.1097/00005053-200011000-00002

Oude Voshaar, R. C., van der Veen, D. C., Kapur, N., Hunt, I., Williams, A. G. J. A., & Pachana, N. A. (2015). Suicide in patients suffering from late-life anxiety disorders; A comparison with younger patients. *International Psychogeriatrics, 27*(7), 1197–1205. https://doi.org/10.1017/S1041610215000125

Owens, G. P., Baker, D. G., Kasckow, J., Ciesla, J. A., & Mohamed, S. (2005). Review of assessment and treatment of PTSD among elderly American armed forces veterans. *International Journal of Geriatric Psychiatry, 20*(12), 1118–1130. https://doi.org/10.1002/gps.1408

Pachana, N. A. (2008). Ageing and psychological disorders. In E. Rieger (Ed.), *Abnormal psychology: Leading researcher perspectives* (pp. 421–457). McGraw-Hill.

Pachana, N. A., Byrne, G. J., Siddle, H., Koloski, N., Harley, E., & Arnold, E. (2007). Development and validation of the Geriatric Anxiety Inventory. *International psychogeriatrics, 19*(1), 103-114.

Petkus, A. J., Gum, A. M., King-Kallimanis, B., & Wetherell, J. L. (2009). Trauma history is associated with psychological distress and somatic symptoms in homebound older adults. *American Journal of Geriatric Psychiatry, 17*(9), 810–818. https://doi.org/10.1097/JGP.0b013e3181b20658

Petkus, A. J., & Wetherell, J. L. (2013). Acceptance and commitment therapy with older adults: Rationale and considerations. *Cognitive and Behavioral Practice, 20*(1), 47–56. https://doi.org/10.1016/j.cbpra.2011.07.004

Pietrzak, R. H., Goldstein, R. B., Southwick, S. M., & Grant, B. F. (2012). Psychiatric comorbidity of full and partial posttraumatic stress disorder among older adults in the US: Results from wave 2 of the National Epidemiologic Survey on Alcohol and Related Conditions. *American Journal of Geriatric Psychiatry, 20*(5), 380–390. https://doi.org/10.1097/JGP.0b013e31820d92e7

Port, C. L., Engdahl, B., & Frazier, P. (2001). A longitudinal and retrospective study of PTSD among older prisoners of war. *American Journal of Psychiatry, 158*(9), 1474–1479. https://doi.org/10.1176/appi.ajp.158.9.1474

Ramos, K., & Stanley, M. A. (2018). Anxiety disorders in late life. *Psychiatric Clinics, 41*(1), 55–64. https://doi.org/10.1016/j.psc.2017.10.005

Remes, O., Brayne, C., Van Der Linde, R., & Lafortune, L. (2016). A systematic review of reviews on the prevalence of anxiety disorders in adult populations. *Brain and behavior, 6*(7), e00497.

Resick, P. A., Monson, C .M., & Chard, K. M. (2017). *Cognitive Processing Therapy for PTSD: A comprehensive manual.* Guilford Press.

Resick, P. A., Nishith, P., Weaver, T. L., Astin, M. C., & Feuer, C. A. (2002). A comparison of cognitive-processing therapy with prolonged exposure and a waiting condition for the treatment of chronic posttraumatic stress disorder in female rape victims. *Journal of Consulting and Clinical Psychology, 70*(4), 867–879. https://doi.org/10.1037/0022-006X.70.4.867

Resnick, H. S., Yehuda, R., Pitman, R. K., & Foy, D. W. (1995). Effect of previous trauma on acute plasma cortisol level following rape. *American Journal of Psychiatry. 152*(11), 1675–1677. https://doi.org/10.1176/ajp.152.11.1675

Reynolds, C. R., Richmond, B. O., & Lowe, P. A. (2003). *The Adult Manifest Anxiety Scale-Elderly Version (AMAS-E).* Western Psychological Services.

Reynolds, K., Pietrzak, R. H., El-Gabalawy, R., Mackenzie, C. S., & Sareen, J. (2015). Prevalence of psychiatric disorders in US older adults: Findings from a nationally representative survey. *World Psychiatry, 14*(1), 74–81. https://doi.org/10.1002/wps.20193

Reynolds, K., Pietrzak, R. H., Mackenzie, C. S., Chou, K. L., & Sareen, J. (2016). Post-traumaticstress disorder across the adult lifespan: Findings from a nationally representative survey. *American Journal of Geriatric Psychiatry, 24*(1), 81–93. https://doi.org/10.1016/j.jagp.2015.11.001

Schnurr, P. P., Spiro, A., Vielhauer, M. J., Findler, M. N., & Hamblen, J. L. (2002). Trauma in the lives of older men: Findings from the Normative Aging Study. *Journal of Clinical Geropsychology, 8*(3), 175–187. https://doi.org/10.1023/A:1015992110544

Schuurmans, J., & van Balkom, A. (2011). Late-life anxiety disorders: A review. *Current Psychiatry Reports, 13*(4), 267–273. https://doi.org/10.1007/s11920-011-0204-4

Seignourel, P. J., Kunik, M. E., Snow, L., Wilson, N., & Stanley, M. (2008). Anxiety in dementia: A critical review. *Clinical Psychology Review, 28*(7), 1071–1082. https://doi.org/10.1016/j.cpr.2008.02.008

Shankar, K. K., Walker, M., Frost, D., & Orrell, M. W. (1999). The development of a valid and reliable scale for rating anxiety in dementia (RAID). *Aging & Mental Health, 3*(1), 39–49. https://doi.org/10.1080/13607869956424

Shapiro, F. (2018). *Eye movement desensitization and reprocessing (EMDR) therapy* (3rd ed.). Guilford Press.

Solomon Z., & Ginzburg K. (1998). War trauma and the aged. In J. Lomranz (Eds.), *Handbook of aging and mental health* (pp. 135–152). Springer. https://doi.org/10.1007/978-1-48 99-0098-2_7

Solomon, Z., Horesh, D., Ein-Dor, T., & Ohry, A. (2012). Predictors of PTSD trajectories following captivity: A 35-year longitudinal study. *Psychiatry Research, 199*(3), 188–194. https://doi.org/10.1016/j.psychres.2012.03.035

Spector, A., Charlesworth, G., King, M., Lattimer, M., Sadek, S., Marston, L., L., Rehill, A., Hoe, J., Qazi, A., Knapp, M., & Orrell, M. (2015). Cognitive-behavioral therapy for anxiety in dementia: Pilot randomised controlled trial. *British Journal of Psychiatry, 206*(6), 509–516. https://doi.org/10.1192/bjp.bp.113.140087

Spiro, A., Schnurr, P. P., & Aldwin, C. M. (1994). Combat-related posttraumatic stress disorder symptoms in older men. *Psychology and Aging, 9*(1), 17. https://doi.org/10.1037/0882-7974.9.1.17

Spitzer, C., Barnow, S., Völzke, H., John, U., Freyberger, H. J., & Grabe, H. J. (2008). Trauma and posttraumatic stress disorder in the elderly: Findings from a German community study. *Journal of Clinical Psychiatry, 69*(5), 693–700. https://doi.org/10.4088/JCP.v69n0501

Spitzer, R. L., Williams, J. B., Gibbon, M., & First, M. B. (1992). The structured clinical interview for DSM-III-R (SCID): Part I: History, rationale, and description. *Archives of General Psychiatry, 49*(8), 624–629. https://doi.org/10.1001/archpsyc.1992.01820080032005

Stanley, M. A., Calleo, J., Bush, A. L., Wilson, N., Snow, A. L., Kraus-Schuman, C., Paukert, A. R., Petersen, N. J., Brenes, G. A., Schulz, P. E., Williams, S. P., & Kunik, M. E. (2013). The Peaceful Mind program: A pilot test of a cognitive-behavioral therapy-based intervention for anxious patients with Dementia. *American Journal of Geriatric Psychiatry, 21*(7), 696–708. https://doi.org/10.1016/j.jagp.2013.01.007

Therrien, Z., & Hunsley, J. (2012). Assessment of anxiety in older adults: a systematic review of commonly used measures. *Aging & mental health, 16*(1), 1–16.

Thomas, R., & Gafner, G. (1993). PTSD in an elderly male: Treatment with eye movement desensitization and reprocessing (EMDR). *Clinical Gerontologist, 14*(2), 57–59.

Thorp, S. R., Sonas, H. M., & Cook, J. M. (2011). Prolonged exposure therapy for older combat veterans in the VA Healthcare System. In K. H. Sorocco & S. Laurderdale (Eds.), *Cognitive behavior therapy with older adults: Innovations across care settings* (pp. 421–442). Springer. https://doi.org/10.1037/e665442011-001

Thorp, S. R., Stein, M. B., Jeste, D. V., Patterson, T. L., & Wetherell, J. L. (2012). Prolonged Exposure Therapy for older Veterans with Posttraumatic Stress Disorder: A pilot study. *American Journal of Geriatric Psychiatry, 20*(3), 276–280. https://doi.org/10.1097/JGP.0b013e3182435ee9

Van Orden, K. A., Talbot, N., & King, D. (2012). Using the interpersonal theory of suicide to inform interpersonal psychotherapy with a suicidal older adult. *Clinical Case Studies, 11*(5), 333–347. https://doi.org/10.1177/1534650112457710

Vega, W. A. (2005). Higher stakes ahead for cultural competence. *General Hospital Psychiatry, 27*(6), 446–450. https://doi.org/10.1016/j.genhosppsych.2005.06.007

Vega, W. A., Kolody, B., Aguilar-Gaxiola, S., Alderete, E., Catalano, R., & Caraveo-Anduaga, J. (1998). Lifetime prevalence of DSM-III-R psychiatric disorders among urban and rural Mexican Americans in California. *Archives of General Psychiatry, 55*(9), 771–778. https://doi.org/10.1001/archpsyc.55.9.771

Wachen, J. S., Patidar, S. M., Mulligan, E. A., Naik, A. D., & Moye, J. (2014). Cancer-related PTSD symptoms in a veteran sample: Association with age, combat PTSD, and quality of life. *Psycho-Oncology, 23*(8), 921–927. https://doi.org/10.1002/pon.3494

Wang, F. L., Tang, Q. Y., Zhang, L. L., Yang, J. J., Li, Y., Peng, H., & Wang, S. H. (2020). Effects of Mindfulness-based Interventions on Dementia Patients: A Meta-analysis. *Western Journal of Nursing Research*, 0193945920916750. https://doi.org/10.1177/0193945920916750

Weathers, F. W., Bovin, M. J., Lee, D. J., Sloan, D. M., Schnurr, P. P., Kaloupek, D. G., Keane, T. M., & Marx, B. P. (2018). The Clinician-Administered PTSD Scale for DSM-5 (CAPS-5): Development and initial psychometric evaluation in military veterans. *Psychological Assessment, 30*(3), 383–395. https://doi.org/10.1037/t71324-000

Wetherell, J. L., Liu, L., Patterson, T. L., Afari, N., Ayers, C. R., Thorp, S. R., Stoddard, J. A., Ruberg, J., Kraft, A., Sorrell, J. T., & Petkus, A. J. (2011). Acceptance and commitment therapy for generalized anxiety disorder in older adults: A preliminary report. *Behavior Therapy, 42*(1), 127–134. https://doi.org/10.1016/j.beth.2010.07.002

Williams, M. T., Beckmann-Mendez, D. A., & Turkheimer, E. (2013). Cultural barriers to African American participation in anxiety disorders research. *Journal of the National Medical Association, 105*(1), 33–41. https://doi.org/10.1016/S0027-9684(15)30083-3

Williamson, V., Stevelink, S. A., Greenberg, K., & Greenberg, N. (2018). Prevalence of mental health disorders in elderly US military veterans: A meta-analysis and systematic review. *American Journal of Geriatric Psychiatry, 26*(5), 534–545. https://doi.org/10.1016/j.jagp.2017.11.001

Wolitzky-Taylor, K., Castriotta, N., Lenze, E., Stanley, M. A., & Craske, M. G. (2010). Anxiety disorders in older adults: A comprehensive review. *Depression and Anxiety, 27*(2), 190–211. https://doi.org/10.1002/da.20653

Woodward, A. T., Taylor, R. J., Bullard, K. M., Aranda, M. P., Lincoln, K. D., & Chatters, L. M. (2012). Prevalence of lifetime DSM-IV affective disorders among older African Americans, Black Caribbeans, Latinos, Asians and Non-Hispanic White people. *International journal of geriatric psychiatry, 27*(8), 816-827.

World Health Organization. (2015). *World report on ageing and health*. World Health Organization.

Yates, J. A., Clare, L., & Woods, R. T. (2013). Mild cognitive impairment and mood: A systematic review. *Reviews in Clinical Gerontology, 23*(4), 317–356. https://doi.org/10.1017/S0959259813000129

Yehuda, R., & Bierer, L. M. (2009). The relevance of epigenetics to PTSD: Implications for the DSM-V. *Journal of Traumatic Stress, 22*(5), 427–434. https://doi.org/10.1002/jts.20448

Yehuda, R., Schmeidler, J., Siever, L. J., Binder-Brynes, K., & Elkin, A. (1997). Individual differences in posttraumatic stress disorder symptom profiles in Holocaust survivors in concentration camps or in hiding. *Journal of Traumatic Stress, 10*(3), 453–463. https://doi.org/10.1002/jts.2490100310

Yoder, M. S., Lozano, B., & Center, K. B. (2013). Effectiveness of prolonged exposure for PTSD in older veterans. *International Journal of Psychiatry in Medicine, 45*(2), 111–124. https://doi.org/10.2190/PM.45.2.b

Yoder, M. S., Tuerk, P. W., & Acierno, R. (2010). Prolonged exposure with a World War II veteran: 60 years of guilt and feelings of inadequacy. *Clinical Case Studies, 9,* 457–467. https://doi.org/10.1177/1534650110386107

Zhang, X., Norton, J., Carrière, I., Ritchie, K., Chaudieu, I., & Ancelin, M. L. (2015). Generalized anxiety in community-dwelling elderly: prevalence and clinical characteristics. *Journal of Affective Disorders, 172,* 24–29. https://doi.org/10.1016/j.jad.2014.09.036

Chapter 6
Working Successfully With Older Persons on the Dementia Continuum, and Their Informal Caregivers

Dolores Gallagher-Thompson
Larry W. Thompson

Introduction

As noted earlier in this book (Chapter 1), now is an exciting time for allied health professionals to provide services to older adults who are living longer as a result of improved health care (overall). Many continue to work and thrive into their 80s and 90s – for example, Pablo Picasso (artist), Ringo Starr (musician), and Nancy Pelosi (politician). However, a potential downside of living that long is the increased likelihood of developing Alzheimer's disease (AD) or a related form of dementia (ADRD). In the total US population, one in 10 people (10%) aged 65 and older has AD. The percentage increases with age: 3% of people aged 65–74, 17% of people aged 75–84, and 32% of people aged 85 and older have AD. People younger than 65 can also develop AD, but it is much less common, and the prevalence rate is uncertain (Alzheimer's Association, 2020). At present, more than 5 million Americans are living with AD, which is now considered the sixth leading cause of death (Alzheimer's Association, 2020). In 2020, it is estimated that ADRD will cost the nation US $305 billion in formal medical care and informal family care. In fact, most care of persons with dementia (PWD) is provided outside established medical and long-term care systems by informal providers (family or friends). About 16 million Americans provide this care, amounting to an estimated 18.6 billion hrs annually. Most informal caregivers (CGs) are not paid for this – although in some states, family members can qualify for a caregiving stipend. These numbers will only increase as baby boomers and subsequent generations reach late adulthood, until a cure and/or preventive interventions are discovered.

AD is a growing global health issue as well, as the World Health Organization (WHO) points out (WHO, 2019). Globally, according to data published in 2015 (Prince et al., 2015), in the most recent systematic review on this topic, regional estimates of dementia prevalence in people aged 60 years and over range from 4.7% in Central Europe to 8.7% in North

Africa and the Middle East, though all other regional estimates lie in a relatively narrow band between 5.6% and 7.6%. This translates into about 47 million persons living with dementia in 2015, with an estimated increase to 75 million in the next decade. Much of this increase will take place in low- and middle-income countries (LMICs): In 2015, 58% of all people with dementia lived in LMICs, which will rise to 63% in 2030 and 68% in 2050. The WHO website contains current information on intervention and prevention, from a global perspective, including details on their global action plan (WHO, 2017; see also https://www.who.int/news-room/fact-sheets/detail/dementia).

Case Example: Treatment for Alzheimer's Disease

> Marie is a 78-year-old widowed African-American woman with hypertension and diabetes and a history of mild stroke 5 years prior, from which she recovered well. She lives with her daughter (Althea, aged 50), two granddaughters (aged 25 and 30), and one great-grandchild (Steph, aged 10) for whom she provides after school care. Marie's complaint to her primary care physician was that of "memory loss" (substantiated by Althea) that was causing problems at home. Marie is not as reliable as she used to be in caring for Steph, forgets things cooking on the stove, and often misidentifies friends who visit. Althea reports this came on gradually over the past year or two but now is concerning since Althea has a new job and needs to be able to count on her mother's help while at work. Both daughters work irregular schedules, and so much of Steph's day-to-day care falls to Marie. Marie's physician refers her to the neurology department where they conclude (based on MRI data) that she "likely" is suffering from Alzheimer's disease with vascular features. Marie is given a prescription for Aricept and told to return in 6 months.

In this chapter four interrelated topics are discussed that will help understand what is happening to Marie in the case example, and what options for care she and Althea have. First, "dementia" and its stages are defined; then selected evidence-based interventions for the PWD are described, followed by a selective review of evidence-based interventions for both the PWD and their primary CGs. Interventions were chosen to be of interest to psychologists and other mental health providers, as well as to those working in interprofessional teams. Finally we will explore cutting edge research on both the promise of technology to mitigate the burden of dementia care and the relevance of lifestyle interventions to either reduce the likelihood of developing dementia in the first place or diminish the severity of its symptoms.

What Do We Mean by the Term "Dementia"?

"Dementia" is an umbrella term that refers not to a specific disease but a group of conditions characterized by impairment of cognitive functions, such as memory, planning, and judgment. Symptoms include forgetfulness, limited social skills, and thinking abilities impaired sufficiently to interfere with the person's daily functioning. The most common form is AD, which accounts for 60–80% of cases. Vascular dementia, which occurs because of microscopic bleeding and blood vessel blockage in the brain, is less common – about 5–10% of cases – though it is more common in those with a history of stroke, diabetes, and poorly controlled hypertension. Lewy body and frontotemporal dementia also account for about 5–10% of cases. Many persons experience brain changes from multiple causes simultaneously and are classified as having mixed dementia (see Alzheimer's Association, 2020, and https://www.alz.org/, for more detailed information on characteristics of dementia subtypes, prevalence rates in various racial and ethnic groups, common risk factors, and current pharmacological and nonpharmacological treatments and interventions).

It is important to note that many medical and psychological conditions can cause dementia-like symptoms, including some that are potentially reversible, such as thyroid problems, medication interactions, vitamin deficiencies, severe depression, and chronic stress (Little, 2018; see also https://GeriatricsCareOnline.org/, sponsored by the American Geriatrics Society). When dementia is suspected, thorough medical and psychological evaluations are necessary first steps to rule out treatable conditions. Referral to a neurology unit often follows for more comprehensive, specialized assessment, and/or to a neuropsychology unit for in-depth assessment of the person's cognitive strengths and weaknesses (Smith & Farias, 2018). Based on both the diagnosis and the symptom profile, various treatments can be initiated to support either or both the PWD and their family (informal) CGs.

AD is characterized on a continuum from preclinical symptoms (referred to as mild cognitive impairment [MCI]) through to clinically significant stages of mild, moderate, and severe, depending on symptom type and severity. Persons with MCI evidence loss of memory for recent events, as well as confusion getting to places, keeping appointments, and/or taking medications on time or as directed. They may also have one or more of the clinical biomarkers used currently (β-amyloid plaques on the outside of cell membranes or protein tau tangles within the cells). But it is very important to note that many older adults report similar issues, and have similar brain changes, so progression from MCI to AD is not automatic but rather depends on a number of factors (Alzheimer's Association, 2020; Kimchi & Lyketsos, 2015).

AD usually starts with learning and memory problems, including reduced executive function: poorer decision making, planning ahead, and organizational skills. These deficits may be noticeable mainly to family and not to outsiders, and they may not yet interfere with carrying out the person's daily activities, but they are concerning or else help seeking would not be occurring. If appropriate psychological and medical evaluations are completed, and the diagnosis of MCI is made, then the older adult has roughly a 38% chance of developing dementia due to AD (Alzheimer's Association, 2020). Others with the same symptoms may revert to near their usual level of functioning or remain stable, depending on what was the cause of the initial changes. For those who do progress to AD, memory loss increases – particularly for recent events such as what the person had for lunch or when their next medical appointment will be. In the mild (or early) stage of AD, confusion also begins to become more evident – the person gets lost on familiar routes and has difficulty sustaining attention (e.g., when reading or watching TV). At this point, many persons function on their own most of the time, still being able to maintain volunteer or paid work, for example, with assistance from supportive social networks. Duration of this phase can vary, but usually within a few years patients move into a moderate (middle) stage of AD, where they will likely experience a variety of behavioral and psychological problems (such as apathy, agitation, wandering, hoarding, depression, sleep problems, disinhibition, and/or delusions and hallucinations). See Aftab and Kim (2020), James (2014), and Kimchi and Lyketsos (2015) for reviews of how to assess and treat these issues. The PWD will definitely need help to carry out more complex activities of daily living, such as decision making, maintaining a regular schedule, and taking care of financial matters. As the inexorable decline of AD progresses, they may also become incontinent at times and have personality changes that affect social relationships, such as being suspicious of others and becoming irritable with family and friends. This phase extends over several years and is generally very stressful for both the PWD and their informal family CGs. In the severe (final) stage of AD, patients lose the ability to recognize family members, need help with nearly all activities of daily living (bathing, dressing, toileting), and may be placed in skilled nursing facilities because family cannot manage them at home any longer. The last consequence varies greatly according to one's cultural values and beliefs about dementia and about caregiving (see Yeo et al., 2019, for information on how dementia is viewed in diverse groups, along with specific recommendations for assessment and intervention strategies).

Recommendations for Working Effectively With the Person with Dementia

At this time, there is no cure for any of the ADRDs, and there are no proven methods to mitigate symptom severity once a diagnosis is made (Alzheimer's Association, 2020). There are medications (e.g., cholinesterase inhibitors such as Aricept) that lessen symptoms in some patients. There are also a number of newer medications in the pipeline being evaluated in clinical trials. For current information on what is being prescribed and for whom, and what the data reveal on effectiveness, see "Medications for Memory" on the Alzheimer's Association website (https://www.alz.org/alzheimers-dementia/treatments/medications-for-memory). Detailed information about National Institute on Aging (NIA)–funded clinical trials on this topic can be found on the NIA website (https://www.nia.nih.gov/research/ongoing-AD-trials/). Mental health professionals need to keep abreast of the latest scientific developments, as it is possible that pharmacological ways to either mitigate symptoms or to cure ADRD will be found in the not-too-distant future.

Meanwhile, most mental health professionals focus on nonpharmacological ways to work with the PWD (and/or their primary CG) to reduce symptoms and improve functioning. Appropriate interventions vary by disease stage, type of problems being experienced, and whether or not the PWD has a primary CG who is willing to participate. For those new to the dementia field, a good introductory text by Mast and Yochim (2017) is recommended for a comprehensive overview and an excellent person-centered practice approach in this area. All of these interventions require a level of professional competence that comes from education, training, and direct experience. Clinicians should familiarize themselves with the Pikes Peak tool (see Appendix 2) to assess their knowledge and skills (as novice, intermediate, advanced, proficient, or expert) regarding dementia itself, and the psychological treatments available for PWD (and/or their CGs), before undertaking this work. For further resources, see GeroCentral website (https://www.gerocentral.org/).

Many studies have been done on a myriad of interventions to improve quality of life of the PWD. They include such nonpsychological interventions such as reminiscence therapy, cognitive stimulation, and music therapy. For reviews, see Gitlin et al. (2012), James (2014), and the main Alzheimer's Association website (https://www.alz.org/). For a carefully done, recent, comprehensive review on this topic, please consult Researchers Against Dementia (2020; https://www.usagainstalzheimers.org/).

Briefly, regarding interventions, in the *early stage* when the PWD is often experiencing depression about the diagnosis and anxiety over the losses ahead, they can usually participate effectively in one or another form of psychotherapy. Successful symptom reduction has been reported for problem-solving therapy (where the patient is taught seven stages of problem solving to use in handling everyday stressful situations; Alexopoulos et al., 2003; Areán et al., 2010); interpersonal psychotherapy (where PWD and CG are often seen together, to promote understanding and improve communication; Miller & Reynolds, 2007; Miller, 2016); and cognitive behavior therapy (CBT), which focuses on questioning unhelpful generalizations about abilities and decline, as well as helping the PWD find satisfying, rewarding activities in their daily lives (Gallagher-Thompson & Thompson, 2010; Teri & Gallagher-Thompson, 1991). Kiosses and Ravdin (2013) briefly review these approaches. Typically modifications are needed in how any of these therapies is implemented so that it is tailored for the cognitive decrements experienced by the patient. These include presenting information multimodally, asking for frequent summaries of what is being discussed, and encouraging the use of memory aids such as recording sessions and writing out home practice assignments.

Some early-stage patients engage in individual therapy; others ask for a family member (often the primary CG) to be included. While this is not typical for most forms of psychotherapy practiced today, the CG's inclusion does seem to improve outcomes since the partner can reinforce what is being discussed and may themselves gain understanding as to what they can do to support the PWD. Being willing to make modifications such as these show respect for the PWD while acknowledging limitations, and exemplifies person-centered care, which has been at the heart of innovative programming in geriatric mental health for some time (Kitwood, 1997; Fazio et al., 2018).

Other modalities of psychotherapy that can be effectively used in the early stages of dementia are family therapy, where the focus is on modifying unhelpful family dynamics (Qualls & Williams, 2013) and couples therapy, when the PWD and the primary CG are spouses (Whitlatch et al., 2006) and the focus is on care planning for the future. See the "Caregiver Briefcase" developed by the American Psychological Association for additional information (https://www.apa.org/pi/about/publications/caregivers/)

For a PWD in the *middle stages*, when insight is reduced, and there are often problems expressing thoughts and feelings accurately, as well as increasing memory and behavior problems to deal with, the focus of treatment may be on the CG–PWD dyad or on the CG alone. Some protocols (but not all) include the PWD; most focus on the CG alone (see the following paragraphs).

There are several successful examples of how training the CG may improve outcomes for the PWD. First, the Seattle protocols or the STAR-C program, based on social learning theory and behavior therapy principles, trains family CGs to reduce sleep disturbances, depression, and anxiety in the PWD by learning a set of appropriate behavior management skills and, in some cases, adding an exercise component to the program (Logsdon et al., 2008; Teri et al., 2003; Teri et al., 1997). For information, or to request manuals, email Dr. Teri (lteri@uw.edu) or see the description on the American Psychological Association's website (https://www.apa.org/).

A second empirically based program that engages both persons in the dyad and is effective in both early and middle stages of dementia is behavioral activation (BA; Bilbrey et al., 2020; Bilbrey et al., 2020). BA methods are first taught to the CG; then once mastered, CGs develop planned everyday positive activities that can be shared together with their care recipient, thus reducing depression in both individuals. This provides welcome relief to most families who are starting to become overwhelmed with tasks to perform for the safety and well-being of the PWD (e.g., restrict them from wandering, hide car keys, and take over financial management). Often precious little of their time together is spent in positive interaction. Since BA is highly individualized, it is designed to be respectful of cultural values and preferences, as well as of the strengths and weaknesses of the PWD. For example, they may no longer retain information about plot and characters from a contemporary movie but may be quite joyful and engaged when watching plots and characters from movies from their past. More information on this approach can be found on the Optimal Aging website (https://www.optimalagingcenter.com/).

A third empirically based program for the dyad facing middle-stage issues is one rooted in both BA and occupational therapy called the tailored activity program (TAP; Gitlin et al., 2009). TAP is an individualized, family-centric program that provides the PWD with activities tailored to their abilities and interests, as determined by an occupational therapist's evaluation, with input from the primary CG. It derives from the theory that engagement is an enduring need throughout the disease process. For detailed information about this and other evidence-based programs' resource materials and training processes, see the website of the Rosalynn Carter Institute for Caregiving (https://www.rosalynncarter.org/resources/).

In the *final stages* of dementia, palliative care protocols are often used to provide comfort (either at home or in inpatient settings), since typically there are multiple other medical problems in addition to the cognitive and behavioral problems related to the dementia itself. If a mental health professional is consulted at this point, it is generally to provide bereavement counseling to family members who may be grappling with unfinished business, experiencing emotional distress, and planning for the final loss of the PWD (Gallagher-Thompson et al., 2020).

Recommendations for Working Effectively With Caregivers of PWD

Caregivers are often referred to as "hidden patients," since their emotional needs are often ignored or relegated to second place, as the medical, psychological, and social needs of the PWD take forefront. This becomes more of an issue as dementia progresses. Schulz and Eden (2016) provide a thorough review of the negative (and positive) impacts of caregiving on CGs' physical and mental health. Although there are positive aspects (such as giving back to one's parent or grandparent, or expressing love to one's spouse "till death do us part"), the negatives far outweigh them in terms of cumulative stress. For most CGs this becomes a new "career" that can last as long as 20+ years, depending on how early in the dementing process their relative (or friend or partner) was diagnosed. With the current press for early diagnosis (so that PWDs can participate in research studies at the point in the process when they are most likely to benefit), this longitudinal commitment is likely to be quite lengthy and draining of psychological, social, and financial resources over time. Providing access to relevant information about dementia and tried-and-true strategies for coping with caregiving stress can be a helpful first step regardless of the specific type of therapy that will be used. For example, CGs can be told how to support memory function in the PWD by creating for them a *recognition* rather than a *recall* world. What this means is that the CG sets up the environment with relevant cues to remind the PWD what they are supposed to be doing – for example, taking out the trash on a certain day. This makes it easier for the PWD to function at a higher level and is empowering for them and the CG who is making this possible. A number of specific recommendations for enhancing *person-centered care* by making environmental modifications can be found in Fazio et al. (2018) and Mast, Shouse, and Camp (2015).

Clinicians wishing to find the latest information about evidence-based programs, therapies, and intervention strategies to use with dementia family CGs are advised to consult a new interactive database called Best Practice Caregiving (https://www.caregiver.org/). It was created by the Benjamin Rose Institute in Cleveland (a long-time leader in the field) and the Family Caregiver Alliance in San Francisco. This is a free online database of effective programs designed for dementia family CGs. It offers a searchable national database of vetted programs that offer much-needed information and support. This is a valuable tool for clinicians to review and, if necessary, from which to seek training or consultation so they can develop the skills required to implement the program(s) of their choice. In the Best Practice Caregiving database, the focus of each program is described (e.g., reducing stress, skill building, health and wellness, etc.), as well as how it is implemented and what any research has found regarding effectiveness. As well, a recently published meta-analysis by Cheng et al. (2020) is worth consulting to decide which intervention(s) might be most effective with each unique CG seeking services.

All of these sources recommend evaluating the CG's depression level (since depression is reported by about 50% of dementia CGs) as well as asking what they do for their PWD and how stressful it is. The Family Caregiver Alliance's website has a downloadable monograph describing a broad range of questionnaires that can be used for a thorough evaluation (https://www.caregiver.org). When time is short, the quick, self-administered Caregiver Self-Assessment Questionnaire can be used. It is downloadable from the Health in Aging website (https://www.healthinaging.org/tools-and-tips/caregiver-self-assessment-questionnaire). It is not dementia-specific but includes questions relevant to making an informed decision as to what treatment to offer the CG. It is available in multiple languages and can be done online or in paper-and-pencil format.

CGs scoring high on stress and depression are likely to benefit from BA (Bilbrey et al., 2020), or a full course of CBT, or a mindfulness-based CBT approach (Whitebird et al., 2013), depending on severity of depression. In contrast, those with relatively poor support networks are likely to benefit from a group experience where they can share feelings and gain support from other CGs. Two examples of the latter (described more on the Best Practice Caregiver website) are the Savvy Caregiver program (Hepburn et al., 2003) and Active Caregiving Empowerment Skills (ACES) program derived from Coping With Caregiving (Cheng et al., 2020). Both focus on skill building (e.g., learning ways to manage stress and question negative thinking patterns), both are delivered in an interactive workshop format to a small group of CGs, and both are effective to reduce depression and improve adaptive coping skills (Cheng et al., 2020).

Finally, if time and resources permit, the Resources for Enhancing Caregivers' Health (REACH II) protocol should be considered. The REACH II program employs home visits to develop individualized action plans to change CGs' behavior. It is considered multicomponent because it addresses negative thinking, stress management, social support, and learning new ways to respond to difficult behaviors of the PWD. A large multisite, multiethnic study found significant results for those in the active versus control conditions (Belle et al., 2006). Further information about the program and its adaptations (e.g., it can be done in office visits, if home visits are prohibitive) can be found on the Best Practice Caregiving website, a partnership between the Benjamin Rose Institute on Aging and the Family Caregiver Alliance (https://bpc.caregiver.org/).

There has been increased interest in the use of online internet facilitated web-based programs and related forms of technology – for example, mobile apps for stress reduction, installation of sensors in the home to decrease wandering, and use of alerts to inform CGs if the PWD took their medications as directed (Astell et al., 2019). Often these are used in combination with psychological treatment in order to enhance effectiveness. Web-based programs, in particular, provide education about dementia, ways to help PWD experience higher life quality, and skills for CGs to deal with the stressful behavioral problems they continually confront. A comprehensive review of web-based programs (Pleasant et al., 2020) highlights positive aspects of research in this relatively new area, along with suggestions to improve the effectiveness of future research. Clearly, the use of online modalities provides opportunities for many CGs to participate in treatment who are not able to attend regular meetings with therapists or instructors, due to scheduling or transportation issues. Another advantage of online programs is that they become a nonconsumable resource, readily available without additional manpower investment, and at no direct cost to CGs.

In sum, based on over 20 years of research, there is now a strong evidence base for the efficacy of a variety of psychological programs and/or psychotherapies to reduce distress, improve self-efficacy, and enhance coping in dementia family CGs. Selection of which approach to use depends on the presenting problems of the CG, available time and resources, and whether the focus of treatment is on the dyad or the CG themselves. Reviewing these programs via the websites and citations provided here should help clinicians make informed decisions about care.

Case Example Revisited and Concluded

It was noted earlier that Marie (the index patient) and her middle-aged daughter Althea (the likely person in the family to become Marie's CG if her condition worsens) were told Marie "likely" had AD following an MRI and neurology consultation – without (apparently) a full medical work-up being conducted to evaluate if depression (or another treatable condition) was responsible for her presenting problems. Lack of comprehensive evaluation and treatment planning are unfortunately common for patients and families of diverse backgrounds – especially African Americans and those of Hispanic and/or Latinx origin (Hargrave, 2019; Chavez-Duenas et al., 2020; see also https://www.ncbi.nlm.nih.gov/books/NBK425844/e).

Although both were very distressed by this news and by the fact that virtually no effort was made to provide or recommend services to assist them (beyond a prescription for Aricept), this worst-case scenario is, unfortunately, not that uncommon (Mast & Yochim, 2017). It is just more likely to occur with families from diverse backgrounds who are often undertreated in the US health care system as it is today (Baciu et al., 2017). If Marie had been a person with insurance beyond basic Medicare (which was all she had), and lived near a major medical center, she likely would have been referred to a specialized geriatrics clinic or memory care program and would been seen by an interprofessional team. That team would have included a psychologist who would have assessed her for depression (which is common at this point in the process) and asked about other issues she was confronting such as difficulty with meal preparation and caring for Steph. The psychologist likely would have also referred Marie for neuropsychological testing, to learn more about her problem-solving skills and executive functioning, since no definitive diagnosis of dementia had been made. It is quite possible that Marie has MCI which may (or may not) advance to full-blown dementia. Marie could also be referred for genetic testing to shed light on this factor, as it is well-known that the APOE-e4 genotype is associated with higher likelihood of AD (Safieh et al., 2019).

In addition, in top-of-the-line practices, Althea would be asked to complete questionnaires about CG stress, burden, and depression – even though this is most likely MCI, Althea is already dealing with some of the effects of her mother's reduced brain function and needs to plan accordingly. At the very least, Marie and Althea should become educated about dementia (by referring them to websites set up for consumers, such as https://www.alz.org/ or https://www.alzheimersla.org/ that have information directed to families and PWD). As well, they should be encouraged to talk with a nurse, social worker, or psychologist about their current situation and figure out what Marie can and cannot be expected to do on an ongoing basis with regard to caring for Steph. They would also benefit from some of the early-stage interventions described above – either as a dyad (e.g., doing BA together to improve mood) or individually, using CBT, interpersonal psychotherapy, or problem-solving therapy to deal with Marie's (likely) feelings of depression, grief, and loss, and/or Althea's feelings of burden, frustration, and depression. Family therapy might be indicated if problems with communication and hurtful family dynamics are present and likely to interfere with effective problem solving. While the clinician is sorting out what to do, when, and with whom, they need to maintain a positive attitude: as Kitwood (1997) says so eloquently – there's still a person in there, no matter how advanced dementia may become in the future.

Of course, if Marie's situation progresses to full-blown dementia, the clinician is advised to review the therapeutic programs described herein and to keep abreast of changing practices in the field by consulting national and international websites and other information sources on a regular basis. This is a rapidly changing field, and clinicians and researchers need to do their best to keep up with new information.

In addition, clinicians would do well to establish a collegial relationship with the primary care physician, since many current and future care decisions will be made by that individual. For example, how long to continue on Aricept, whether to do repeat neurological evaluations, and whether to prescribe additional medications should there be a significant increase in behavior problems over time. Of course, Marie's consent is needed for this, and as long as she is in the MCI (or perhaps early dementia) phase, she would be considered competent to provide written informed consent. In addition, at this stage, future care planning is encouraged, as well as taking the opportunity to put legal and financial affairs in order – before cognitive decline becomes so pervasive that competence is called into question. Clinicians may find that guiding families through this kind of decision making is a valuable component of any therapeutic intervention.

In Marie's case, unfortunately, MCI did progress to full-blown dementia. Althea participated in several programs to empower her and enhance her self-efficacy, as described above, and at the website of the National Brain Health Center for African Americans (http://brainhealthcenterforafricanamericans.org/caregiving/). Various treatment decisions for both Marie and Althea were made at different points along the trajectory of caregiving (Gallagher-Thompson et al., 2020) and in the end, after about 5 years of follow up and intermittent treatment by one of the authors (D.G.-T.), Marie succumbed to vascular complications and passed away. Althea returned for short-term grief counseling related to her mother's death, which was completed in six follow-up sessions. Althea expressed gratitude to the therapist for "sticking with her" over the years and for providing help at critical times.

In our opinion this case illustrates the long-term commitment generally required when working with persons with any form of dementia and their family CGs. It is possible, of course, for clinicians to go in and out of the trajectory – only being called upon to assist at certain pivotal points in the process. Or it is possible for clinicians to be there throughout the process, providing interventions as appropriate at different points along the way. At this time, there is no road map for what to do, when, and with whom, to maximize quality of life for the PWD and/or their family CGs. Hopefully, future research will provide guidance for these treatment decisions.

Lifestyle Interventions to Reduce the Likelihood of Dementia

Lifestyle interventions to reduce the likelihood of dementia are a fast-moving area of active research at present, since robust data were published in 2015 reporting on the Finnish Geriatric Intervention Study to Prevent Cognitive Impairment and Disability (FINGER) study (Ngandu et al., 2015). This multidomain 2-year randomized clinical trial with over 1,200 participants was the first to study whether a lifestyle modification program reduced the risk of cognitive decline in elderly persons at risk for dementia. They found that a combination of exercise, brain games, diet, and social activity synergistically prevented decline in cognitive function for those in the active versus the control arm of the study. Attempts to replicate these promising results are now ongoing in 25 countries around the world, including the US. In the US, there is the US Study to Protect Brain Health Through Lifestyle Intervention to Reduce Risk (POINTER) study, which was launched in January 2019 and aims to enroll 2,000 participants using similar lifestyle modifications but tailored to the more heterogeneous American public. Older adults interested to see if they qualify for POINTER should consult the website (https://www.alz.org/us-pointer/).

Further support for the validity of this approach comes from two independent sources: First, the National Academies of Sciences, Engineering, and Medicine in 2017 published an entire volume on preventing cognitive decline and dementia that addressed the importance of knowing and reducing potential risk factors, and second, there is work done by the Lancet Commission in the UK, which was first published by Livingston et al. (2017). That group identified nine potentially modifiable risk factors for development of dementia: less education, hypertension, hearing impairment, smoking, obesity, depression, physical inactivity, diabetes, and low social contact. They concluded that modification of these risk factors during one's lifespan would reduce incident cases by about 35%!

Of these, four domains had been included in the FINGER study: exercise, brain games, diet, and physical activity, with very good results. There is every reason to think that the replication studies now underway (which vary to some extent in which domains they are modifying) will further support the immense value of making specific lifestyle changes throughout the lifespan, but particularly in later life.

Recently, the Lancet Commission updated these risk recommendations to include three new factors: alcohol consumption, traumatic brain injury (at any age), and air pollution. (Livingston et al., 2020). Taken together, these 12 modifiable risk factors account for around 40% of worldwide dementias which could theoretically be prevented or delayed. This report also contains specific recommendations for protecting people with dementia, such as providing holistic postdiagnostic care that encourages lifestyle modification, if applicable, to potentially reduce symptom severity as dementia progresses.

One might now ask, How is this information relevant to mental health providers – specifically psychologists? The answer lies in the fact that many older adults who are not experiencing dementia but who are worried that they "might" develop AD as they age will seek psychological assistance for these concerns. It would be a disservice for practitioners to say there is nothing that can be done to prevent the onset of dementia, given the data just reviewed and the new data that will likely emerge in the next few years. Being well-informed as to what lifestyle changes would be appropriate for a given client (which can be determined through careful assessment of the domains noted, done in collaboration with the older adults primary care physician) will enable you to work with them on a brain health program – possibly in the role of coach rather than therapist, depending on the extent of their overall psychological distress. Psychological coaching is reviewed in depth by Lowman (2016), which contains a variety of resources for further professional development along these lines. In addition, a novel program that purports to reverse AD is described by Bredesen and colleagues (2016). Although a randomized controlled trial has not yet been completed to test the efficacy of Bredesen's approach, case reports are exciting and encouraging.

Taken together these findings as to potential value of targeted lifestyle changes in the domains specified provide rays of hope to older adults fearful about getting AD, as well as those now struggling with dementia, and their family caregivers. Think of the suffering that could be reduced or prevented entirely if this type of program proves viable in multiple countries and with heterogeneous populations! In the opinion of the chapter authors, it would be an honor and a privilege to be part of that solution.

Recommendations and Future Directions

In this chapter we describe common signs and symptoms of dementia, how these change over time, and what kinds of psychological interventions can be used successfully with persons with dementia– either by themselves, with their primary family caregiver, or with the caregiver alone. Knowledge of the range of effective interventions is particularly important since, at present, there is no cure for any of the dementias, and their relentless downhill course is very debilitating for both the patient and the family caregiver. Thus, psychologists have a key role to play, given their breadth of training and expertise with a variety of forms of psychological interventions.

Throughout the progression of dementia a "person-centered approach" is strongly recommended in which effort is made to customize whatever form of treatment is selected, so that there is a good "fit" between the person and the intervention. Many studies have pointed out that there is no "one size fits all" when it comes to working with patients and family members (Gallagher-Thompson et al., 2020). Their needs vary according to a number of factors such as: current cognitive and psychological status; extent of concurrent medical problems and functional disabilities; availability and access to health care systems and supportive community resources; and strength of their informal support system (other relatives, friends, neighbors). Detailed assessment of the cognitive status and psychological and social strengths and weaknesses of both the person with dementia and their family caregiver is strongly recommended, as described in Afab and Kim (2020). Details for what to include in caregiver assessments can be found in the American Psychological Association's comprehensive "caregiver briefcase for psychologists" which is available by searching this website: www.apa.org.

A related construct relevant to this discussion is the notion of "stages" of dementia. These are well-described for AD though not as clear for other forms of dementia. For persons with AD in the early stages, treatments such as family or couples therapy, interpersonal therapy, and CBT can be very helpful to reduce distressing emotions and aid in problem-solving and planning for the future. In the middle stage, when behavioral problems begin to surface and cognitive function decreases, most clinicians opt to work directly with the caregiver, even though there are some forms of treatment that can still be effectively done with the dyad (such as behavioral activation). Programs that engage the caregiver are many and include individual therapies of various kinds as well as psychoeducational programs such as Savvy Caregiving and Coping with Caregiving that use small groups and a workshop format to educate the caregiver and teach relevant coping skills. As noted above, selection of which form of treatment to employ should be made after a thorough assessment is completed, whenever possible.

In the final stages, palliative care is often used with the person with dementia and at that time, caregivers are coping with significant grief and loss and can benefit from psychotherapeutic approaches that focus on those dimensions.

To understand and appreciate the breadth and depth of extant evidence-based programs for caregivers, the reader is referred to the website of the Benjamin Rose Institute on Aging Best Practice Caregiving (https://bpc.caregiver.org/). This curated resource is updated as new studies become available and is an excellent starting point for those desiring to learn more about this topic. In addition, in this chapter we provide a detailed case example of an African-American patient and her daughter/caregiver that highlights some of the barriers to access and care experienced by racial and ethnic minorities at this time in this country. It is hoped that raising awareness of these issues will sensitize clinicians to their possible presence and will encourage all of us to examine our own beliefs and practices, and make modifications as needed, so that all patients and caregivers receive the best possible care we can provide.

Finally, the chapter concludes with a brief section on what is known about the importance of lifestyle interventions to reduce the likelihood of becoming cognitively impaired. This is valuable information to incorporate into work with caregivers so that they themselves can maintain their cognitive acuity. Clinicians need to keep abreast of this fast-emerging literature so that as knowledge increases, they will be more confident about the value of incorporating elements of lifestyle modifications into treatment programs. There is also promising early research on the impact of these lifestyle changes on persons with dementia themselves – in some cases, disease progression was slowed, which correlates with improved well-being for both the index patient and their family.

Conclusions and Implications

In sum, the field has made tremendous progress in the past 20 years, but there is still much to learn. For example, there is a small but growing body of research on the use of dyadic and family therapies with these populations. As well, many families share caregiving responsibilities yet most intervention research focuses on the primary caregiver alone. Finally, there is much that we do not know about effective interventions for caregivers from diverse socio-cultural backgrounds. Most treatment efficacy research has been conducted with Caucasian/white/middle class participants so generalization to groups with other salient characteristics is difficult to do. Treatments that are developed by and for these marginalized groups are sorely needed, as is community-based participatory research so that key stakeholders can participate, from the ground up, in program design and implementation. It is hoped that future research will broaden its scope and begin to address some of the issues noted here.

Suggested Resources for Working With Older Persons on the Dementia Continuum and Their Informal Caregivers

Alzheimer's Disease International. (2020). *World Alzheimer Report 2020: Design, Dignity, and Dementia.* Alzheimer's Disease International.

Bilbrey, A., Laidlaw, K., Cassidy-Eagle, E., Thompson, L. W., & Gallagher-Thompson, D. (2020). Cognitive-behavioral therapy for late-life depression: Evidence, issues and recommendations. *Cognitive and Behavioral Practice.* https://doi.org/10.1016/j.cbpra.2020.03.003

Cheng, S-T., Li, K-K., Losada, A., Zhang, F., Au, A., Thompson, L. W., & Gallagher-Thompson, D. (2020). The effectiveness of nonpharmacological interventions for informal dementia caregivers: An updated systematic review and meta-analysis. *Psychology and Aging, 35*(1), 55–77. https://doi.org/10.1037/pag0000401

Mast, B. T., Shouse, J. N., & Camp, C. (2015). Person-centered assessment and intervention for people with dementia. In P. A. Lichtenberg & B. T. Mast (Eds.), *Handbook of clinical geropsychology.* American Psychological Association. https://doi.org/10.1037/14459-012

Mast, B. T., & Yochim, B. P. (2017). *Alzheimer's disease and dementia.* Hogrefe.

Yeo, G., Gerdner, L. A., & Gallagher-Thompson, D. (Eds.). (2019). *Ethnicity and the Dementias* (3rd ed.). Routledge.

References

Aftab, A., & Kim, D., (2020). Behavioral and psychological symptoms of dementia. In L. B. Dunn & E. L. Cassidy-Eagle (Eds.), *Practical strategies in geriatric mental health: Cases and approaches* (pp. 265–285). American Psychiatric Publishing.

Alexopoulos, G. S., Raue, P., & Arean, P., (2003). Problem-solving therapy in geriatric major depression with executive dysfunction. *American Journal of Geriatric Psychiatry, 11,* 46–52. https://doi.org/10.1097/00019442-200301000-00007

Alzheimer's Association. (2020). *Alzheimer's disease: Facts and figures.* https://doi.org/org/10.1002/alz.12068

Areán, P. A., Raue, P., Mackin, R. S., Kanellopoulos, D., McCulloch, C., & Alexopoulos, G. S. (2010). Problem-solving therapy and supportive therapy in older adults with major depression and executive dysfunction. *American Journal of Psychiatry, 167*(11), 1391–1398. https://doi.org/10.1176/appi.ajp.2010.09091327

Astell, A. J., Bouranis, N., Hoey, J., Lindauer, A., Mihailidis, A., Nugent, C., & Robillard, J. M., (2019). Technology and dementia: The future is now. *Dementia and Geriatric Cognitive Disorders, 47,* 131–139. https://doi.org/10.1159/000497800

Baciu A, Negussie Y, Geller A, & Weinstein, J. (Eds.). (2017). *Communities in action: Pathways to health equity.* National Academies Press.

Belle, S. H., Burgio, L., Burns, R., Coon, D., Czaja, S., Gallagher-Thompson, D., Gitlin, L., Klinger, J., Koepke, K. M., Lee, C. C., Martindale-Adams, J., Nichols, L., Schulz, R., Stahl, S., Stevens, A., Winter, L., & Zhang, S. (REACH investigators presented in alphabetical order). (2006). Enhancing the quality of life of dementia caregivers from different ethnic or racial groups: A randomized, controlled trial. *Annals of Internal Medicine, 145,* 727–738.

Bilbrey, A. C., Cassidy-Eagle, E. L., & Gallagher-Thompson, D. (2020). In L. B. Dunn & E. L. Cassidy-Eagle (Eds.), *Practical strategies in geriatric mental health: Cases and approaches* (pp. 31–41). American Psychiatric Publishing.

Bilbrey, A., Laidlaw, K., Cassidy-Eagle, E., Thompson, L. W., & Gallagher-Thompson, D. (2020). Cognitive-behavioral therapy for late-life depression: Evidence, issues and recommendations. *Cognitive and Behavioral Practice.* https://doi.org/10.1016/j.cbpra.2020.03.003

Bredesen, D., Amos, E. C., Canick, J., Ackerley, M., Raji, C., Fiala, M., & Ahdidan, J. (2016). Reversal of cognitive decline in Alzheimer's disease. *Aging, 8,* 1250–1258. https://doi.org/10.18632/aging.100981

Chavez-Duenas, N., Adames, H. Y.., Perez-Chavez, J., & Smith, S. N. (2020). Contextual, cultural and sociopolitical issues in caring for Latinxs with dementia: When the mind forgets and the heart remembers. In H. Y. Adames & Y. N. Tazeau (Eds.), *Caring for Latinxs with dementia in a globalized world* (pp. 17–35). Springer. https://doi.org/10.1007/978-1-0716-0132-7_2

Cheng, S-T., Li, K.-K., Losada, A., Zhang, F., Au, A., Thompson, L. W., & Gallagher-Thompson, D. (2020). The effectiveness of nonpharmacological interventions for informal dementia caregivers: An updated systematic review and meta-analysis. *Psychology and Aging, 35*(1), 55–77. https://doi.org/10.1037/pag0000401

Fazio, S., Pace, D., Flinner, J., & Kallmyer, B. (2018). The fundamentals of person-centered care for individuals with dementia. *Gerontologist, 58*(S1), S10–S19. https://doi.org/10.1093/geront/gnx122

Gallagher-Thompson, D., Bilbrey, A. C., Apesoa-Varano, E. S., Ghatak, R., Kim, K. K., & Cothran, F. A. (2020). Conceptual framework to guide intervention research across the trajectory of dementia caregiving. *Gerontologist, 60*(1), S29–S40. https://doi.org/10.1093/geront/gnz157

Gallagher-Thompson, D., & Thompson, L. W. (2010). Effectively using cognitive/behavioral therapy with the oldest old: Case examples and issues for consideration. In N. A. Pachana, K. Laidlaw, & B. Knight (Eds.), *Casebook of clinical geropsychology: International perspectives on practice* (pp. 227–241). Oxford University Press. https://doi.org/10.1093/med/9780199583553.003.0014

Gitlin, L. N., Kales, H. C., & Lyketsos, C. G. (2012). Managing behavioral symptoms in dementia using nonpharmacologic approaches: An overview. *JAMA, 308*(19), 2020–2029. https://doi.org/10.1001/jama.2012.36918

Gitlin, L. N., Vinter, L., Earland, T. V., Herge, E. A., Chernett, N. L., Piersol, C. V., & Burke, J. P. (2009). *The tailored activity program to reduce behavioral symptoms in individuals with dementia: Feasibility, acceptability, and replication potential, Gerontologist, 49*(3), 428–439. https://doi.org/10.1093/geront/gnp087

Hargrave, R. (2019). Dementia assessment in African Americans. In G. Yeo, L. Gerdner, & D. Gallagher-Thompson (Eds.), *Ethnicity and the dementias* (3rd ed., pp. 91–107). Routledge. https://doi.org/10.4324/9781315161358-4

Hepburn, K. W., Lewis, M., Sherman, C. W., & Tornatore, J. (2003). The savvy caregiver program: Developing and testing a transportable dementia family caregiver training program. *Gerontologist, 43*(6), 908–915. https://doi.org/10.1093/geront/43.6.908

James, I. A. (2014). The use of CBT for behaviors that challenge in dementia. In N. A. Pachana & K. Laidlaw (Eds.), *Oxford handbook of clinical geropsychology* (pp. 753–775). Oxford University Press.

Kimchi, D., & Lyketsos, C. (2015). Dementia and mild neurocognitive disorders. In D. C. Steffens, D. G. Blazer, & M. E. Thakur (Eds.), *Textbook of geriatric psychiatry* (5th ed., pp. 177–242). American Psychiatric Press. https://doi.org/10.1176/appi.books.9781615370054.ds08

Kiosses, D. N., & Ravdin, L. D. (2013). Psychosocial interventions for depressed older adults with cognitive impairment and disability: strategies to improve everyday functioning and quality of life. *Psychiatric Times, 30*(5), 34–34.

Kitwood, T. (1997). *Dementia reconsidered: The person comes first.* Open University Press.

Little, M. O. (2018). Reversible dementias. *Clinics in Geriatric Medicine, 34,* 537–562. https://doi.org/10.1016/j.cger.2018.07.001

Livingston, G., Huntley, J., Sommerlad, A., Ames, D., Ballard, C., Banerjee, S., Brayne, C., Burns, A., Cohen-Mansfield, J., Cooper, C., Costafreda, S. G., Dias, A., Fox, N., Gitlin, L. N., Howard, R., Kales, H. C., Kivimäki, M., Larson, E. B., Ogunniyi, A., Sampson, E. L., Samus, Q., Schneider, L. S., Selbæk, G., Teri, L., & Mukadam, N. (2020). Dementia prevention, intervention, and care: 2020 Report of the Lancet Commission. *The Lancet Commissions, 396*(10248), P413–446. https://doi.org/10.1016/S0140-6736(20)30367-6

Livingston, G., Sommerlad, A., Ortega, V., Costafreda, S. G., Huntley, J., Ames, D., Ballard, C., Banerjee, S., Burns, A., Cohen-Mansfield, J., Cooper, C., Fox, N., Gitlin, L. N., Howard, R., Kales, H. C., Larson, E. B., Ritchie, K., Rockwood, K.L., Samus, Q., Schneider, L. S., Selbæk, G., Teri, L., & Mukadam, N. (2017). Dementia prevention, intervention, and care. *Lancet, 390,* 2673–2734. https://doi.org/10.1016/S0140-6736(17)31363-6

Logsdon, R. G., McCurry, S. M., & Teri, L. (2008). Assessment and treatment of dementia-related affective disturbances. In K. Laidlaw & B. Knight (Eds.), *Handbook of emotional disorders in later life: Assessment and treatment* (pp. 345–362). Oxford University Press. https://doi.org/10.1093/med:psych/9780198569459.003.0014

Lowman, R. L. (2016). *The psychologist as managerial coach.* Oxford Handbooks on line: https://www.oxfordhandbooks.com. https://doi.org/10.1093/oxfordhb/9780199935291.013.27

Mast, B. T., Shouse, J. N., & Camp, C. (2015). Person-centered assessment and intervention for people with dementia. In P. A. Lichtenberg & B. T. Mast (Eds.), *Handbook of clinical geropsychology.* American Psychological Association. https://doi.org/10.1037/14459-012

Mast, B. T., & Yochim, B. P. (2017). *Alzheimer's disease and dementia.* Hogrefe. https://doi.org/10.1027/00503-000

Miller, M. D. (2016). Using interpersonal therapy (IPT) with older adults today and tomorrow: A review of the literature and new developments. *Current Psychiatry Report, 10,* 16–22. https://doi.org/10.1007/s11920-008-0005-6

Miller, M. D., & Reynolds, C. F., 3rd. (2007). Expanding the usefulness of interpersonal therapy (IPT) for depressed elders with co-morbid cognitive impairment. *International Journal of Geriatric Psychiatry, 22,* 101–105. https://doi.org/10.1002/gps.1699

National Academies of Sciences, Engineering, and Medicine. (2017). *Preventing cognitive decline and dementia: A way forward.* National Academies Press. https://doi.org/10.17226/24782

Ngandu, T., Lehtisalo, J., Solomon, A., Levälahti, E., Ahtiluoto, S., Antikainen, R., & Lindström, J. (2015). A 2 year multidomain intervention of diet, exercise, cognitive training, and vascular risk monitoring versus control to prevent cognitive decline in at risk elderly people (FINGER): A randomized controlled trial. *Lancet, 385*(9984), 2255–2263. https://www.sciencedirect.com/science/article/pii/S0140673615604615 https://doi.org/10.1016/S0140-6736(15)60461-5

Pleasant, M., Molinari, V., Dobbs, D., Meng, H., & Hyer, K. (2020). Effectiveness of online dementia caregivers training programs: A systematic review. *Geriatric Nursing, 41*(6), 921–935. https://doi.org/10.1016/j.gerinurse.2020.07.004

Prince, M. J., Wu, F., Guo, Y., Robledo, L. M. G., O'Donnell, M., Sullivan, R., & Yusuf, S. (2015). The burden of disease in older people and implications for health policy and practice. *The Lancet, 385*(9967), 549–562. https://doi.org/10.1016/S0140-6736(14)61347-7

Qualls, S. H., & Williams, A. A. (2013). *Caregiver family therapy: Empowering families to meet the challenges of aging.* American Psychological Association. https://doi.org/10.1037/13943-000

Researchers Against Alzheimer's. (2020). *Non-pharmacological therapies in Alzheimer's disease: A systematic review.* https://UsAgainstAlzheimers.org

Safieh, M., Korczyn, A. D., & Michaelson, D. M. (2019). ApoE4: An emerging therapeutic target for Alzheimer's disease. *BMC Medicine, 17,* 64. https://doi.org/10.1186/s12916-019-1299-4

Schulz, R., & Eden, J. (2016). *Families caring for an aging America: A report of The National Academies of Sciences, Engineering & Medicine.* National Academies Press.

Smith, G. E., & Farias, S. T. (Eds.). (2018). *APA handbook of dementia: Part of the APA Handbooks in Psychology Series and APA Reference Books Collection.* American Psychological Association.

Teri, L., & Gallagher-Thompson, D. (1991). Cognitive-Behavioral interventions for treatment of depression in Alzheimer's patients. *Gerontologist, 31,* 413–416. https://doi.org/10.1093/geront/31.3.413

Teri, L., Gibbons, L., McCurry, S. M., Logsdon, R. G., Buchner, D. M., Barlow, W. E., Kukull, W. A., LaCroix, A. Z., McCormick, W., & Larson, E. B. (2003). Exercise plus behavioral management in patients with Alzheimer Disease: A randomized controlled trial. *JAMA, 290*(15), 2015–2022. https://doi.org/10.1001/jama.290.15.2015

Teri, L., Logsdon, R. G., Uomoto, J., & McCurry, S. M. (1997). Behavioral treatment of depression in dementia patients: A controlled clinical trial. *Journal of Gerontology, B, Psychological and Social Science, 52,* 159–166. https://doi.org/10.1093/geronb/52B.4.P159

Whitebird, R. R., Kreitzer, M., Crain, A. L., Lewis, B. A., Hanson, L. R., & Enstad, C. J. (2013). Mindfulness-based stress reduction for family caregivers: a randomized controlled trial. *The Gerontologist, 53*(4), 676–686. https://doi.org/10.1093/geront/gns126

Whitlatch, C.J., Judge, K., Zarit, S. H., & Femia, E. (2006). Dyadic intervention for family caregivers and care receivers in early-stage dementia. *Gerontologist. 46*(5), 688–694.

World Health Organization. (2017). *Global action plan on the public health response to dementia 2017–2025.* https://www.who.int/health-topics/dementia

World Health Organization. (2019). *The epidemiology and impact of dementia: Current state and future trends.* https://www.who.int/mental_health/neurology/dementia/en/

Yeo, G., Gerdner, L. A., & Gallagher-Thompson, D. (Eds.). (2019). *Ethnicity and the dementias* (3rd ed.). Routledge.

Chapter 7
Working With Older Adults in Long-Term Care Settings

Hillary J. Rouse
Victor Molinari

Introduction

By 2050, 85.7 million people in the US (22% of the population) will be 65 or older (Vespa et al., 2018). Recent estimates suggest that of these older adults, 19 million will require long-term care (LTC) due to cognitive and functional limitations (Spetz et al., 2015). An increasing concern about this demographic shift is the mounting unmet mental health needs of this older population who require LTC services. On average, between 60% and 90% of older adults in institutional LTC (e.g., nursing homes, assisted living facilities) meet diagnostic criteria for a mental health disorder (Li, 2010); however only 28% of these settings provide regular mental health services (Carney & Norris, 2017). The demand for high-quality mental health services in LTC will continue to grow alongside this population, thereby highlighting the necessity of understanding how to work with older adults across a range of LTC settings. Indeed, LTC is described as a "specific environmental context where psychologists increasingly provide services" (Knight et al., 2009, p. 207), and the delivery of services in LTC settings is recognized as a competency in the Pikes Peak model for training in professional geropsychology (Competency III.E.5; see Appendix 1).

The term "long-term care" refers to comprehensive services and support for persons who require assistance with activities of daily living or instrumental activities of daily living, due to chronic physical or mental disorders, or frailty. The services offered may include housing, medical care, or social services, and be provided within either the community or an institution (Harris-Kojetin et al., 2016). Not surprisingly 75% of LTC users receive these services in their home, due to a desire to "age in place" within their own community (Nguyen, 2017; Spetz et al., 2015), but when the needs of these individuals can no longer be met, a move to an institutional setting is necessary. Demographic risk factors that increase the likelihood of needing institutional LTC services include older age, female sex, and White race. Additional risk factors include poor diet, sedentary lifestyle, family history, living alone, disability, and chronic conditions such as diabetes, incontinence, stroke, and dementia (Andel et al., 2007; Department of Health & Human Services, 2017).

The dynamic of LTC settings has continuously evolved, and there is a persistent blurring of lines between assisted living facilities and nursing homes. This has altered the demographics of LTC residents. Currently nursing homes are incorporating more acute care for rehabilitation, and assisted living facilities are offering more memory care services. This translates into an extensive heterogenic LTC population, challenging the abilities of the staff within these facilities to care for residents who are in need of an array of services. Central to these challenges are the turnover rates of nurses within LTC, as well as the limited training for professionals in geriatric mental health care. Turnover rates are currently estimated at 74.5% for certified nursing assistants, 51.0% for licensed practical nurses, and 56.1% for registered nurses. The dearth of mental health professionals specializing in geriatrics has resulted in a "geriatric workforce crisis" (Jeste et al., 1999), with scarce opportunities to receive even minimal training. Recent research suggests that this crisis is growing, as only 1.2% of psychologists indicate that their primary specialty is geropsychology, although just over a third of psychologists report that they frequently or very frequently work with older adults (Moye et al., 2019). The staff turnover rates, coupled with limited graduate training of geriatric mental health professionals, and the inability to even fill all geriatric medicine slots, bode poorly for the mental health needs of the frail oldest-old being met (Donoghue, 2010). Further it should be noted that as detailed below, to be optimally effective, mental health services need to be delivered in a planned person-centered organizational environment that attends to the unique needs of each older adult.

Similarities and Differences in Mental Health Across LTC Settings

The growing concern for older adults' mental health as society continues to age is heightened by the high rates of suicide among older adults both within the community (Conwell et al., 2011) and within institutional LTC settings (Mezuk et al., 2015). Older adults living in the community are also found to have high rates of substance abuse, while those in institutional LTC have disproportionately higher levels of serious mental illness and adjustment disorders (Muralidharan et al., 2019). Regardless of one's living situation, psychotherapy can be largely beneficial for older adults in LTC settings. While the basic principles of psychotherapeutic assessment and intervention for these mental health disorders can be applied to a wide range of mental health concerns across LTC settings (Molinari & Ellis, 2016), there are unique features of how one delivers care in these settings. When conducting evaluations and implementing interventions for older adults, it is essential that one take into consideration any comorbid illnesses and medications prescribed. Those in LTC institutions typically have more comorbid physical and psychological illnesses compared with those living in the community, and not surprisingly, more complex medication regimens (Koeller et al., 2014). The comorbidities and medication regimens of those in LTC institutions are found to increase the likelihood of one having symptoms of mental illness (Litchenberg & Duffy, 2000), which is most likely also a contributing factor as to why the person had to be institutionalized (Molinari & Ellis, 2016).

The most significant difference between working with frail older adults in the community and in institutionalized settings is the move into a new residential location (Brownie et al., 2014). The process of transitioning into LTC can be quite challenging, as new residents have to reconceptualize what "home" means to them. During the transition process, a primary challenge is the loss of control experienced, and the fear of losing autonomy and independence. Most of the time, relocation to LTC institutional settings occurs during a crisis period when the person involuntarily locates because there are no other community options available to manage essential medical care. New residents may be acutely ill and confused in their new surroundings, and family members often feel guilt-ridden because they believe that they have failed their loved one (Brownie et al., 2014; Wiles et al., 2012).

Along with the reinterpretation of what home means, older adults transitioning into institutionalized LTC have to reconceptualize their community. Typically, older adults have strong social ties and connections to their communities, and these can change once a move is required (Wiles et al., 2012). With this comes the obvious concern of social isolation, particularly when the reason for placement is the death of a family member or an already strained social support system. For this reason, it is critical that the older adult is helped to understand that home is not so much the actual physical dwelling, but rather can be defined through relationships, personal hobbies, and continued ability to access familiar things (Brownie et al., 2014; Wiles et al., 2012). The staff of LTC facilities play an important role during the transitioning process, and will help to determine how much individuals will thrive during their time spent living there. Staff should be encouraged to cultivate relationships with the new resident, and to facilitate the development of new friendships between residents. Research has established that these meaningful relationships, regardless of their being with staff or other residents, are strong predictors of how well older residents will adjust to their new environment. These relationships lower the stress of the transition and increase the older adult's sense of security (Brownie et al., 2014). While LTC personnel can influence the transitioning process, their ability to do so is often limited due to a lack of resources and staffing (Donoghue, 2010). These issues will consistently arise when it comes to incorporating staff into the treatment plan of both short- and long-stay residents.

A major difference between life in community versus institutional settings are the rules and restrictions imposed in facilities. Facilities typically have regulations that do not allow residents the same freedom they had when they lived at home, which can limit their ability to participate in preferred activities. Further, conflicts among family members, formal caregivers, and the older adult may arise if there is concern for the older adult's ability to consent and make decisions on their own in LTC settings (American Psychological Association, 2014). Psychologists should adhere to their ethical principles by ensuring the safety and well-being (beneficence) of residents, and by recognizing their right to make their own decisions (autonomy). Regardless of whether a family member or formal caregiver requests treatment for the older adult, psychologists should always try to get informed consent from the person with whom they are working. This includes respecting the desires of an individual who is cognitively impaired as much as possible – that is, garner geriatric assent. Additionally, confidentiality issues can arise due to pressure from the family or formal caregivers to share information. Before any treatment begins, one should inform all active parties about the levels of confidentiality that must be maintained in an attempt to mitigate future inappropriate requests for information.

It should be noted that there are obligatory times when psychologists have to break confidentiality for safety issues. Examples of this most relevant to LTC include if the person, with or without cognitive impairment, is a threat to themselves or others; or if the person is a victim of abuse or neglect (American Psychological Association, 2014). Further, when working with older adults living in institutional LTC settings, there are unique challenges in complying with the privacy regulations required by HIPPA (Health Insurance Portability and Accountability Act). A lack of privacy is a concern in LTC facilities because two beds to a room is commonly found to be the rule rather than the exception. Privacy considerations must be managed, especially in situations when one is trying to provide psychological services at bedside where the threat of interruption by a bedridden roommate or ministering health professional is very real.

Theoretical Models of Long-Term Care

There are fundamental conceptual models that guide psychologists who work with older adults across the gamut of LTC settings where compromised older adults are displaying symptoms of mental illness or challenging behaviors. These models are complementary to one another because each was designed with the understanding that one should always attend to the context of the situation at hand, as well as the person's background. Such considerations direct clinicians regarding how to assess if, or when, an older adult should be placed in an institutionalized setting, and also how the desires of each person can be met within LTC in a variety of situations. A subset of these models focuses solely on attempting to understand any inappropriate behavior that occurs due to physical or psychological distress, or through circumstances surrounding their occurrence (Lawton, 2001). While some of these models emphasize the overall environment and how it can foster mental health and quality of life, others are specifically designed to aid staff and psychologists in understanding undesirable behavioral and psychological symptoms.

Person–Environment Model

The first person–environment model, formulated by Lawton & Nahemow (1973), proposes that the environment should match the needs of individuals in order for them to function at their highest level. One's environment, encompassing the physical, social, small group, and personal domains, has consistently been found to influence thoughts and feelings (Lawton, 1983). This person–environment model stresses the importance of having a *home-like* environment that will minimize undesirable behavioral and psychological symptoms, and encourage desirable behaviors that will foster quality of life (Lawton, 2001). To achieve a high-quality psychological milieu across each environmental domain, it is important to understand how each individual resident subjectively defines and evaluates well-being and quality of life (Lawton, 1983). Understanding the unique aspects of what one deems desirable will allow staff to match four overarching needs within the person–environment model to the unique aspects of the resident (Lawton, 2001). The four needs according to Lawton

(2001) are increasing activity levels, increasing social behaviors, increasing the ratio of positive to negative feelings, and decreasing behaviors that are not desired. In addition to meeting these needs, helping one maintain dignity, privacy, autonomy, individuality, relationships, comfort, spiritual well-being, safety, and functional abilities can increase quality of life and influence one's perception of the environment. Evaluating all of these needs and factors helps a mental health professional to identify what environmental features will maximize a resident's quality of life and lessen distressing symptoms that are present.

In summary, properly modifying the environment toward individual preferences and greater familiarity can drastically improve mental health symptoms and yield better outcomes. This can result in a reinterpretation of the LTC setting for the new resident, with it no longer being seen as *institutional*, but instead being viewed as home.

Antecedent-Behavior-Consequence Model

There are a variety of models that specifically attempt to understand challenging behaviors that present in older adults, especially those with dementia (Bird & Moniz-Cook, 2008; Volicer & Hurley, 2003). (See Chapter 6 for a comprehensive discussion of dementia.) When applying these models, it is essential that geriatric mental health professionals take into consideration the diverse nature of presenting signs and symptoms, along with their multifaceted causes (Bird & Moniz-Cook, 2008). The first model, the antecedent-behavior-consequence (ABC) model, uses a learning-based framework that attempts to understand behavior (Volicer & Hurley, 2003). This framework provides guidance on how to describe the behavior, identify antecedents triggering behavior, while simultaneously determining the consequences that may maintain the behavior. When applied to a particular behavior, the *antecedent* part of the framework emphasizes the need to assess how frequent and severe the behavior is, as well as how long it has occurred. The *consequences* part of the framework stresses the importance of documenting how the person is affected by the behavior. This model has clear benefits in allowing a mental health professional to identify a strategy that may help to prevent the behavior. An added benefit is that rather than directly modifying the person's behavior if the behavior is not found to be particularly distressing, an intervention to modify the environment (e.g., building a walking path to redirect rather than stop wandering) might be all that is necessary, reflecting the interconnectedness between this framework and the person–environment model (Volicer & Hurley, 2003). A limitation of the ABC model is its oversimplistic nature, as one is not always able to identify the trigger for the behavior, or manipulate its consequences (Bird & Moniz-Cook, 2008).

Behavioral Models Specific to Older Adults With Dementia

Additional behavioral models focus on what is going on within the person with dementia. Two of these models include the need-driven dementia-compromised behavior (NDB) model, and the progressively lowered stress threshold (PLST) model. The NDB model is grounded on the idea that challenging behaviors are the consequence of unmet needs (Cohen-Mansfield & Werner, 1995). These unmet needs are the result of a variety of background factors, some of which may be stable, such as neurological, cognitive, health, and psychosocial ones. In conjunction with these more enduring influences, this model postulates that the immediate causes of these behaviors also may be related to a mix of fluctuating variables. These variables are the personal environment (e.g., emotional and physiological needs), the physical environment, (e.g., light and noise), and the social environment (e.g., atmosphere and staff behavior). This model, also closely intertwined with the person-environment framework, implies that one has little control over stable factors, and therefore interventions should work at targeting the fluctuating factors. Specifically, when applied to an older adult with dementia, this model hypothesizes that as one sees greater cognitive decline, modifying the environment to provide more supports (e.g., monitoring nutritional intake, toileting, sleep needs) will be the optimal way to promote the highest level of function, while also preventing behavioral symptoms (Volicer & Hurley, 2003).

The PLST model is based on the appreciation that older adults with dementia typically have lower thresholds for stress, and the presentation of challenging behavioral or psychological symptoms are the result of excess environmental stress (Bird & Moniz-Cook, 2008; Volicer & Hurley, 2003). This model has identified five common stressors: fatigue; misleading or inappropriate stimuli; demands that exceed ability; change in environment, routine, or caregiver; and physical stressors like pain, discomfort, and depression. These can lead to behaviors such as agitation, wandering, confusion, repetitive behaviors, and nighttime awakenings. The PLST model, also strongly aligned with the person-environment model, assumes that if environmental stress is reduced, and routines are followed, challenging behavioral and psychological symptoms can be prevented (Volicer & Hurley, 2003). A major limitation of the NDB and PLST models are that they tend to focus on external stimuli such as the environment when deciding on the best intervention approaches (Bird & Moniz-Cook, 2008).

One final *hybrid model* was formulated by Volicer and Hurley (2003), which indicates that agitated behaviors result from lack of stimulation, while aggressive behavior is provoked by poor caregiving technique. Perhaps the best way to proceed as a LTC mental health professional is to be guided by Kunik and colleagues' (2003) broad integrative conceptualization of mutable versus immutable determinants of challenging behaviors. The psychologist needs to recognize that certain causative factors associated with challenging behaviors such as male sex, higher degree of dementia, and high staff–resident ratio would be difficult to change, but that other more mutable factors such as delirium, pain, anxiety, and psychosis are amenable to interventions. Increasingly innovative strategies by professionals with expertise in LTC, which are grounded in theoretical frameworks, will continue to contribute to the evidence base of high-quality interventions as discussed below to address challenging behaviors and mental illness within this population.

Treatment Within Long-Term Care

With the number of people relying on LTC growing, effective interventions to target challenging behaviors and mental illness are of obvious necessity. Although the above theoretical models can assist with understanding and interpreting behaviors and symptoms, it is essential that implementation of all interventions be consistent with best practices and training in LTC (Molinari, 2018) guided by the individual person's values and preferences. This is the core of person-centered care, which focuses on promoting choice, purpose, and meaning in one's life and health care (The American Geriatrics Society Expert Panel on Person-Centered Care, 2015). Person-centered care is especially important when developing treatment plans because it encourages residents to express their goals and desires, as well as preserves their sense of dignity and personhood.

It must be emphasized that the only way to provide person-centered care is for the LTC administration to instill in the staff the ethos and importance of understanding incoming residents by giving them the time to comprehensively assess the resident's full gamut of bio-psycho-social needs, with periodic reevaluations. Screenings for cognitive impairment, mood problems, and behavioral difficulties are just the early stages of getting to know the resident, and should be supplemented by in-depth life history interviews, and appraisals of meaningful activities and old hobbies that promote quality of life. Activities should only be designed in ways that are tailored to individual residents and that generate meaning in their lives, instead of being utilized for distraction (Trahan et al., 2014). Indeed, activity preference scales for use in LTC have been developed (Feliciano et al., 2009). Interviews with family members are also recommended to gauge a baseline for the person's physical and mental health status. When evidence-based interventions validated in LTC settings, such as reminiscence therapy, cognitive behavior therapy (CBT), and Staff Training in Assisted Living Residences – Veterans Affairs (STAR-VA) are implemented in a thoughtful person-centered way, older adults have the opportunity not only to have their needs satisfied and symptoms reduced, but also to thrive.

Reminiscence Therapy

Reminiscence therapy, the discussion of memories and past events using an array of prompts, has consistently been proven to be effective in treating a variety of older adults with challenging behaviors or mental illness, including those residing in LTC settings (Woods et al., 2018). Reminiscence serves several important functions for older adults, including both intrapsychic and interpersonal functions. From an intrapsychic, self-integrative perspective, reminiscence helps to reinforce a sense of self-continuity, to find meaning and coherence in life, and to promote resilience (Bohlmeijer et al., 2007). It does this by allowing residents in LTC the opportunity to share their positive memories by specific queries about the past or activities that encourage reminiscence. In the life review variant of reminiscence, older adults are asked to evaluate their lives more systematically in an attempt to synthesize both pleasant and unpleasant memories. This furnishes the person with the opportunity to resolve any past conflicts to transform negative memories into more positive ones, as well as with the prospect of using life strategies that were successful in the past to resolve any current problems (Bohlmeijer et al., 2007). From an interpersonal perspective, reminiscence and life review also allows residents, who may feel isolated and depressed, the opportunity to connect with staff and residents in their new communal living situation, or to reconnect with, or maintain a connection to, loved ones who are not as present in their lives anymore (Henkel et al., 2016). Reminiscence therapy can be implemented in an individual or group format (Molinari, 1999), and has been found to be very successful in reducing boredom and feelings of social isolation, as well as in increasing conversation between residents that may lead to the development of friendships (Henkel et al., 2016). Indeed, simple reminiscence activities such as games of trivia or remembering the names of old songs may improve the current mood of residents with cognitive impairment (Cotelli et al., 2012).

Cognitive Behavior Therapy

Evidence for the use of CBT in older adults within the community and LTC has grown. CBT allows challenging behaviors and symptoms of mental illness to be satisfactorily addressed by emphasizing how clients can change their current perceptions to modify undesired behaviors or emotions (Gallagher-Thompson et al., 2017). Older adults tend to have the most success with CBT when skills are taught to help them identify unhelpful thought patterns, and to learn different techniques to help modify these thoughts. A limitation of CBT is that it has been largely validated with people who are cognitively healthy, and is not as effective for people with cognitive impairment. However, some researchers have used simplified materials to address the cognitive component of CBT in those with mild dementia (Snow et al., 2006). A branch of CBT found to be particularly useful in LTC settings is behavioral activation, which entails a systematic approach for identifying situations, people, and activities that will help to maintain a positive mood for a specific individual (Gallagher-Thompson et al., 2017). Behavioral activation can be effectively applied to older adults with dementia by offering them engaging activities to occupy their time gainfully. Such activities have consistently been found to reduce problematic behaviors (Camp et al., 2002; Cohen-Mansfield, 2013), but may be more limited in their ability to influence psychiatric symptoms associated with anxiety (Brown-Wilson et al., 2019). Regardless of their implementation in an individualized or group setting, meaningful activities may provide those with dementia with social contact and necessary stimulation (Cohen-Mansfield, 2013).

Staff Training in Assisted Living Residences – Veterans Affairs

STAR-VA is a multicomponent approach to addressing challenging behaviors in people with dementia (Karlin et al., 2014). The central component of STAR-VA is the individualized nature of the interventions used, as well as the structured design of the program. STAR-VA attempts to reduce undesirable behaviors by addressing both intrapersonal and environmental triggers, through the development of an activity schedule specially tailored for that specific person (Karlin et al., 2014). The STAR-VA intervention was found to be extremely valuable in reducing problematic behaviors in older adults with dementia, significantly reducing the severity and frequency of targeted behaviors across a range of behavioral issues (Karel et al., 2016; Karlin et al., 2014). A *nurse champion* also plays an important role in encouraging staff at every level to become more involved with activity planning as well as to listen and communicate better with the residents (Karel et al., 2016).

Interdisciplinary Facilitators of and Barriers to Treatment in LTC

Interdisciplinary care models for behavioral health care interventions are critical to patient outcomes and quality of life. The quality of care received by older adults in LTC is directly related to the ability of the multidisciplinary treatment team to coordinate and integrate their care (Bartels et al., 2002). Collaboration between staff about treatment plans and goals is essential to the well-being of the resident (Litchenberg & Duffy, 2000). Indeed, research has found that when care within LTC is integrated, there is less hospital utilization (Beswick et al., 2008), including a reduction in the number of emergency room visits (Hernandez et al., 2015) and time spent in the hospital (Meret-Hanke, 2011). At the patient-level, integrated care can lower mortality rates and enhance the quality of life for the person (Hernandez et al., 2015). Further, studies have also found that integrated care improves the residents' ability to function on a daily basis, reduces levels of depression (Hernandez et al., 2015), and potentially lowers the risk of falls (Beswick et al., 2008). It is important that psychologists working in LTC settings understand their roles within the integrated care team, as well as understand the organizational structure of the LTC.

Team integration is preferable to the lone consultant model (Bartels et al., 2002) of writing detailed notes on charts which may or may not be understood or even read by staff. Team integration requires respect for the roles of varied disciplines in the care of residents (Litchenberg & Duffy, 2000). Central to the team concept are the direct care workers themselves, as studies have consistently stressed the impact they have on the short- and long-term outcomes of residents. This underlines the importance of training staff on the psychological needs of residents in their particular LTC setting. Psychologists should take the initiative to train direct care workers on how to detect symptoms of mental illness, convey their concerns to the appropriate staff, implement supervised interventions guided by evidence-based protocols to reduce the frequency and severity of psychological and behavioral symptoms, and most importantly, take measures to prevent psychological and behavioral symptoms from developing (Bartels et al., 2002). However, systemic buy-in from the administration is a necessity for the provision of training and consultation services to transcend piecemeal and solitary efforts, and to create a person-centered environment that is maintained by an informed workforce that can carry out treatment plans (Bartels et al., 2002; Burgio et al., 2002).

It should be noted that a significant barrier for the optimal effectiveness of any psychological intervention is often the lack of provider cultural competency. Most evidence-based interventions for older adults are geared toward the White population, with findings less applicable to minority groups. However, researchers developing caregiving interventions for older adults are now highlighting ethnic diversity considerations (Dilworth-Anderson et al., 2004; Elliott et al., 2010; Ta Park et al., 2019). It is necessary that these interventions be sensitive to all aspects of diversity (Hinrichsen, 2006), including sexual orientation (Beaudreau et al., 2019; Hinrichsen, 2010) and spirituality, which can be central to one's person (Koenig & Cohen, 2006). The effectiveness of the intervention plan can be reduced if one is not willing to address such core lifelong aspects of a person's identity. Within LTC populations, there is an especial need for more effective culturally considerate intervention options. Research has established that there are health care disparities, and a reduced quality of care, for older adults in LTC who are of ethnic minority status

(Chisholm et al., 2013) and/or who are lesbian, gay, bisexual, or transgender (Smith et al., 2019). With multiple barriers to care already present in these populations, it will be even more important that LTC staff become aware of how to intervene in the most ethically sensitive way that allows these individuals to maintain the highest level of psychological and physical functioning.

Case Example: Older Adult in LTC

Mrs. J. is an 85-year-old widowed White woman who was admitted to the nursing home 6 months ago after she had a left hemispheric stroke and was no longer able to live independently in the community even after intensive rehabilitation. Since her stroke, she has had right-sided weakness and needs daily supervision. She has had minor residual cognitive impairment, problems paying her bills, repeated falls, and been unable to drive. Her only daughter lives in the neighborhood but travels regularly for her job and is unable to provide the necessary support for her mother to continue to live in her own home.

Mrs. J. had owned her own commercial art business until she retired when she was 75, and was described by her daughter as a fiercely independent woman who always made her own decisions. Her initial adjustment to the nursing home was slow, but the supportive staff and management worked with her to allow flexibility about when and what she ate, and at what time she went to bed and got up in the morning. Her daughter also visited regularly but tapered her visits as her mother felt better. Mrs. J. gradually began to view the nursing home as her new home. She particularly enjoyed reading, crocheting, and oil painting classes which the nursing home offered. Two weeks prior to her mental health consultation she had another stroke which caused her additional significant memory problems and right-sided damage. She was now unable to hold things in her hand, and exhibited behavior problems by staying in bed and becoming verbally aggressive with the staff when they urged her to attend rehabilitation. The day before, Mrs. J. had slapped one of the nursing assistants when she tried to get her up from her bed to take a bath. This nursing assistant was new and had had problems with other residents to whom she had been assigned. A referral was made to the psychologist (Dr. P.) who consults in the nursing home facility for him to make an assessment and intervene.

Dr. P. is a well-trained geropsychologist. He had taken one course in graduate school on aging, in addition to the required developmental psychology course; did internship rotations on rehabilitation and geropsychiatric units; and had worked in LTC facilities for years – the first year of which he was supervised weekly for licensure by a psychologist experienced in LTC. He has also attended APA seminars on aging and geropsychology to meet the annual continuing education requirement for licensure in his state, making him a strong potential candidate for credentialing as a specialist in geropsychology (ABGERO) with a focus in LTC. Given Dr. P.'s expertise regarding the varied presentations and effects of cognitive impairment in LTC settings, he was aware that Mrs. J. might become disinhibited if he pushed her too hard to respond to his entreaties. He found her asleep and gently tapped on her bed railing. Although at first quite angry that Dr. P. had woken her up for the psychological evaluation, she did warm up to him after he queried her about her prior work history and told her that he himself had been an aspiring but alas failed artist. He performed a cognitive assessment and determined that Mrs. J. had moderate memory impairment, which reflected a decline from her prior cognitive level before the second stroke. Her tearfulness and sad affect also suggested that she might be depressed because she believed that due to the right-sided weakness from her second stroke, she will never be able to practice her art again and that she was now just waiting to die. Dr. P. also determined that her depression was contributing to her cognitive difficulties as well as possibly precipitating her inappropriate behavior.

Dr. P. developed a treatment plan that included psychotherapy sessions whereby Mrs. J. could process her losses and frustration within a broad discussion of her overall life history and values. These therapy sessions also included relatively simple discussions regarding how rehabilitation might forestall what she feared and offer her the opportunity of recovering some function and thereby continuing to do some of her beloved artwork. They also included a plan of behavioral activation whereby attendance at rehabilitation and social activities would be rewarded by additional visits from her daughter. Indeed, a family meeting with the daughter and Mrs. J. was scheduled to brainstorm alternate activities that she had enjoyed in the past but could no longer recall. Attendance at team planning meetings gave Dr. P. additional valuable information about what times of the day or evening Mrs. J. did better so that encouragement was geared toward when she was most receptive to becoming active and engaged with others. Consultation with a psychiatrist regarding psychotropic medications was considered as well, particularly if the depression became more severe and if the resident voiced suicidal ideation.

Discussions with the head nurse were initiated by Dr. P. to provide the new nursing assistant additional training in person-centered care for those residents with cognitive and mental health issues so that she would be more patient with Mrs. J. and the other residents. Online staff training geared for caregivers allowed for convenient scheduling of her training sessions (Pleasant et al., 2017). As Dr. P. gained the trust of staff and administration, he set the stage for championing mental health throughout the nursing home by advocacy that would foster resident well-being and maximize the chances of not only reducing an impaired resident's mental health symptoms but also fostering more fulfilling, flourishing lives for all residents.

In LTC, psychologists are faced with complex situations such as in this case example where psychological symptoms are comorbid with medical problems (stroke) and rehabilitation (slower recovery time), social considerations (family involvement), psychological distress (belief that one can no longer lead a fulfilling life), and personality characteristics (independent traits). They frequently need to have an understanding not only of geropsychology, but also of rehabilitation, health psychology, palliative care, and neuropsychology (Molinari et al., 2018). These psychologists must not only conduct traditional psychotherapy and behavior therapy, but also arrange family meetings and consult with staff in the LTC setting. Attendance at interdisciplinary team meetings will allow the psychologist to gather important discipline-specific information from registered nurses, nursing aides, social workers, activities directors, and rehabilitation specialists (e.g., occupational therapists and physical therapists) to coordinate treatment efforts better. Interventions should aim not only to reduce symptoms, but also to improve quality of life, and perhaps even target systemic change such as regular consultation with the nursing home administration on the need for person-centered care and consistent monitoring of the well-being of the residents for immediate referral to geriatric mental health professionals.

Resources for Psychologists Working in LTC Settings

Psychologists just entering the LTC field should recognize that there are organizations, Listservs, guidelines, books, and websites to assist them with the task of providing optimal services to LTC residents. In the early 1980s, the group Psychologists in Long-Term Care (PLTC) was formed and continues to be the primary psychology organization that promotes quality practice, research, and training in LTC settings. It has a very lively and informative Listserv, with members addressing payment, training, and best practice issues. The journal *Clinical Gerontologist* has an affiliation with PLTC, with a designated LTC editor to keep the readership informed about the latest research in this neglected area. In 1998, PLTC sponsored a workgroup to develop standards of practice in LTC, culminating in the seminal publication "Standards for Psychological Services in Long-Term Care Facilities" (Lichtenberg et al., 1998). These standards outlined the growing presence of psychologists in LTC settings and the necessity for an understanding of the basic aspects of the provision of psychological services and ethical practice in LTC settings. The standards were divided into sections on providers, referrals, assessment, treatment, and ethical issues. Recently, these standards were revised into guidelines (Molinari et al., in press) to emphasize their educational and training value so psychologists and students would be able to identify their weaknesses as well as strengths, to fine-tune their professional approaches and remedy their deficits. The revised guidelines also acknowledge and address the changing demographics of LTC, especially the increasing number of younger residents with chronic medical and psychiatric problems such as traumatic brain injury and serious mental illness, short-stay residents admitted for rehabilitation, and those requiring palliative care and hospice. Such changes necessitate an expanded skill set not only encompassing geropsychology and neuropsychology, but also rehabilitation, health psychology, and death and dying. Guidelines in these other areas of practice should be consulted on an as-needed basis, especially for some psychologists working in specialty LTC settings.

However, it must be emphasized that the Pikes Peak model remains foundational for LTC, and the Pikes Peak Geropsychology Knowledge and Skills Assessment Tool (see Appendix 2; Karel et al., 2012) should be considered an important guide for LTC practice. Supervisors, students, and licensed psychologists interested in LTC can rate themselves as novice, intermediate, advanced, proficient, or expert, based on anchor items reflecting the varied Pikes Peak competencies. These include general knowledge about adult development, aging, and the older adult population; foundations of professional general practice; and assessment, intervention, and consultation. A couple of items within these competencies specifically address LTC settings.

There are a number of edited books on mental health in LTC, such as *Professional Psychology in Long Term Care: A Comprehensive Guide* (Molinari, 2000); *Emerging Trends in Psychological Practice in Long Term Care* (Norris et al., 2002); *Caring for People With Challenging Behaviors: Essential Skills and Successful Strategies in Long-Term Care* (Long, 2005); *Geropsychological Interventions in Long-Term Care* (Hyer & Intrieri, 2006); *Geropsychology and Long-Term Care* (Rosowsky et al., 2009); and *Transforming Long-Term Care: Expanded Roles for Mental Health Professionals* (Carney & Norris, 2017). A manual that outlines an evidence-based approach to managing difficult behaviors in LTC settings in a systematic manner has also been published (Karlin et al., 2017). The GeroCentral website provides an extensive list of current geropsychology resources (https://gerocentral.org/), and the PLTC website also has information dedicated specifically to LTC (https://www.pltcweb.org/index.php).

Conclusions and Implications

The number of older adults is steadily growing, and with this will come an increased demand for psychological services and interventions. It is projected that at least half of older adults will need to reside in a LTC setting at some point in their later years (Favreault & Dey, 2016), and for this reason, it is critical for one to fully understand the differences in how to care for older adults living in these settings. When providing assessments and interventions for older adults, it is essential to take their life stories into one's perspective, as this will be critical to the types of interventions developed and their outcomes. Theoretical models guided by a person-centered approach will allow one to contextualize undesirable behavioral and psychological symptoms by understanding patients and their history across their lifespan, and deciding on which treatment intervention may work best.

Major limitations in providing LTC services revolve around barriers that are encountered when working in different LTC settings. In the community, older adults may neither have access to, nor the ability to obtain, mental health services, due to the dearth of LTC professionals in the geographical area where they live (e.g., a rural area), because of physical limitations (e.g., unable to drive due to sensory impairment), or due to their community not meeting age-friendly standards (e.g., lack of public transportation). Older adults in institutionalized LTC may not have access to high-quality mental health services due to lack of expert consultants. These residents also may be unable to receive the full benefits of their therapy due to restrictions within their care setting or insurance plans. Telepsychiatry offers the promise of allowing older adults in LTC the opportunity to have easier access to high-quality mental health care. Recent studies have found this modality to be efficient, yielding outcomes that are similar to those found for in-person psychiatric sessions (Choi et al., 2014; Khatri et al., 2014; Rabinowitz et al., 2010).

There are a number of emerging roles for psychologists in LTC. One nontraditional responsibility psychologists are encouraged to assume is advocacy for better quality of LTC. For example, a psychologist could assist LTC administrators with the design of new units of assisted living facilities and nursing homes to foster culture change. The Pioneer Network, the Eden Alternative, and the Green House Project initiatives promote person-centered care and autonomy for residents. Psychologists can marshal substantiating evidence for their effect on the quality of life of residents (Lum et al., 2008), and perhaps even conduct site-specific program evaluations. Given the aforementioned workforce shortages plaguing LTC, mental health care professionals must also find systematic ways of supporting family members in remaining involved with their loved one's care. Although research has demonstrated that many families maintain emotional bonds with residents after nursing home placement (Gaugler, 2005), there are no clear-cut expectations for family members in LTC institutional settings. Offering orientation groups, encouraging family attendance at treatment planning meetings, and conducting traditional family therapy may elevate quality of life for caregivers as well as reduce the likelihood of perceived abandonment by residents. Along these lines, offering cutting-edge mental health services to minister to the psychological needs of residents and their relatives in palliative or hospice care would fulfill a great familial need across the spectrum of LTC. Regardless of care in community or institutional LTC settings, the demographics of increasing numbers of frail older adults who will continue to need mental health care services that help them to achieve maximal functioning and enhance their quality of life reflects a societal imperative that must be realized.

Suggested Resources for Working With Older Adults in Long-Term Care Settings

Mast, B. T., & Yochim, B. P. (2017). *Alzheimer's disease and dementia.* Hogrefe. https://doi.org/10.1027/00503-000

Rosowsky, E., & Casciani, J. M. (2010). *Geropsychology and long term care: A practitioner's guide.* Springer.

References

American Psychological Association (2014). Guidelines for psychological practice with older adults. *American Psychological Association, 69*(1), 34–65. https://doi.org/10.1037/a0035063

Andel, R., Hyer, K., & Slack, A. (2007). Risk factors for nursing home placement in older adults with and without dementia. *Journal of Aging and Health, 19*(2), 213–228. https://doi.org/10.1177/0898264307299359

Bartels, S., Moak, G., & Dums, A. (2002). Models of mental health services in nursing homes: A review of the literature. *Psychiatric Services, 53*(11), 1390–1396. https://doi.org/10.1176/appi.ps.53.11.1390

Beaudreau, S. A., Gallagher-Thompson, D., & Pachana, N. (2019). Two, four, six, eight, don't assume your grandma's straight: The intersectionality of aging and sexual minority status. *Clinical Gerontologist, 42*(2), 135–136. https://doi.org/10.1080/07317115.2019.1565644

Beswick, A., Rees, K., Dieppe, P., Ayis, S., Gooberman-Hill, R., Horwood, J., & Ebrahim, S. (2008). Complex interventions to improve physical function and maintain independent living in elderly people: A systematic review and meta-analysis. *Lancet, 371*(9614), 725–735. https://doi.org/10.1016/S0140-6736(08)60342-6

Bird, M., & Moniz-Cook, E. (2008). Challenging behaviour in dementia: A psychosocial approach to intervention. In B. Woods & L. Clare (Eds.), *Handbook of the clinical psychology of ageing* (2nd ed., pp. 571–594). John Wiley & Sons. https://doi.org/10.1002/9780470773185.ch33

Bohlmeijer, E., Roemer, M., Cuijpers, P., & Smit, F. (2007). The effects of reminiscence on psychological well-being in older adults: A meta-analysis. *Aging and Mental Health, 11*(3), 291–300. https://doi.org/10.1080/13607860600963547

Brownie, S., Horstmanshof, L., & Garbutt, R. (2014). Factors that impact residents' transition and psychological adjustment to long-term aged care: A systematic literature review. *International Journal of Nursing Studies, 51*(12), 1654–1666. https://doi.org/10.1016/j.ijnurstu.2014.04.011

Brown-Wilson, C., Arendt, L., Nguyen, M., Scott, T., Neville, C., & Pachana, N. (2019). Nonpharmacological interventions for anxiety and dementia in nursing homes: A systematic review. *Gerontologist, 59*(6), e731-e742. https://doi.org/10.1093/geront/gnz020

Burgio, L., Stevens, A., Burgio, K., Roth, D., Paul, P., & Gerstle, J. (2002). Teaching and maintaining behavior management skills in the nursing home. *Gerontologist, 42*(4), 487–496. https://doi.org/10.1093/geront/42.4.487

Camp, C., Cohen-Mansfield, J., & Capezuti, E. (2002). Mental health services in nursing homes: Use of nonpharmacologic interventions among nursing home residents with dementia. *Psychiatric Services, 53*(11), 1397–1401. https://doi.org/10.1176/appi.ps.53.11.1397

Carney, K., & Norris, M. (2017). *Transforming long-term care: Expanded roles for mental health professionals.* American Psychological Association.

Chisholm, L., Weech-Maldonado, R., Laberge, A., Lin, F., & Hyer, K. (2013). Nursing home quality and financial performance: Does racial composition of residents matter? *Health Services Research, 48,* 2060–2080. https://doi.org/10.1111/1475-6773.12079

Choi, N., Marti, N., Bruce, M., Hegel, M., Wilson, N., & Kunik, M. (2014). Six-month post-intervention depression and disability outcomes of in-home telehealth problem-solving therapy for depressed low-income homebound older adults. *Depression and Anxiety, 31,* 653–663. https://doi.org/10.1002/da.22242

Cohen-Mansfield, J. (2013). Nonpharmacologic treatment of behavioral disorders in dementia. *Current Treatment Options in Neurology, 15*(6), 765–785. https://doi.org/10.1007/s11940-013-0257-2

Cohen-Mansfield, J., & Werner, P. (1995). Environmental influences on agitation: An integrative summary of an observational study. *American Journal of Alzheimer's Care and Related Disorders & Research, 10*(1), 32–39. https://doi.org/10.1177/153331759501000108

Conwell, Y., Van Orden, K., & Caine, E. (2011). Suicide in older adults. *Psychiatric Clinics of North America, 34*(2), 451–468. https://doi.org/10.1016/j.psc.2011.02.002

Cotelli, M., Manenti, R., & Zanetti, O. (2012). Reminiscence therapy in dementia: A review. *Maturitas, 72*(3), 203–205. https://doi.org/10.1016/j.maturitas.2012.04.008

Department of Health & Human Services. (2017, November 14). *Who needs care?* https://longtermcare.acl.gov/the-basics/who-needs-care.html

Dilworth-Anderson, P., Goodwin, P. Y., & Williams, S. W. (2004). Can culture help explain the physical health effects of caregiving over time among African American caregivers? *Journals of Gerontology B: Psychological and Social Sciences,* 59*B*, S138–S145. https://doi.org/10.1093/geronb/59.3.S138

Donoghue, C. (2010). Nursing home staff turnover and retention: An analysis of national level data. *Journal of Applied Gerontology, 29*(1), 89–106. https://doi.org/10.1177/0733464809334899

Elliott, A. F., Burgio, L. D., & DeCoster, J. (2010). Enhancing caregiver health: Findings from the Resources for Enhancing Alzheimer's Caregiver Health II Intervention. *Journal of the American Geriatrics Society, 58*(1), 30–37. https://doi.org/10.1111/j.1532-5415.2009.02631.x

Favreault, M., & Dey, J. (2016, February). *Long-term services and supports for older Americans: Risks and financing brief.* https://aspe.hhs.gov/basic-report/long-term-services-and-supports-older-americans-risks-and-financing-research-brief

Feliciano, L., Steers, M. E., Elite-Marcandonatou, A., McLane, M., & Arean, P. A. (2009). Applications of preference assessment procedures in depression and agitation management in elders with dementia. *Clinical Gerontologist, 32*(3), 239–259. https://doi.org/10.1080/07317110902895226

Gallagher-Thompson, D., Cassidy-Eagle, E., & Dunn, L. (2017). Cognitive behavioral therapy for treatment of late-life depression. *Today's Geriatric Medicine, 10*(1), 22.

Gaugler, J. (2005). Family involvement in residential long-term care: A synthesis and critical review. *Aging and Mental Health, 9*(2), 105–118. https://doi.org/10.1080/13607860412331310245

Harris-Kojetin, L., Sengupta, M., Park-Lee, E., Valverde, R., Caffrey, C., Rome, V., & Lendon, J. (2016). *Long-term care providers and service users in the United States: Data from the National Study of Long-Term Care Providers,* 2013–2014. *Vital and Health Statistics, 3*(38), 1–105.

Henkel, L., Kris, A., Birney, S., & Krauws, K. (2016). The functions and value of reminiscence for older adults in long-term residential care facilities. *Memory, 25*(3), 425–435. https://doi.org/10.1080/09658211.2016.1182554

Hernandez, C., Alonso, A., Garcia-Aymerich, J., Serra, I., Marti, D., Rodriguez-Roisin, R., Narsavage, G., Gomez, M., & Roca, J. (2015). Effectiveness of community-based integrated care in frail COPD patients: A randomised controlled trial. *Primary Care Respiratory Medicine, 25*(1502), 1–6. https://doi.org/10.1038/npjpcrm.2015.22

Hinrichsen, G. (2006). Why multicultural issues matter for practioners working with older adults. *Professional Psychology: Research and Practice, 37*(1), 29–35. https://doi.org/10.1037/0735-7028.37.1.29

Hinrichsen, G. (2010). Sexual orientation issues in the context of interpersonal psychotherapy in late-life depression. In N. Pachana, K. Laidlaw, & B. Knight (Eds.), *Casebook of clinical geropsychology: International perspectives on practice* (pp. 1–16). Oxford University Press. https://doi.org/10.1093/med/9780199583553.003.0001

Hyer, L., & Intrieri, R. (Eds.). (2006). *Geropsychological interventions in long-term care.* Springer.

Jeste, D., Alexopoulos, G., Bartels, S., Cummings, J., Gallo, J., Gottlieb, G., Halpain, M., Palmer, B., Patterson, T., Reynolds, C., & Lebowitz, B. (1999). Consensus statement on the upcoming crisis in geriatric mental health: Research agenda for the next 2 decades. *Archives of General Psychiatry, 56*(9), 848–853. https://doi.org/10.1001/archpsyc.56.9.848

Karel, M. J., Holley, C. K., Whitbourne, S. K., Segal, D. L., Tazeau, Y. N., Emery, E. E., Molinari, V., Yang, J., & Zweig, R. A. (2012). Preliminary validation of a tool to assess knowledge and skills for professional geropsychology practice. *Professional Psychology: Research and Practice, 43*(2), 110–117. https://doi.org/10.1037/a0025788

Karel, M., Teri, L., McConnell, E., Visnic, S., & Karlin, B. (2016). Effectiveness of expanded implementation of STAR-VA for managing dementia-related behaviors among veterans. *Gerontologist, 56*(1), 126–134. https://doi.org/10.1093/geront/gnv068

Karlin, B. E., Teri, L., McGee, J. S., Sutherland, E. S., Asghar-Ali, A., Crocker, S. M., Smith, T. L., Curyto, K., Drexler, M., & Karel, M. J. (2017). *STAR-VA intervention for managing challenging behaviors in VA community living center residents with dementia: Manual for STAR-VA behavioral coordinators and nurse champions.* U.S. Department of Veterans Affairs.

Karlin, B., Viscnic, S., McGee, J., & Teri, L. (2014). Results from the multisite implementation of STAR-VA: A multicomponent psychosocial intervention for managing challenging dementia-related behaviors of veterans. *Psychological Services, 11*(2), 200–208. https://doi.org/10.1037/a0033683

Khatri, N., Marziali, E., Tchernikoc, I., & Shepard, N. (2014). Comparing telehealth-based and clinic-based group cognitive behavioral therapy for adults with depression and anxiety: A pilot study. *Clinical Interventions in Aging, 9,* 765–770. https://doi.org/10.2147/CIA.S57832

Knight, B. G., Karel, M. J., Hinrichsen, G. A., Qualls, S. H., & Duffy, M. (2009). Pikes Peak model for training in professional geropsychology. *American Psychologist, 64*(3), 205–214. https://doi.org/10.1037/a0015059

Koeller, D., Schon, G., Schafer, I., Glaeske, G., van den Bussche, H., & Hansen, H. (2014). Multimorbidity and long-term care dependency: A five year follow-up. *BMC Geriatrics, 14*(70), 1–9. https://doi.org/10.1186/1471-2318-14-70

Koenig, H., & Cohen, H. (2006). Spirituality across the lifespan. *Southern Medical Journal, 99*(10), 1157–1158. https://doi.org/10.1097/01.smj.0000242796.62483.de

Kunik, M., Lees, E., Snow, A., Cody, M., Rapp, C., Molinari, V., & Beck, C. (2003). Disruptive behavior in dementia: A qualitative study to promote understanding and improve treatment. *Alzheimer's Care Today, 4*(2), 125–136.

Lawton, M. (1983). Environment and other determinants of well-being in older people. *Gerontologist, 23*(4), 349–357. https://doi.org/10.1093/geront/23.4.349

Lawton, M. (2001). The physical environment of the person with Alzheimer's disease. *Aging & Mental Health, 5*(S1), S56–S64. https://doi.org/10.1080/713650004

Lawton, M., & Nahemow, L. (1973). Ecology and the aging process. In C. Eisdorfer & M. Lawton (Eds.), *The psychology of adult development and aging* (pp. 619–674). American Psychological Association https://doi.org/10.1037/10044-020

Li, Y. (2010). Provision of mental health services in U.S. nursing homes: 1995–2004. *Psychiatric Services, 61*(4), 349–355. https://doi.org/10.1176/ps.2010.61.4.349

Litchenberg, P., & Duffy, M. (2000). Psychological assessment and psychotherapy in long-term care. *Clinical Psychology: Science and Practice, 7,* 317–328. https://doi.org/10.1093/clipsy.7.3.317

Lichtenberg, P. A., Smith, M. C. Frazer, D., Molinari, V., Rosowsky, E., Crose, R., Stillwell, N., Kramer, N., Hartman-Stein, P., Quails, S., Salamon, M., Duffy, M., Parr, J., & Gallagher-Thompson, D. (1998). Standards for psychological services in long-term care facilities. *Gerontologist, 38*(1), 122–127.

Long, S. W. (2005). *Caring for people with challenging behaviors: Essential skills and successful strategies in long-term care.* Health Professions Press.

Lum, T. Y., Kane, R. A., Cutler, L. J., & Tzy-Chyi, Y. (2008). Effects of Green House® nursing homes on residents' families. *Health Care Financing Review, 30*(2), 35–51.

Meret-Hanke, L. A. (2011). Effects of the program of all-inclusive care for the elderly on hospital use. *Gerontologist, 51*(6), 774–785. https://doi.org/10.1093/geront/gnr040

Mezuk, B., Lohman, M., Leslie, M., & Powell, V. (2015). Suicide risk in nursing homes and assisted living facilities: 2003–2011. *American Journal of Public Health, 105*(7), 1495–1502. https://doi.org/10.2105/AJPH.2015.302573

Molinari, V. (1999). Using reminiscence and life review as natural therapeutic strategies in group therapy. In M. Duffy (Ed.), *Handbook of counseling and psychotherapy with older adults* (pp. 154–165). John Wiley & Sons.

Molinari. V. (Ed.). (2000). *Professional psychology in long term care: A comprehensive guide.* Hatherleigh Press.

Molinari, V., Edelstein, B. A., Gibson, R., Lind, L., Norris, M., Carney, K., Bush, S., Heck, A., Moye, J., Gordon, H., & Hiroto, K. {PLTC Guidelines Revision Task Force}. (2018). *PLTC guidelines for psychological and behavioral health services in long-term care settings.* http://www.pltcweb.org/cms/uploads/documents/PLTC%20Guidelines%20for%20Psychological%20and%20Behavioral%20Health%20Services%20-%20revisedLL.pdf

Molinari, V., Edelstein, B., Gibson, R., Lind, L., Norris, M., Carney, K., Bush, S. S., Heck, A. L., Moye, J., Gordon, B. H., & Hiroto, K. (in press). Guidelines for psychological and behavioral health services in long term care settings. *Professional Psychology: Research and Practice.* Advance online publication. http://dx.doi.org/10.1037/pro0000298

Molinari, V., & Ellis, M. (2016). Psychological interventions in long-term care settings. In N. A. Pachana (Ed.), *Encyclopedia of geropsychology* (pp. 1926–1931), Springer. https://doi.org/10.1007/978-981-287-080-3_58-2

Moye, J., Karel, M., Stamm, K., Qualls, S., Segal, D., Tazeau, Y., & DiGilio, D. (2019). Workforce analysis of psychological practice with older adults: Growing crisis requires urgent action. *Training and Education in Professional Psychology, 13*(1), 46–55. https://doi.org/10.1037/tep0000206

Muralidharan, A., Mills, W., Evans, D., Fujii, D., & Molinari, V. (2019). Preparing long-term care staff to meet the needs of aging persons with serious mental illness. *JAMDA, 20,* 683–688. https://doi.org/10.1016/j.jamda.2019.03.018

Norris, M., Molinari, V., & Ogland-Hand, S. (Eds.). (2002). *Emerging trends in psychological practice in long term care.* Haworth Press.

Nguyen, V. (2017). Long-term support and services. *AARP Public Policy Institute*, 1–4.

Pleasant, M., Molinari, V., Hobday, J., Fazio, S., Cullen, N., & Hyer. K. (2017). An evaluation of the CARES® Dementia Basics Program caregivers. *International Psychogeriatrics, 29*(1), 45–56. https://doi.org/10.1017/S1041610216001526

Rabinowitz, T., Murphy, K., Amour, J., Ricci, M., Caputo, M., & Newhouse, P. (2010). Benefits of a telepsychiatry consultation service for rural nursing home residents. *Telemedicine and E-Health, 16*(1), 34–40. https://doi.org/10.1089/tmj.2009.0088

Rosowsky, E., Casciani, J., & Arnold, M. (Eds.). (2009). *Geropsychology and long-term care: A practitioner's guide.* Springer.

Smith, R., Altman, J., Meeks, S., & Hinrichs, K. (2019). Mental health care for LGBT older adults in long-term care settings: Competency, training, and barriers for mental health providers. *Clinical Gerontologist, 42*(2), 198–203. https://doi.org/10.1080/07

Snow, A., Powers, D., & Liles, D. (2006). Cognitive-behavioral therapy for long-term care patients with dementia. In L. Hyer & R. Intrieri (Eds.), *Geropsychological interventions in long-term care* (pp. 265–294). Springer.

Spetz, J., Trupin, L., Bates, T., & Coffman, J. (2015). Future demand for long-term care workers will be influenced by demographic and utilization changes. *Health Affairs, 34*(6), 936–945. https://doi.org/10.1377/hlthaff.2015.0005

Ta Park, V. M., Ton, V., Tiet, Q. Q., Vuong, Q., Yeo, G., & Gallagher-Thompson, D. (2019). Promising results from a pilot study to reduce distress in Vietnamese American dementia and memory loss caregivers.

Alzheimer's & Dementia: Translational Research & Clinical Interventions, 5, 319–327. https://doi.org/10.1016/j.trci.2019.05.006

The American Geriatrics Society Expert Panel on Person-Centered Care (2015). Person-centered care: A definition and essential elements. *Journal of the American Geriatrics Society, 64*(1), 15–18. https://doi.org/10.1111/jgs.13866

Trahan, M., Kuo, J., Carlson, M., & Gitlin, L. (2014). A systematic review of strategies to foster activity engagement in persons with dementia. *Health, Education, & Behavior, 41*(1), 70S–83S. https://doi.org/10.1177/1090198114531782

Vespa, J., Armstrong, D., & Medina, L. (2018). Demographic turning points for the United States: Population projections for 2020 to 2050. *United States Census Bureau,* 1–15.

Volicer, L., & Hurley, A. (2003). Management of behavioral symptoms in progressive degenerative dementias. *Journals of Gerontology: Medical Sciences, 58A*(9), 837–845. https://doi.org/10.1093/gerona/58.9.M837

Wiles, J., Leibing, A., Buberman, N., Reeve, J., & Allen, R. (2012). The meaning of "aging in place" to older people. *Gerontologist, 52*(3), 357–366. https://doi.org/10.1093/geront/gnr098

Woods, B., O'Philbin, L., Farrell, E., Spector, A., & Orrell, M. (2018). Reminiscence therapy for dementia. *Cochrane Database of System Reviews, 2018*(3), 1–130. https://doi.org/10.1002/14651858.CD001120.pub3

Chapter 8

Determining Decisional Capacity Across Settings and Clinical Presentations: A Systematic Approach

Shane S. Bush
Stacey Wood

Introduction

Concerns commonly emerge about the ability of older adults to continue functioning independently or continue making the decisions that govern their lives. Personal autonomy is a deeply held value in Western societies. With few exceptions, such as where suicidal or homicidal plans are involved, competent adults have the right to live their life as they choose, even when their choices seem poor to others. However, despite the importance afforded to personal autonomy, Western societies also place value on helping or protecting those who cannot, due to compromised mental abilities, act in their own best interests. A primary challenge in the case of some older adults lies in determining whether they retain the ability to function or make certain decisions independently. Given the increased prevalence of progressive neurocognitive disorders and other medical risk factors that tend to occur in older adults, questions of capacity are commonly raised by family members, health care providers, and others who interact with older adults.

The American Psychological Association (APA, 2014) *Guidelines for Psychological Practice with Older Adults* state that "psychologists strive to understand the functional capacity of older adults in the social and physical environment" (Guideline 8, p. 44). Psychologists who have experience evaluating and treating older adults are well-positioned to provide valuable information regarding decisional and functional capacities. The assessment of capacity is a foundational competency for geropsychologists (Knight et al., 2009). "Undue influence" refers to an interpersonal dynamic based on trust where a stronger party improperly influences or persuades a weaker party in order to benefit financially. Vulnerable older adults are more susceptible to undue influence as a class, and as a result, undue influence assessments may be part of a capacity assessment.

The following are a few scenarios that can trigger a referral for a capacity evaluation.

- A 79-year-old woman residing in a skilled nursing facility is found in her room having sex with her roommate's 40-year-old son.
- An 83-year-old man invests $20,000 with a pleasant young man who has called offering a guaranteed way to secure his savings for his family.
- A 65-year-old woman with a history of uncontrolled type 2 diabetes and gangrenous ulcers on her lower extremities refuses a right below-knee amputation which is needed to save her life.
- A 70-year-old man with a history of impulsivity and poor judgment resulting from a significant traumatic brain damage involving the prefrontal lobes, who resides in a long-term care facility, requests a motorized wheelchair; however, his treatment team is concerned about his safety and that of other residents and staff.

Despite the numerous contexts in which decisional capacity questions arise, the goal of the present chapter is to focus on general decision-making capacity, the principles and methods of which can be tailored to meet the needs of diverse situations.

Incapacity Defined

The criteria for incapacity are defined by varying statutes in each US state (Demakis, 2012; Dudley & Edmonds, 2018). The core of the definition in many states is that persons lack capacity if they are unable to manage their own affairs in their best interest, cannot make decisions independently, or are unable to meet their essential needs because of a disabling condition (Dudley & Edmonds, 2018). Such definitions tend to be broader than the more focused clinical questions that target specific decisions or behaviors. In addition to statutes, case law can be used to inform the understanding of incapacity.

Traditionally, different terms have been used in clinical and legal contexts (Dudley & Edmonds, 2018). "Capacity" or "incapacity" has been used clinically, and "competency" or "incompetency" has been used in forensic contexts. "Incapacity" is used clinically until a person has been deemed legally "incompetent" by a court. This distinction has changed over time, with a majority of states now preferring the less pejorative term "incapacitated" instead of "incompetent" (Demakis, 2012; Dudley & Edmonds, 2018). The term "incapacitated" is also considered to reflect a state that is more amenable to restorative efforts.

"Capacity" is not an all-encompassing construct; it is situationally dependent (American Bar Association [ABA] Commission on Law and Aging & American Psychological Association [APA], 2008). For example, someone who does not have the capacity to make financial decisions may retain the capacity to make medical decisions, drive, and engage independently in other aspects of life. Capacity is not static. Some medical and psychiatric conditions that affect decisional and functional capacity are temporary or reversible. A person may lack capacity while affected by the condition and then regain capacity once the condition has resolved. Similarly, capacity can fluctuate as the medical or psychiatric condition fluctuates. Table 8.1 provides a nonexhaustive list of capacities commonly encountered by psychologists who work with older adults.

Table 8.1. Common decisional, functional, and legal capacities and competencies

Clinical or civil	Criminal
Decisional	Competence to stand trial
Financial decisions (including avoiding exploitation)	Competence to be executed
Health care decisions / treatments	
Contractual	
Functional	
Independent living	
Sexual activity	
Driving	
Testamentary (of or relating to one's will)	

The Influence of Culture and Family

The older adult population is very diverse, and it is anticipated that the heterogeneity will continue to increase for the foreseeable future (APA, 2014). Cultural differences exist in (a) the value placed on autonomy, (b) the role of the community or family in the lives of persons with diminished capacity, and (c) the trust placed in, or acceptance of intervention by, psychologists and other health care professionals (APA, 2017a; Blackhall et al., 1995; Palzer, 2018). Demographic differences exist in the approach to, and performance on, cognitive and emotional testing (Byrd & Manly, 2005; Tan et al., 2020). Lack of awareness of such differences by clinicians can result in inaccurate or inappropriate capacity determinations, and in decisions that are not in the best interests of the older adult with diminished capacity.

Family conflict and greed can result in undue influence on vulnerable older adults and sway decision making in a manner that is inconsistent with the older adult's longstanding values and preferences (Hoffman, 2018; Peisah et al., 2006; Quinn, 2002). Undue influence is the unfair persuasion of a party who is under the domination of the person exercising the persuasion or who by virtue of the relation between them is justified in assuming that that person will not act in a manner inconsistent with his welfare (American Law Institute, 1981). Undue Influence is most frequently evoked in cases involving wills or trusts; however, it can bear on other types of decisional capacity as well.

There have been a number of conceptual models developed in psychology to explain the power dynamic of undue influence in general (ABA & APA, 2008; Borchard Foundation Center for Law and Aging, 2010). The Borchard Foundation Center for Law and Aging (2010) reviewed these clinical models as well as state definitions of undue influence across the country, and concluded, "Despite wide variations in the contexts and circumstances in which undue influence and coercive persuasion in general have been explored, the findings are remarkably similar in terms of the salient features. Psychologists, sociologists, criminologists, victimologists, legal experts, and courts have focused on the following" (p. 10):

A. Characteristics of the victim that may be contributing to a vulnerability: These can include medical, cognitive, psychological, and functional vulnerabilities.
B. Descriptions of the influencer's power: Undue influence occurs in a relationship where the influencer has power and has a confidential or trusting relationship. The authority can be formal such as a physician or financial advisor, or informal such as a caregiver or neighbor.
C. Improper action or tactics: Influencers often take steps to actively take advantage of the alleged influenced individual. These may range from isolating the older person from others, reinforcing dependency, initiating and/or actively procuring legal documents, and many others. There may also be an element of secrecy or inappropriate timing (same day as a hospitalization, shortly after a loss) that favors the influencer.
D. Unfair, unequal, or "unnatural" financial outcomes: Undue influence results in financial losses for the victim and financial gain for the influencer. An unfair outcome may be a transaction that is below market value, benefiting the influencer. An unequal outcome may refer to impact on beneficiaries, and an unnatural outcome may refer to the disinheritance of a natural heir in favor of a non-family member. Undue influence occurs when a powerful person with a confidential relationship with a vulnerable individual takes advantage of that relationship to financially benefit themselves at the expense of the vulnerable older person through improper influence or persuasion.

Frequency of Capacity Assessment Referrals in Clinical Practice

The frequency and type of referrals for capacity evaluations vary considerably with the practice context. For example, in inpatient medical settings, questions about the ability to make decisions regarding advance directives and medical procedures occur frequently, whereas in outpatient settings, questions regarding the ability to drive, continue managing finances or medications, or live independently are more likely to be encountered. An informal online survey of practicing neuropsychologists found that capacity issues occurred in up to 75% of cases, with executive functions being the cognitive domain of most relevance for determining capacity (Moberg & Kniele, 2006). A survey of consultation–liaison psychiatrists revealed that nearly 20% of referrals were for decision-making capacity assessments (Seyfried et al., 2013). For those psychiatrists, dementia and delirium were the most common diagnoses among the persons assessed for capacity issues. Thus, to address these questions, family members, clinicians, and legal professionals are increasingly turning to psychologists to provide empirically supported capacity determinations (Moye et al., 2013).

Competencies Required for Capacity Evaluations

Numerous medical, psychological, pharmacological, and situational factors can have temporary or long-term impacts on cognitive functioning and the ability to make sound decisions independently. Such factors can have wide ranging etiologies and interact in complex ways, leading to challenges in the ability to make correct capacity determinations, particularly for early-career professionals and others with limited experience in this aspect of practice. Because of the challenging and complex nature of capacity determinations and the importance of their outcomes for the lives of patients, their families, treatment teams, and others, specialist knowledge and skills are required.

The performance of effective and useful capacity evaluations requires knowledge of, and skills relevant to, psychological and neurological pathologies that have a greater prevalence in later life. The Pikes Peak model for training in professional geropsychology (see Appendix 1; Knight et al., 2009) describes the foundational and functional competencies required for effective psychological practice with older adults in general. In the context of capacity evaluations more specifically, the model's sections on assessment and consultation are particularly informative. Sections II C and D describe the knowledge foundations necessary for assessment and consultation, and Sections III B and D describe the skill competencies needed for assessment and consultation. Included among the various skills are the ability to (a) select and use psychometrically sound screening instruments, (b) adapt instruments and make test administration accommodations, (c) make accurate diagnostic determinations, and (d) communicate assessment results clearly and concisely to the relevant stakeholders, including treatment teams when indicated. The ability to "evaluate decision-making and functional capacities (e.g., for managing finances, independent living, driving, making health care decisions)" is a specific assessment skill competency (Section III.B.5.; Knight et al., 2009, p. 213; see Appendix 1). Given the necessary technical skills and clinical judgment involved, determination of decisional capacity is often quite challenging for early-career psychologists. It is recommended that clinicians seek consultation when these issues arise in clinical practice, until sufficient expertise has been accumulated.

Ethical and Legal Considerations

A primary ethical challenge in capacity evaluations involves balancing the importance of respecting and protecting patient autonomy with the need to protect vulnerable patients and others from harmful decisions that they may make if their capacity is compromised (Bush et al., 2015; Bush et al., 2017; Karel, 2011). The ethical principle of *beneficence* guides psychologists and other health care professionals to take actions that promote the well-being of patients and protects their interests. The principle of *respect for autonomy* directs psychologists and other health care professionals to defend the right of competent adult patients to make the decisions that govern their lives – that is, psychologists support decisions made by patients that are consistent with their long-held values and preferences, even when such decisions are considered by others to be "bad" decisions. For example, a competent older adult with a long history of uncontrolled diabetes may choose to forego a life-sustaining amputation of a gangrenous lower extremity, despite strong pressure from medical professionals or family members to have the procedure and prolong life. Similarly, a competent older adult may choose to give away large sums of money to non-family members, despite considerable opposition from family members and arguments from family members that such behavior must be a sign of incompetence. The principle of respect for autonomy involves an appreciation that competent adults can, within legal limits, make decisions or engage in behaviors that others consider to be bad decisions or inappropriate behaviors.

The principle of respect for autonomy underlies informed consent, including consent for the capacity evaluation. Demakis and Mart (2018) noted, "Perhaps one of the most vexing ethical issues in capacity evaluations is how to obtain informed consent – a key ethical feature of psychological practice – from those individuals who may not possess the capacity to provide such consent" (p. 331). In such instances, clinicians nevertheless provide the same information as would otherwise be provided, seek the patient's assent, consider the patient's preferences and best interests, and obtain consent from a legally authorized representative if possible. In the absence of a legally authorized representative, the clinician keeps the patient's rights and welfare as the foremost priority (APA, 2017b). Because negotiating competing ethical responsibilities can be a complex endeavor that affects the lives of others, psychologists need to be aware of their own values and how their values impact the ethical and clinical decisions that are made (Bush, 2012).

The 2017 Uniform Guardianship, Conservatorship and Other Protective Arrangements Act (UGCOPPA) is a comprehensive guardianship statute that promotes person-centered planning that incorporates a person's values and preferences in a guardianship order. The act further requires courts to order the least-restrictive means necessary to protect those who are not fully able to care for themselves. *Supported decision making* (SDM) is one option that is less restrictive than guardianship for persons who have disabilities. SDM is an approach to supporting persons with compromised capacity to make and communicate their own decisions about their lives, rather than having a legally appointed person make the decisions for them without their involvement (see https://www.supportmydecision.org/assets/tools/DRM-SDM-Handbook-Rev.-7.19.19.pdf). SDM focuses on abilities rather than disability, and reflects a model of support over one of protection (ABA Commission on Law and Aging, 2016; Kohn et al., 2013). SDM's emphasis on the individual's values, wishes, and self-determination reflects a shift from the substitution of decisions by a guardian to the support of the alleged incapacitated person's preferences (Glen, 2014). Proponents of SDM view the "right to fail" as an important freedom. The opponents of SDM (e.g., Voice of Reason, https://www.vor.net/) note that while SDM may be of value to those who need guardianship the least (if at all), it weakens protections for those who are most vulnerable. Psychologists tasked with making determinations about capacity benefit from considering the concept of decision support in the pursuit of a balance between beneficence and respect for patient autonomy.

Systematic Capacity Assessment Process

Capacity typically comprises four abilities: understanding, appreciation, reasoning, and expressing a choice. The clinician's task is to determine whether the patient has the ability to understand the relevant information, appreciate the likely consequences of different courses of action, reason about the information in the context of their own situation, and express a choice regarding their options (Grisso & Appelbaum, 1998).

Capacity evaluations tend to be challenging. Seyfried et al. (2013) surveyed experienced consultation psychiatrists and found that approximately 60% judged capacity assessments to be both more challenging and more time-consuming than other types of assessments, and that there is often disagreement among professionals regarding the capacity of patients (Kim et al., 2011; Marson et al., 1997). Such disagreements may arise from different (1) emphases placed on different information, (2) interpretation of responses, and (3) thresholds for risk. For example, in a case involving an individual with early Alzheimer's disease, all parties may agree with the specific diagnosis but have different opinions regarding the extent that the diagnoses impacts the individuals ability to make a specific decision.

The clinician's ability to obtain the necessary information and to arrive at an optimal clinical decision about the patient is maximized by having a *systematic capacity assessment process* (SCAP). The ABA/APA guide (ABA & APA, 2008) provides a nine-part framework for the assessment of capacity. In this present chapter, Box 8.1 presents a 10-part model that offers additional guidance to clinicians. Despite the value of such frameworks, the authors of the ABA/APA guide note that "there is no equation, cookbook, or test battery for the assessment of capacity. A one-size fits all approach is doomed to failure..." (ABA & APA, p. 23). Ultimately, decisions about a person's capacity come down to the clinician's judgment, with the clinician taking the steps deemed necessary to adequately inform that judgment.

Box 8.1. Systematic capacity assessment process (SCAP)

Preassessment considerations
Informed consent or assent
Record review
Interviews and observations
Assessment
Values
Diagnosis and prognosis
Capacity opinion
Recommendations
Report results and final steps

Preassessment Considerations

Establishing the parameters of the evaluation is the first step in the SCAP. Prior to performing the evaluation, the clinician must determine (a) the specific purpose of the evaluation, (b) the relevant legal standards, (c) the functional capacities to be assessed, (d) the characteristics of the patient, (e) what other parties are involved, (f) the context of the evaluation, (g) the urgency of the request, and (h) the overall appropriateness of the referral. The clinician must also determine whether they have any conflicts of interest in the case that could bias the results and conclusions and that would warrant a referral to a different clinician.

Informed Consent or Assent

At the outset of the assessment, the clinician explains to the patient the purpose and process of the evaluation, the anticipated risks and benefits, and the use of the results, in language appropriate for the patient. Commonly, brief statements, supported by written materials, can be helpful in promoting the patient's understanding of the information. Additionally, having the patient repeat back in their own words the information can help demonstrate their understanding. For patients who may, or clearly do, lack capacity to provide informed consent, the clinician provides the person with the same information about the assessment process and seeks their willingness (i.e., assent) to undergo the assessment and seeks consent from the legally authorized decision maker, if available.

Record Review

Considerable information about a person's functional abilities can be found in relevant records (e.g., medical, legal, and financial records). Clinicians should review such records with a focus on issues of relevance to the capacity in question. Reviewing the records prior to interviewing and testing the patient can help identify issues to be covered and questions to be asked during the assessment. Also reviewing the records after meeting with the patient can help to fill in gaps or clarify inconsistencies in the information provided by the patient.

Interviews and Observations

Interview questions include obtaining the patient's understanding of their strengths and weaknesses in general, as well as regarding the specific issue in question. Obtaining relevant information from family members, other caregivers, facility staff, other health care providers, and others as needed further helps the clinician understand the patient's functioning regarding the capacity in question. Direct observation of the patient's behaviors and interactions during the evaluation, including with others, provides an important piece of the emerging understanding of the patient's ability to manage certain aspects of their life.

Assessment

Although all steps in the SCAP are important, the quantitative assessment of cognition, emotional state, and functioning sets psychologists apart from many of the other health care professionals who are asked to provide capacity determinations. Moye et al. (2007) noted,

> Although a clinician's opinion is currently the accepted standard for capacity determination – there is no "gold" standard – clinical opinion can be inaccurate, unreliable, and invalid. Thus, understanding capacity requires a construct validation approach, where multiple lines of reliability and validity evidence are interwoven to establish knowledge about the nature, workings, and measurement of the construct. (p. 5)

The complexity of the capacity assessment process can be illustrated from the literature on financial decision making. Pinsker et al. (2010) report that financial capacity requires three underlying abilities: (1) declarative knowledge (the ability to describe financial concepts), (2) procedural knowledge (how to complete a financial task such as writing a check), and (3) a minimally sufficient level of judgment to make sound financial decisions. O'Brien (2013) propose a need for evidence of financial incapacity that, instead of self-neglect, insufficient resources, or a (poor) reasoned choice, reflects a clear pattern of inability to manage funds. Lichtenberg et al. (2015) add that (1) awareness of the risk factors for financial exploitation or abuse, (2) an understanding financial knowledge and skills, and (3) financial judgment are all components of a good financial capacity evaluation.

A multimethod approach to assessing decisional capacity is typically employed to understand the constructs of interest. Cognitive abilities and psychopathology are assessed via interviews, observations, and psychometric measures. Functional assessment occurs via interviews, home visit, observations, and use of standardized measures of functional abilities if they exist for the specific capacity. Many measures and techniques exist to help clinicians better understand these components of decisional capacity.

Commonly used, commercially available psychological and cognitive tests often form the core of the psychometric aspect of the evaluation, sometimes supplemented by specific measures of capacity assessment and functional assessments. Accommodations (e.g., sensory, motor) are provided as needed to help obtain a reliable and valid understanding of the constructs of interest.

There are two general types of capacity assessment measures: those that are vignette-based and those that are structured or semistructured interviews. Some measures allow for generalization of findings across capacities, whereas others address one type of capacity (e.g., financial). Although no specific "capacimeter" (Kapp & Mossman, 1996) exists to readily meet the needs of all evaluations, numerous measures have been developed to aid clinicians in this process. A comprehensive review of capacity assessment measures is beyond the scope of this chapter (Demakis, 2012). Dudley and Edmonds (2018) note that despite the existence of measures of decision-making capacity, the use of such measures is not required and may not be the best choice for some evaluations. It is the clinician's responsibility to select the assessment measures that can help answer the question at issue.

Values

The clinician strives to understand the patient's values and preferences about autonomy, openness to information or assistance from others, and the specific issue in question, in the context of their cultural identity. The clinician also identifies and discusses risks of different courses of action, or inaction, regarding the issue in question. The clinician seeks consistency between choices and values. Understanding the caregiver's values and any discrepancies between the values of the patient and caregiver informs the clinician about whether substituted judgments are truly in the patient's best interests. Bush (2009) has created a questionnaire to assist clinicians with gathering information about caregivers' values. Clinicians who also consider their own values about the issue in question reduce the impact of their biases on the conclusions reached.

Diagnosis and Prognosis

Clinicians integrate various sources of data and information to arrive at an evidence-based diagnosis, if relevant. The prognosis, including possibility for improvement, is described when relevant. Clinicians who perform capacity assessments should understand that neurocognitive and psychiatric disorders in and of themselves do not indicate incapacity. Moberg and Gibney (2005) note that "a person's inability to complete a task may reflect executional rather than decisional incapacity" (p. 493). For example, a person's difficulty managing their finances may result from an inability to see bank statements or small details in a checkbook rather than poor financial decision making per se. In such instances, identifying and recommending assistive devices or environmental adaptations becomes essential.

Capacity Opinion

The clinician provides an opinion regarding capacity to make the decision or engage in the behavior in question, with the understanding that a diagnosis does not imply impaired capacity. Ideally, the information and data obtained from the multimethod evaluation converge to clarify the patient's capacity, allowing the clinician to conclude that the patient *retains* capacity or *lacks* capacity. Clear statements regarding whether the patient retains or lacks capacity are most helpful to referral sources and decision makers. Statements such as "the patient demonstrates *diminished* capacity" are less helpful and sometimes add to the confusion. However, it is appropriate for the clinician to note fluctuating capacity when applicable. It is also important to note the decisional domain at issue. For example, a statement such as "the patient lacks the capacity to manage their finances" is clearer than a plenary statement, such as "the patient 'lacks capacity.'" When the information and data obtained appear to be contradictory or inconclusive, clinicians should consider whether (1) additional information or clarification should be obtained, (2) consultation with a colleague would be helpful, and/or (3) their self-confidence in rendering an opinion is lacking. Considering these options and obtaining the additional information, assistance, or clarity can help the clinician transition to a more confident and useful conclusion.

Recommendations

Clinicians consider whether medications or other treatments or environmental changes could improve capacity or clinical care and make such recommendations as indicated.

Report Results and Final Steps

Depending on the purpose and context of the evaluation, the clinician provides a written report, verbal feedback, or other follow-up services to the referral source, patient, and/or other involved parties. Clinicians document the process for their own records.

Complex Medicolegal Case Example

Mr. C. is a 78-year-old man currently living on his own in California. His neighbors have reported concerns that he wanders in the evenings and appears confused at times, but other times appears lucid. There has also been a report from his bank that his account has shown some unusual activity, including multiple US $500 ATM withdrawals and liquidation of some investment accounts. Mr. C is a diabetic. He is a retired professor, widower, with two adult children who live out of the area. He was hospitalized a few months ago because of a urinary tract infection (UTI).

When you met with Mr. C. you found that he was mostly oriented and able to walk and complete basic activities of daily living (ADLs). His home was a bit cluttered and somewhat disorganized. His personal care appeared to be adequate. You asked him specifically about his recent suspicious transactions, and he denied awareness of these, claiming he never uses his ATM card. He no longer drives, so you asked him how he is getting groceries, etc. He reported that his lovely neighbor, Ms. J., has been helping him out, including taking him to the store, the doctor, and the bank. In fact, he recently made Janice his Power of Attorney (POA) for finances in case he becomes incapacitated.

Subsequently, Mr. C. contracted the flu and was admitted to the hospital. There was a question about whether or not he could be discharged home. He was insisting he was "OK" and could hire help if needed. He reported that he prefers to manage his diabetes with "diet."

You were asked to conduct a capacity assessment. The legal capacity issues involve medical decision making, care planning, and financial decision making. Each of these capacity issues must be considered in turn following the SCAP. While the psychological and cognitive assessments would be the same, the specific legal standards and functional components would differ depending upon the legal question, capacity issue, and the jurisdiction in which the evaluation was performed.

In this case, the preassessment concerns involved awareness of the legal issues in question. In terms of informed consent, Mr. C. did not have a Healthcare Power of Attorney (HPOA), and capacity was presumed, with the safeguards from the APA Ethics Code considered. Mr. C. reported that he understood the purpose and procedure of the capacity assessment and gave both written permission and verbal assent to continue. The next step, record review, documented his medical history which included diabetes, UTIs, and two hospitalizations in the past year for a fall and the flu. In the interview, Mr. C. did not have awareness of any suspicious financial transactions.

Overall, the neuropsychological findings indicated that Mr. C. had moderate cognitive impairment with performance on the Montreal Cognitive Assessment (MoCA; Nasreddine et al., 2005) at 15 out of 30 (more than 2 standard deviations below the mean; Rossetti et al., 2011). Further neurocognitive assessment indicated deficits primarily in the domains of memory and executive functioning, with intact language. The results of other cognitive domains were more mixed.

Performance on self-report measures of emotional state did not indicate depression or anxiety. In terms of his functional abilities, Mr. C. retained the ability to manage ADLs for personal care but struggled with instrumental ADLs (IADLs) including money management, medication management, and driving. Mr. C. was also asked about his values and preferences regarding his decision making. He reported that he had a strong preference to involve his adult children in his decision making and intended to leave his estate to his children equally. He also indicated a preference to use diet rather than medications to manage his diabetes.

In terms of diagnosis, Mr. C.'s presentation included memory impairment and deficits in executive functioning in the context of relatively spared language and social skills, consistent with major neurocognitive disorder due to Alzheimer's disease.

Given the above findings from the clinical assessment, the assessment of the capacity issues had to be considered next. In this matter, the first issue considered was his ability to manage his medical care. Decisional capacity requires that an individual have the ability to understand, appreciate, reason, and express a choice. Poor memory and executive functioning can impact understanding, appreciation, and reasoning. There was evidence that he was not able to actively manage his medications and that he would need formal assistance to manage his health, including maintaining a healthy diet. Further, his impairments in memory and executive functioning diminished awareness of his finances and his ability to manage them in his best interest. In this case, his neighbor was removed as POA, and his adult son stepped in to serve as conservator.

Conclusions and Implications

Making decisions about possibly limiting another person's freedoms and right to self-determination can be as challenging as it is significant. Multiple constructs must be considered and evaluated when making capacity determinations. Psychologists play an essential role in the assessment of capacity. Use of standardized assessment measures enhances the multimethod assessment process by helping to establish an empirical evidence base for the opinion that is ultimately rendered. It is the clinician's responsibility to select the assessment measures to best meet the needs of the specific evaluation and context. A systematic approach to the evaluation process allows the clinician to arrive at an opinion that reflects a balance between beneficence and respect for patient autonomy, and serves the needs of the parties involved.

Suggested Resources on Decisional Capacity

American Bar Association Commission on Law and Aging & American Psychological Association. (2008). *Assessment of older adults with diminished capacity: A handbook for psychologists.*

American Psychological Association Office on Aging. (2012). *Capacity assessment training needs.*

Demakis, G. J. (Ed.) (2012). *Civil capacities in clinical neuropsychology.* Oxford University Press.

Lichtenberg, P. A., Teresi, J. A., Ocepek-Welikson, K., & Eimicke, J. P. (2017). Reliability and validity of the Lichtenberg Financial Decision Screening Scale. *Innovation in aging, 1*(1), igx003. https://doi.org/10.1093/geroni/igx003

References

American Bar Association Commission on Law and Aging. (2016). *Role of clinical evaluation professionals in adult guardianship proceedings: Survey of state statutes.* http://www.americanbar.org/content/dam/aba/administrative/law_aging/chartclinicaleval.authcheckdam.pdf

American Bar Association Commission on Law and Aging & American Psychological Association. (2008). *Assessment of older adults with diminished capacity: A handbook for psychologists.*

American Law Institute. (1981). *Restatement of the law second, contracts.*

American Psychological Association. (2014). Guidelines for psychological practice with older adults. *American Psychologist, 69,* 34–65. https://doi.org/10.1037/a0035063

American Psychological Association. (2017a). *Multicultural guidelines: An ecological approach to context, identity, and intersectionality.* http://www.apa.org/about/policy/multicultural-guidelines.pdf

American Psychological Association. (2017b). Ethical principles of psychologists and code of conduct (2002, Amended June 1, 2010 and January 1, 2017). http://www.apa.org/ethics/code/index.aspx

Blackhall, L. J., Murphy, S. T., Frank, G., Michel, V., & Azen, S. (1995). Ethnicity and attitudes toward patient autonomy. *JAMA, 274,* 820–825. https://doi.org/10.1001/jama.1995.03530100060035

Borchard Foundation Center for Law and Aging. (2010). *Undue influence definitions and applications: Final report.* http://www.courts.ca.gov/documents/UndueInfluence.pdf.

Bush, S. S. (2009). *Geriatric mental health ethics: A casebook.* Springer.

Bush, S. S. (2012). Ethical considerations in the psychological evaluation and treatment of older adults. In S. J. Knapp (Ed.), *APA handbook of ethics in psychology: Vol. 2. Practice, teaching, and research* (pp. 15–28). American Psychological Association. https://doi.org/10.1037/13272-002

Bush, S. S., Allen, R. S., Heck, A. L., & Moye, J. (2015). Ethical issues in geropsychology: Clinical and forensic perspectives. *Psychological Injury and Law, 8,* 348–356. https://doi.org/10.1007/s12207-015-9242-2

Bush, S. S., Allen, R. S., & Molinari, V. A. (2017). *Ethical practice in geropsychology.* American Psychological Association. https://doi.org/10.1037/0000010-000

Byrd, D. A., & Manly, J. J. (2005). Cultural considerations in the neuropsychological assessment of older adults. In S. S. Bush & T. A. Martin (Eds.), *Geriatric neuropsychology: Practice essentials* (pp. 115–139). Psychology Press.

Demakis, G. J. (2012). Introduction to basic issues in civil capacities. In G. J. Demakis (Ed.), *Civil capacities in clinical neuropsychology: Research findings and practical applications* (pp. 3–16). Oxford University Press.

Demakis, G. J., & Mart, E. G. (2018). Civil capacities. In S. S. Bush, G. J. Demakis, & M. L. Rohling (Eds.), *APA handbook of forensic neuropsychology* (pp. 309–339). American Psychological Association.

Dudley, K. C., & Edmonds, N. (2018). Psychology's role in guardianship and conservatorship evaluations. In S. S. Bush & A. L. Heck (Eds.), *Forensic geropsychology: Practice essentials* (pp. 257–279). American Psychological Association.

Glen, K. B. (2014, May-June). The perils of guardianship and the promise of supported decision-making. *Clearinghouse Review Journal of Poverty Law and Policy*, 17–22.

Grisso, T., & Appelbaum, P. S. (1998). *MacArthur competency assessment tool for treatment (MacCAT-T)*. Professional Resource Press.

Hoffman, N. (2018). The assessment of testamentary capacity and undue influence in the older adult. In S. S. Bush & A. L. Heck (Eds.), *Forensic geropsychology: Practice essentials* (pp. 213–234). American Psychological Association.

Kapp, M. B., & Mossman, D. (1996). Measuring decisional capacity: Cautions of the construction of a "capacimeter." *Psychology, Public Policy, and Law, 2,* 73–95. https://doi.org/10.1037/1076-8971.2.1.73

Karel, M. J. (2011). Ethics. In V. Molinari (Ed.), *Specialty competencies in geropsychology* (pp. 115–143). Oxford University Press. https://doi.org/10.1093/med:psych/9780195385670.003.0009

Kim, S. Y. H., Appelbaum, P. S., Kim, H. M., Wall, I. F., Bourgeois, J. A., Frankel, B., Hails, K. C., Rundell, J. R., Seibel, K. M., & Karlawish, J. H. (2011). Variability of judgments of capacity: Experience of capacity evaluators in a study of research consent capacity. *Psychosomatics, 52,* 346–353. https://doi.org/10.1016/j.psym.2011.01.012

Knight, B. G., Karel, M. J., Hinrichsen, G. A., Qualls, S. H., & Duffy, M. (2009). Pikes Peak model for training in professional geropsychology. *American Psychologist, 64,* 205–214. https://doi.org/10.1037/a0015059

Kohn, N. A., Blumenthal, J. A., & Campbell, A. T. (2013). Supported decision-making: A viable alternative to guardianship. *Penn State Law Review, 117,* 1111–1157. https://doi.org/10.2139/ssrn.2161115

Lichtenberg, P. A., Qualls, S. H., & Smyer, M. A. (2015). Competency and decision-making capacity: Negotiating health and financial decision making. In P. A. Lichtenberg, B. T. Mast, B. D. Carpenter, & J. Loebach Weatherall (Eds.), *APA handbook of clinical geropsychology: Vol. 2. Assessment, treatment, and issues of late life* (pp. 553–578). American Psychological Association. https://doi.org/10.1037/14459-021

Marson, D. C., McInturff, B., Hawkins, L., Bartolucci, A., & Harrell, L. E. (1997). Consistency of physician judgments of capacity to consent in mild Alzheimer's disease. *Journal of the American Geriatrics Society, 45,* 453–457. https://doi.org/10.1111/j.1532-5415.1997.tb05170.x

Moberg, P. J., & Gibney, M. (2005). Decision-making capacity in the impaired older adult. In S. S. Bush & T. A. Martin (Eds.), *Geriatric neuropsychology: Practice essentials* (pp. 491–506). Psychology Press.

Moberg, P. J., & Kniele, K. (2006). Evaluation of competency: Ethical considerations for neuropsychologists. *Applied Neuropsychology, 13,* 101–114. https://doi.org/10.1207/s15324826an1302_5

Moye, J., Karel, M. J., Edelstein, B., Hicken, B., Armesto, J. C., & Gurrera, R. J. (2007). Assessment of the capacity to consent to treatment. *Clinical Gerontologist, 31,* 37–66. https://doi.org/10.1080/07317110802072140

Moye, J., Marson, D. C., & Edelstein, B. (2013). Assessment of capacity in an aging society. *American Psychologist, 68,* 158–171. https://doi.org/10.1037/a0032159

Nasreddine, Z. S., Phillips, N. A., Bedirian, V., Charbonneau, S., Whitehead, V., Colin, I. Cummings, J. L., Chertkow, H. (2005). The Montreal Cognitive Assessment, MoCA: A brief screening tool for mild cognitive impairment. *Journal of the American Geriatrics Society, 53,* 695–699. https://doi.org/10.1111/j.1532-5415.2005.53221.x

O'Brien, R. C. (2013). Attorney responsibility and client incapacity. *The Journal of Contemporary Health Law and Policy, 30,* 59–95.

Palzer, J. Y. (2018). Assessment of age-related cognitive changes and dementia in Chinese and Chinese American older adults. In G. E. Smith (Ed.), *APA handbook of dementia* (pp. 125–140). American Psychological Association. https://doi.org/10.1037/0000076-007

Peisah, C., Brodaty, H., & Quadrio, C. (2006). Family conflict in dementia: Prodigal sons and black sheep. *International Journal of Geriatric Psychiatry, 21,* 485–492. https://doi.org/10.1002/gps.1501

Pinsker, D. M., Pachana, N. A., Wilson, J., Tilse, C., & Byrne, G. J. (2010). Financial capacity in older adults: A review of clinical assessment approaches and considerations. *Clinical Gerontologist: The Journal of Aging and Mental Health, 33*(4), 332–346. https://doi.org/10.1080/07317115.2010.502107

Quinn, M. J. (2002). Undue influence and elder abuse: Recognition and intervention strategies. *Geriatric Nursing, 23,* 11–16. https://doi.org/10.1067/mgn.2002.122560

Rossetti, H. C., Lacritz, L. H., Cullum, C. M., & Weiner, M. F. (2011). Normative data for the Montreal Cognitive Assessment (MoCA) in a population-based sample. *Neurology, 77,* 1272–1275. https://doi.org/10.1212/WNL.0b013e318230208a

Seyfried, L., Ryan, K. A., & Kim, S. Y. H. (2013). Assessment of decision-making capacity: Views and experiences of consultation psychiatrists. *Psychosomatics, 54,* 115–123. https://doi.org/10.1016/j.psym.2012.08.001

Tan, Y. I., Burgess, G. H., & Green, R. J. (2020). The effects of acculturation on neuropsychological test performance: A systematic literature review. *Clinical Neuropsychologist.* Advance online publication. https://doi.org/10.1080/13854046.2020.1714740

Chapter 9
Elder Abuse: Navigating Ethical and Legal Responsibilities

Kyle S. Page
Nabeel T. Yehyawi

Introduction

Elder abuse is a complex issue and requires a coordinated response to address its multifaceted impact. In 2017, the World Health Organization (WHO) estimated that one in six older adults were experiencing some form of abuse (Yon et al., 2017), with current estimates widely recognized to underrepresent the scope of the problem (Jackson, 2018; Pillemer et al., 2016). Identification of elder abuse will become increasingly important as the number of adults over the age of 60 is expected to increase globally to 2.1 billion by 2050, including a threefold increase in persons over the age of 80 (United Nations, 2017). In concert with these growing concerns, legal professionals are increasing protections for vulnerable older adults. For example, in the US, the Elder Justice Act (as part of the Patient Protection and Affordable Care Act, P.L. 111-148) and the Elder Abuse Prevention and Prosecution Act (P.L. 115-70) serve to coordinate a federal response to understanding and addressing abuse. With increasing social and legal awareness, our understanding of elder abuse is benefiting from collaborative efforts to define, recognize, and develop cultural-specific conceptualizations and interventions.

Psychologists encountering older adults in their clinical practice will need to know how to identify and respond to elder abuse. Indeed, the importance of addressing this topic clinically, particularly identifying and acting upon the risk of elder abuse, is reinforced in professional practice guidelines and recommendations for the development of geropsychology competencies (e.g., American Psychological Association, 2014; Knight et al., 2009), acknowledging the unique legal and ethical situations surrounding elder abuse. Referrals for psychological services may be related to abuse or suspicion of abuse, or more likely, suspicion may arise in the course of another unrelated clinical encounter. This chapter serves as an introduction to the topic of elder abuse, to the challenges clinicians face when addressing this issue, and to possible courses of action in practice.

Defining Elder Abuse

Many definitions of elder abuse exist due to the involvement of various stakeholders, including researchers, federal agencies, and state and federal jurisdictions. In fact, this creates a barrier to standardizing research, not only among organizations within the US, but also across countries (Hall et al., 2016). Depending on the intended scope, elder abuse may also be referred to as elder mistreatment (National Research Council, 2003), incorporating a broader view on the experiences of later life, including but not limited to, loss of respect and dignity and ageist practices. In this chapter, we will use the definition proposed by WHO:

> a single or repeated act, or lack of appropriate action, occurring within any relationship where there is an expectation of trust, which causes harm or distress to an older person (aged 60 years and older). It includes physical, sexual, psychological/emotional abuse, financial and material abuse, abandonment, neglect, and serious loss of dignity and respect. (WHO, 2018)

Importantly, no single definition has emerged as the standard, but most specify the presence of a relationship of trust. The Centers for Disease Control and Prevention recently proposed definitions for elder abuse and related variables in an effort to advance standardization (Hall et al., 2016).

Psychologists should not confuse organizational and research definitions of elder abuse with those outlined in their specific jurisdictions of practice. State statutes defining elder abuse vary greatly, and may incorporate specific examples of abuse, different benchmarks for what constitutes an "elder," criteria for vulnerability, and potential mandatory actions for the public and professionals. For these reasons, it is important to be familiar with your local region or state's definition, as this will ultimately determine how you respond clinically to suspected abuse. For example, the state of Wyoming includes photographing vulnerable adults, in their definition of elder abuse (Wyo. Stat. § 35-20-102), whereas the state of Illinois does not specifically mention this, although this action could be conceptualized as causing mental injury (320 ILCS 20).

Across the various definitions of elder abuse in use today, there are five generally recognized forms: (a) physical abuse (intentional use of physical force that results in distress, pain, injury, or a person's death); (b) sexual abuse (any unwanted sexual activity, including verbal and physical acts); (c) abandonment or neglect (failure to protect a dependent older adult from harm or to provide for their essential needs); (d) emotional and psychological abuse (verbal and nonverbal behavior that results in distress, fear, or anguish); and (e) financial abuse and exploitation (improper use of an older adult's money or assets for the benefit of another) (Hall et al., 2016; National Research Council, 2003; Roberto, 2016).

While these organizational and legal definitions of elder abuse offer us one point of reference in understanding this complex issue, we recognize that most definitions in the US were developed largely from a European-American perspective (Patterson & Malley-Morrison, 2006). Enguidanos et al. (2014) have argued for more inclusivity in how we understand and define elder abuse, joining calls for the development of a culture-specific understanding (e.g., Moon, 2000). Cultural background may influence perceptions of (un) acceptable behavior, what constitutes abusive behavior, and what steps are appropriate to take to address the issue (Jackson, 2018; Moon, 2000; Roberto, 2016). Unfortunately, less is known about the impact of racial, ethnic, and cultural perspectives on one's understanding of abuse. Nevertheless, Moon (2000) cautions that a broader perspective from non-professionals (i.e., older adults) is needed to increase our understanding of abuse in the context of the diversity found in later life.

Several studies have offered cultural-specific conceptualizations of abuse, including disrespect, discrimination, and lack of recognition (Cadmus et al., 2015; Enguidanos et al., 2014; Tam & Neysmith, 2006). One project focusing on developing countries identified common themes of violation (e.g., social isolation, exclusion), neglect, and deprivation (e.g., of choices, status, respect) as community-identified abusive situations (WHO & International Network for the Prevention of Elder Abuse, 2002). However, data are still lacking for certain areas of the world, including Africa and South America (Dong, 2015), as well as an understanding of within-group variability and generational differences. Hernandez-Tejada and colleagues (2013) have highlighted that studies focused on race and ethnicity have yielded mixed results, likely due to confounding variables. Language and level of acculturation have emerged as variables warranting consideration. Importantly, clinicians working with older adults need to understand the relational context, including traditional norms for how family members interact with one another. In summary, these findings have brought attention to how current legal conceptualizations of elder abuse may not align with the diverse reality of older adults. When we include more relevant stakeholders, our professional and societal understanding of elder abuse will undoubtedly shift, forcing a reconceptualization of abuse on various levels.

Prevalence of Elder Abuse

In his 1975 letter to the *British Medical Journal*, G. R. Burston (1975) first called upon the scientific literature to identify elder abuse as a pressing social issue that warranted further study and intervention. Since that time, the research on elder abuse has indeed found it to be a considerable public health problem (Eslami et al., 2016), yet its prevalence has varied across studies depending on the country in which the study took place (Pillemer et al., 2016), and the type of elder abuse being assessed (Burnes et al., 2015; Peterson et al., 2014; Laumann et al., 2008). Internationally, research has found that the prevalence rate of elder abuse ranges from 2.2% to 14%, with the highest rates being reported in India (14%), the US (7.6%), and Europe (6.03%; Pillemer et al., 2016). Further complicating epidemiological matters, many older adults suffer from multiple types of abuse simultaneously (i.e., polyvictimization; Hamby et al., 2016), and current estimates of the prevalence of all types of elder mistreatment may underestimate the scope of the problem as a result of multiple factors.

First, older adults may be less likely to share issues of personal conflict or violence with others (Bonnie & Wallace, 2003). Second, in relying largely on the self-report of community-dwelling older adults who are able to take part in such surveys, many prevalence studies may inadvertently exclude older adults with dementia, a condition that has been found to increase one's risk of abuse and/or mistreatment (Dong et al., 2014). Third, due to methodological factors, such studies often do not take into account those older adults who reside in residential care facilities, which has made estimating the prevalence of elder abuse in this specific population quite challenging (McDonald et al., 2012).

Despite these limitations, a 2015 review article in the *New England Journal of Medicine* suggested that, after considering the available evidence, a reasonable estimate of the overall prevalence of elder abuse in the US is approximately 10% (Lachs & Pillemer, 2015). This is important for any psychologist who works with older adults to recognize, as it means that they are likely to regularly encounter individuals suffering from elder abuse in their practice. Moreover, given the rapidly increasing older adult population, it also means that psychologists will likely encounter cases of elder abuse even more often in the future, such that improving their ability to identify and address this important social problem becomes ever more important.

Risk Factors and Barriers

Over the past 20 years, there has been a considerable amount of empirical research identifying the risk factors associated with the victims of elder abuse (Storey, 2020). An international review of the scientific literature on the subject found substantial evidence that functional dependence and/or disability, poor physical health, cognitive impairment or dementia, mental health problems, and low socioeconomic status all increased the risk of an older adult being susceptible to elder abuse or mistreatment, with only potential, mixed evidence to suggest that female gender and financial dependence also did so (Pillemer et al., 2016). There have also been indications that, compared with individuals suffering from a single type of abuse, older adults suffering from multiple types of abuse simultaneously experience greater fear, longer durations of abuse, and have poorer outcomes (Jackson & Hafemeister, 2012).

Research has produced mixed results with regard to the effects of racial and ethnic variations in both the susceptibility to elder abuse and the different level of risk for different types of elder abuse, such that further research is needed to clarify the differences between and within these groups (Burnes et al., 2015). For example, some studies have found that African-American older adults are more at risk for financial and psychological and/or emotional abuse than European-American older adults. Further, there have also been some studies that have found Hispanic older adults to have a lower risk of abuse and neglect than other racial or ethnic groups (Laumann et al., 2008), which may reflect the close family bonds and respect for older people that are often strong cultural values within the Hispanic community (Montoya, 1998). Research on protective factors against victimization, including studies of individuals in the US, Canada, Europe, India, and Israel, have indeed found strong evidence that greater social support and connectedness to one's social network/community lower one's risk of elder abuse. However, it is important to recognize that such connections do not make older adults immune to elder abuse or mistreatment, as research has also found that some older adults may be more vulnerable to abuse because they are less likely to report mistreatment to those who do not share their language, community, or culture (DeLiema et al., 2012).

Unfortunately, while research on the factors that place older adults at risk of victimization has been burgeoning in recent decades, there have been far fewer studies designed to increase our understanding of the risk factors associated with the perpetrators of elder abuse (Pillemer et al., 2016). Despite the comparative dearth of literature on this group, there have been several studies sufficient to provide at least a preliminary risk factor profile of those likely to victimize older adults. Pillemer and colleagues (2016) observed that individuals with mental health problems, who misuse alcohol and/or drugs, or who are dependent on an older adult for support (i.e., emotional, financial, and housing), are at increased risk of being a perpetrator of elder abuse. Another recent review examined the characteristics of professionals who are likely to abuse older adults within institutions and found that male gender, being front-line work staff member, having limited qualifications and/or professional skills, and the stress level of the institution work environment were all related to an increased risk of an individual becoming an abuser (Kamavarapu et al., 2017). In any case, while these risk factors may be helpful in preventing elder abuse, the literature does suggest that elder abuse perpetrators represent a heterogeneous group and that research aimed at better understanding the factors that increase risk of both victims and perpetrators is still needed (Jackson, 2016).

Ethics and Elder Abuse

Psychologists aspire to ethical practice in accordance with the American Psychological Association's (APA) Ethical Principles of Psychologists and Code of Conduct (hereafter referred to as the APA ethics code; APA, 2017), though the complexity of the ethical considerations associated with elder abuse can be challenging (Scheiderer, 2012; Saghafi et al., 2019). While the APA ethics code does not specifically mention elder abuse per se, many of the general principles and ethical standards clearly apply to this important issue (APA, 2017). Indeed, the APA ethics code calls on psychologists to respect the rights and dignity of others (Principle E; APA, 2017), which includes both being aware of the importance of a person's right to autonomy and self-determination, and being aware that special safeguards may be needed to protect the rights of vulnerable individuals in circumstances that may impair their ability to make autonomous decisions for themselves. Further, psychologists also ethically strive both to do no harm and to benefit those with whom they work (Principle A: Beneficence and Non-Malfeasance; APA, 2017). The ethical complexities of elder abuse perhaps are most easily recognized when these principles come into conflict with the need to maintain the confidentiality of patients (Standard 4.01; APA, 2017), which is why it is important for psychologists to know the mandatory reporting laws in their state or area of jurisdiction, and to discuss how such laws may place limits on confidentiality, at the beginning of any professional relationship with a patient (Standards 4.02 & 4.05; APA, 2017). Yet, perhaps the APA ethical standard that is most often overlooked in the context of elder abuse is the requirement that psychologists practice only within the boundaries of their competence (Standard 2.01; APA, 2017). After all, Guideline 19 of the APA "Guidelines for Psychological Practice with Older Adults" (APA, 2014) calls on psychologists to strive to understand the special ethical and/or legal issues entailed in providing services to older adults. Therefore, it can be argued that those who choose to work with older adults have an ethical duty to acquire the training, continuing education, and professional experiences necessary to competently identify and address elder abuse in their clinical practice (Scheiderer, 2012).

Screening for Elder Abuse

There are multiple factors that may contribute to elder abuse being both underidentified and underreported, which is why it is important for psychologists who work with older adults to become more adept at identifying and addressing these concerns. Yet, elder abuse can be difficult to identify even for those professionals trained to do so. Many older adults have chronic medical conditions and physical traits that can mask the signs of elder abuse or cause others to dismiss them as merely being due to aging (Dyer et al., 2003). The physical signs of abuse may also be quite subtle or may even diminish to subclinical levels by the time the victim interacts with someone trained to identify them (Burnett et al., 2014). For this reason, it is important for psychologists who work with those at risk of elder abuse to have some time to speak alone with the older adult during sessions, in the absence of caregivers. Doing so allows the psychologist the opportunity to directly ask nonthreatening questions about any indicators of possible abuse that are identified. Further, psychologists should also be alert to other signs of elder abuse, such as older adult patients frequently deferring questions to their caregivers, increasing isolation from friends and family, presenting with poor hygiene (i.e., neglect or self-neglect), nonadherence to their medication regimen, and/or having difficulties paying bills, as all may be suggestive of possible abuse (Lachs & Pillemer, 2015).

In addition to the signs and symptoms of elder abuse that may be detected during clinical visits, there has been a call in the literature for the development and use of structured screening tools to better aid providers in identifying elder abuse in their clients and patients (Cohen, 2011). According to National Center on Elder Abuse (NCEA, 2016), there is currently no gold standard screening measure to identify elder abuse, but many such screening tools have been developed for use by health care providers. One type of screening tool provides a guide of direct questions for a health care provider to ask an older adult to encourage disclosure of any current abusive experiences. These measures include the Hwalek-Sengstock Elder Abuse Screening Test (H-S/EAST; Neale et al., 1991), the Vulnerability to Abuse Screening Scale (VASS; Schofield & Mishra, 2003), and the Elder Abuse Suspicion Index (EASI; Yaffe et al., 2008). These measures are perhaps best suited for use with cognitively intact older adults (Cohen, 2011); however, in cases of cognitive decline or dementia, interviewing the caregiver becomes even more important. In designing screening tools for caregivers, it is essential that such measures involve asking direct questions in a nonconfrontational manner to increase the likelihood of identifying a potentially abusive situation. The Caregiver Abuse Screen (CASE) is an example of one such measure designed for this purpose (Reis & Nahmiash, 1995).

There are also a host of other elder abuse screening tools available, though opinions vary as to their utility. The US National Center on Elder Abuse (2016) points out that screening by professionals may help to identify or prevent elder abuse earlier without noticeable harm. However, there are also concerns that such screenings may not detect financial abuse and neglect as well as other forms of abuse, may further burden the already underresourced US Adult Protective Services agencies, and in cases of false negatives may result in even fewer reports of elder abuse by health care providers. Indeed, the US Preventative Services Task Force (2018) concluded that there was currently insufficient evidence to recommend that all older and vulnerable adults be screened for elder abuse and neglect. Thus, while brief screening measures have many benefits, they also have many weaknesses, such that further research is warranted to meet the call of health care providers who continue to seek a valid, concise, and user-friendly screening tool to more quickly identify and aid elder abuse victims (see Brijnath et al., 2020; Jackson, 2018).

Reporting Elder Abuse

Whenever there is a reasonable suspicion of elder abuse, it is important to report it to the appropriate agency to ensure that potential victims are able to get the help they need as soon as possible. Since the 1980s, many US states have passed legislation to help protect and assist older adults being abused, neglected, or exploited (McPherson & Koltai, 2018). However, state laws differ with regard to when and how to report suspected abuse of older adults to the appropriate adult protective services agency. The website of the US NCEA provides state resources to assist health care providers, including a listing of the laws specific to each state, which, at the time of this writing, can be found at https://ncea.acl.gov/Resources/State.aspx. Another resource that may be beneficial is the Eldercare Locator (https://eldercare.acl.gov/public/index.aspx), which can be used to find the locations and contact information of local agencies and organizations that focus on older adult services and elder abuse prevention. Interventions may range from supportive community assistance to appointment of surrogate decision makers; however, it is worth noting that even in these instances, appointing from abuse is not guaranteed (e.g., United States Government Accountability Office, 2016).

The Role of Capacity

Clinicians who encounter an older adult in a potentially abusive or exploitative situation will undoubtedly find themselves needing to consider and address issues of capacity (i.e., decision-making capacity, or the older adult's ability to safely make their own decisions, and functional capacity, or their ability to perform tasks that allow them to be in such a situation). Psychologists are uniquely qualified to inform others about what an older adult is still able to do independently and/or what supports may still need to be put in place to ensure their safety. As it relates to suspected elder abuse, adult protection agencies (or their equivalents depending on the jurisdiction) may request a psychologist's clinical opinion about an alleged victim's vulnerability, their cognitive status, their functional status, and their capacity status, as all of these issues may affect if and how to best move forward to aid the individual at risk.

Historically, the legal and clinical conceptualizations of capacity have been viewed much more broadly than they are currently. Thanks to advocacy and reform efforts, our clinical conceptualization of capacity has been transformed over the last several decades and continues to evolve today. Whereas capacity statements in the past may have used global terms to describe an individual as "incompetent" to care for themselves or their affairs, today we respect that people have multiple *capacities* and that the conceptualization and evaluation of these must be tailored to the individual (Moye & Wood, 2020). The American Bar Association and American Psychological Association's *Handbook for Psychologists* (2008) encourages psychologists to consider multiple aspects of an individual's values, history, and abilities, while also taking into account the urgency and risks, available supports, and the specific situation, as they attempt to balance an individual's safety with the individual's right to self-determination and autonomy. See Chapter 8 in the current work for an expanded discussion of capacity and its assessment.

While medical and financial decisions are common referral questions for capacity evaluations, perhaps more challenging is determining if an individual has the capacity to decide to remain in an abusive or exploitative situation. Given the emphasis on self-determination in Western societies, adults in abusive or exploitative situations can and do turn down assistance from clinicians, law enforcement, and protection agencies. Psychologists will find little practical guidance in evaluating capacity to remain in a suspected abusive relationship or situation, especially when there is concomitant evidence of cognitive and functional decline. It is important to recognize that while the purpose of such evaluations is not to determine if abuse has indeed occurred, which is a legal matter, a capacity evaluation may still be beneficial in determining an older adult's understanding of the situation, and their level of functioning given their current context. An evaluation may take or borrow perspectives from other areas of the capacity literature, such as the capacity for independent living (managing their home environment, medical needs, finances, and general personal safety practices), or be tailored to specific concerns such as financial capacity if questions about financial abuse arise. While each type of capacity has its own unique history, literature, and research, several core components have emerged over the years and have been applied to diverse areas such as medical decision making, financial capacity, and independent living. These components are understanding the information relevant to the decisions, appreciating the risks/benefits and likely outcomes of a choice, reasoning through the decision, and being able to express that choice (Grisso & Appelbaum, 1998). Some areas, such as financial capacity, have accrued a substantial literature on assessment approaches (Pinsker et al., 2010), including innovative client-centered approaches for those living with dementia (Lichtenberg et al., 2015).

If a person is clinically determined to lack capacity in a certain area or for a certain task, you must follow local regulations on reporting. If they do not lack capacity for the situation you are evaluating, offer help with safety planning, emergency phone numbers, supportive services, and resources in these situations (Lachs & Pillemer, 2004). Ideally, with sufficient rapport, clinicians can keep the conversation going and monitor an older adult's risk over time during future visits.

Consideration of Undue Influence

While not a type of elder abuse as defined in this chapter, undue influence can certainly be used as a tool to commit elder abuse, making it an important concept to understand when working with older adults. Undue influence is a coercive or exploitative situation where a relationship is used deceptively to undermine the free will of another individual. These instances may also involve creating an environment of duress or fear to gain control of a vulnerable individual's decision-making process, ultimately suppressing self-determination (Stiegel & Quinn, 2017). The concept of undue influence has long been recognized in legal theory but is also found in psychological and sociological research (Wood & Liu, 2012). Therefore, like elder abuse, undue influence can be understood in terms of legal, research, and clinical applications. Statutory definitions of undue influence, if available at all, vary from state to state, but may include conditions of a confidential relationship, a susceptible individual, a power differential, and coercion (Marson et al., 2004). Given the variability, this is another reason it is important for psychologists to be both knowledgeable and current regarding specific legislation and policy in their area.

Legal professionals often turn to mental health clinicians for an evaluation of cognition, mental health, and capacity to help with the conceptualization of vulnerability. Clinicians are well-positioned to use interview and standardized assessment skills to understand patient and situational factors. Some legal professionals encourage clinicians to assist with describing the individual and vulnerabilities, rather than deciding whether undue influence occurred – a process for a court to decide (Spar et al., 1995). Importantly, undue influence is a related but separate construct to capacity. When evaluating a specific capacity, concern about undue influence may arise. However, someone does not necessarily need to lack decision-making capacity to be unduly influenced. Under the right conditions, it is argued, all persons are vulnerable (Quinn, 2001). Several conceptual models exist but lack widespread application and empirical support (ABA & APA, 2008). Across these models, specific social conditions (e.g., isolation from friends), individual factors (e.g., cognitive impairment), or risks (e.g., change of a will inconsistent with previous wishes) are identified and may assist in increasing awareness of when to assess further. Increased social engagement may protect an older adult from undue influence (Quinn, 2000).

Most research examining undue influence and capacity relates to financial and testamentary capacity, but such manipulative interpersonal activity can occur in other forms of abuse (e.g., sexual) and capacities (e.g., medical). Few tools exist to assist a clinician in identifying undue influence. In contrast to a capacity evaluation, which often assesses the abilities of an older adult at a specific point in time, an evaluation of undue influence focuses on a process over time. In one translational project, Quinn et al. (2017) developed a screening tool for adult protective service employees, matching their tool to state-specific definitions. Using a checklist approach, reviewers identify potential client vulnerabilities (e.g., problems with memory, language or literacy barriers, living in a dysfunctional environment), influencer's authority and power factors (e.g., an individual standing in a position of trust or authority, access to documents or private information), specific actions or tactics that may have transpired (e.g., influencer controls access to information, changes the address, solicits loans), and for any unfair or improper outcome (e.g., economic loss, identity theft, negative emotional changes). Clinicians new to the assessment of undue influence will want to seek out professional consultation, given the many ethical and legal challenges involved.

Self-Neglect and Crimes Against Older Adults

Given that most definitions of elder abuse conceptualize the involvement of a relationship of trust (either through family, formal caregiving, or legal representation), older adults who are exhibiting signs of self-neglect or are victims of certain crimes are often not included in these statistics and discussions. These are beyond the scope of this chapter but are referred to here due to their importance. Self-neglect involves an adult who is unable to meet basic needs to ensure their own welfare and safety to such an extent that there is a risk for injury, illness, or death. This is often a factor in long-term care placement (Lachs et al., 2002) and requires special attention. Psychologists may also encounter confirmed or suspected crimes committed against older adults, such as those perpetrated by individuals unknown to the person. The US Senate Special Committee on Aging, which hosts a national fraud hotline, has estimated that nearly US $3 billion were lost in 1 year due to financial scams alone (United States Senate Special Committee on Aging, 2019), including IRS impersonations or lottery scams. Psychologists involved in these situations may need to consider clinical ramifications of cognitive decline and questionable financial capacity (Wood & Lichtenberg, 2017).

Case Example: Elder Abuse

Mrs. H. is a 78-year-old Salvadoran-American woman with a history of hypertension, mild cognitive impairment, and gait instability who presented to a primary care appointment accompanied by her 35-year-old grandson, Ray, who lives with her and serves as her primary caregiver. English is Mrs. H.'s second language, and she is much more comfortable communicating in Spanish when possible, such that Ray often serves as her translator during health care visits. Records showed that whereas she had always regularly attended her physical therapy appointments in the past, she had neither attended nor cancelled such appointments over the past 6-month period. It seemed that her driver's license had been revoked approximately 6 months ago, and that she now depended on her grandson for transportation and to run various errands for her, as she was not able to ambulate for long periods of time even when using her walker. She apparently called to schedule the current appointment due to concerns about an injury she sustained during a recent fall.

As the psychologist in the primary care clinic, you receive a consultation from Mrs. H.'s primary care physician. The doctor informs you that during her examination, she noticed that Mrs. H. was quite a bit thinner than is typical and that she was not as eager to engage in conversation as she had been in the past, often deferring to her grandson to answer any question posed. The physician added that, when discussing if Mrs. H. had completed an advance directive or had identified a power-of-attorney for health care, Mrs. H. had asked, "And I can name anyone I want?" to serve as her power-of-attorney. However, the physician was surprised when her grandson interrupted and sternly told Mrs. H., "You are going to name me," which again caused Mrs. H. to become quiet and to look at the floor. Her physician informed Mrs. H. that she could indeed identify anyone she wanted to serve as her power-of-attorney for health care decisions, but this did little to reengage Mrs. H. in the conversation.

The primary care physician explained that she then asked Ray to leave the exam room so she could conduct a physical examination on Mrs. H., only to find that he became irritated and objected to leaving the room. Mrs. H. sheepishly told her grandson, "it's fine," which caused him to give her a very stern look before leaving the exam room as the physician had requested. During the exam, Dr. S. was concerned that Mrs. H.'s blood pressure had increased considerably since her last visit. Mrs. H. stated she had been taking her blood pressure medication as prescribed, but in reviewing the records, Dr. S. discovered that Mrs. H. had not recently reordered or refilled her medications with the hospital pharmacy as she always had previously. After the exam, a nurse escorted Mrs. H. back to the exam room. When the nurse returned, she related to the physician that she had discovered Ray already filling out the health care surrogate forms himself. The physician acknowledged that she discovered no signs of physical abuse during her exam, but has asked to consult with you to determine what, if any, additional steps need to be taken.

Before reading on, take a moment and consider the following questions. Should the psychologist be concerned about elder abuse? If so, what type(s)? Do you suspect Mrs. H. is being subjected to undue influence regarding the completion of an advance directive? Why or why not? Does Mrs. H. present with any risk factors that place her at a higher risk of abuse? Are there any cultural factors that are important to recognize in determining if abuse is taking place? What steps might you take next to address your concerns?

In this case example, the psychologist was concerned about psychological abuse and possible neglect, as well as the possibility of undue influence. Ray's demand that he be named her health care surrogate, his eagerness to complete the paperwork on his own, and Mrs. H.'s reaction during the visit all raised concerns about undue influence. Ray was in a position of power, as Mrs. H. was dependent on him for both transportation and caregiving. She may perceive pressure to acquiesce to his demands in order to avoid moving to a care facility. The psychologist recognized Mrs. H.'s physical limitations, her dependence on others, and her gender may all potentially raise her susceptibility to elder abuse. The psychologist also recognized that Mrs. H.'s weight loss and her atypical failure to reorder or refill her prescriptions might represent neglect due to her caregiver not effectively assisting her to meet her needs.

In planning the next steps forward, the psychologist should consider how Mrs. H.'s cultural background may both potentially serve as a protective factor against elder abuse, while also potentially making it less likely that she will involve authorities or report abuse to others who do not share her primary language. To avoid making inaccurate assumptions about Mrs. H.'s cultural background, the psychologist should discuss Mrs. H.'s unique background with her, particularly with regard to her perspectives on family interactions and her expectations of her health care providers. In addition to conducting the interview in the language Mrs. H. is most comfortable with, the psychologist might also consider administering a formal screening measure, recognizing that such a measure may not fully capture the different experiences of abuse across various cultures. In this instance, the psychologist should not rely on the grandson to serve as a translator, but rather a hospital translator should be called to assist in the session. If sincere concerns about elder abuse are indeed suspected, the psychologist may need to review the state statutes on mandatory reporting requirements and discuss these issues with Mrs. H. Of course, ideally, the limitations of confidentiality would have already been shared and reviewed with Mrs. H. at the very beginning of the encounter.

Conclusions and Implications

As we hope is evident, elder abuse represents a considerable global public health issue. Given its prevalence and the expected increasing population of older adults, elder abuse is likely to be a problem frequently encountered by any psychologist who works with the older adult population. Due to the various cultural and societal factors reviewed in this chapter, it should be apparent that psychologists working with older adults need to obtain the appropriate training, continuing education, and clinical experience to be able to identify and address cases of elder abuse that arise in their clinical practice and to be familiar with the tools and measures designed to help them to do so. It is also important for psychologists to stay abreast of the burgeoning literature on elder abuse. While the research thus far has demonstrated the impact an individual's race, culture, and language can have on the occurrence and/or reporting of elder abuse, it remains unclear to what degree these factors contribute to the clinical picture, such that further research is clearly warranted. Finally, issues related to capacity, undue influence, and potential mandatory reporting of suspected abuse vary across jurisdictions, and as such, psychologists will need to review their local regulations and consult with peers.

Suggested Resources on Elder Abuse

Literature

For additional reading on developing a culturally informed perspective on elder abuse:

Horsford, S. R., Para-Cardona, J. R., Post, L. A., & Schiamberg, L. (2010). Elder abuse and neglect in African American families: Informing practice based on ecological and cultural frameworks. *Journal of Elder Abuse and Neglect, 23,* 75–88. https://doi.org/10.1080/08946566.2011.534709

Joseph, J., & Gonzalez, A. (2018). Elder abuse in communities of color in the United States: A literature review. In P. C. Kratcoski & M. Edelbacher (Eds.), *Perspectives on elderly crime and victimization* (pp. 125–139). Springer. https://doi.org/10.1007/978-3-319-72682-3_7

Pérez-Cárceles, M. D. (2017). Elder abuse and culture: Latino anthropological and ethnographic experience. In X. Dong (Ed.), *Elder abuse: Research, practice and policy* (pp. 495–522). Springer.

For additional reading on expanding conceptualizations of elder abuse and recommendations for working with this population:

Beckman, R., Levin, M., Mantrone, L., & Solomon, J. (2020). *The things they carry: Advancing trauma-informed responses to elder abuse.* The NYC Elder Abuse Center at Weill Cornell Medicine; the Harry and Jeanette Center for Elder Justice at the Hebrew Home at Riverdale.

Roberto, K. A., & Teaster, P. B. (2017). Theorizing elder abuse. In X. Dong (Ed.), *Elder abuse: Research, practice and policy* (pp. 21–41). Springer.

Online Resources

The US National Center on Elder Abuse (NCEA) provides state resources to assist health care providers, including a listing of the laws specific to each state, which at the time of this writing, can be found at https://ncea.acl.gov/Resources/State.aspx

Eldercare Locator (http://eldercare.acl.gov/public/index.aspx), which can be used to find the locations and contact information of local agencies and organizations that focus on older adult services and elder abuse prevention.

World Health Organization (WHO) provides data, publications, and resources on elder abuse from a global and public health perspective: https://www.who.int/violence_injury_prevention/violence/elder_abuse/en/

References

American Bar Association & American Psychological Association Assessment of Capacity in Older Adults Project Working Group. (2008). *Assessment of older adults with diminished capacity: A handbook for psychologists.*

American Psychological Association. (2014). Guidelines for psychological practice with older adults. *American Psychologist, 69,* 34–65. https://doi.org/10.1037/a0035063

American Psychological Association. (2017). *Ethical principles of psychologists and code of conduct.* https://www.apa.org/ethics/code/

Bonnie, R. J., & Wallace, R. B. (2003). *Elder mistreatment: Abuse, neglect and exploitation in an aging America.* Committee on National Statistics and Committee on Law and Justice, Division of Behavioral and Social Sciences and Education, National Research Council.

Brijnath, B., Gahan, L., Gaffy, E., & Dow, B. (2020). "Build rapport, otherwise no screening tools in the world are going to help": Frontline service providers' views on current screening tools for elder abuse. *Gerontologist, 60,* 472–482. https://doi.org/10.1093/geront/gny166

Burnes, D., Pillemer, K., Caccamise, P. L., Mason, A., Henderson, C. R., Berman, J., Cook, A. M., Shukoff, D., Brownell, P., Powell, M., Salamone, A., & Lachs, M. S. (2015). Prevalence of and risk factors for elder abuse and neglect in the community: A population-based study. *Journal of the American Geriatrics Society, 63*(9), 1906–1912. https://doi.org/10.1111/jgs.13601

Burnett, J., Achenbaum, W. A., & Murphy, K. P. (2014). Prevention and early identification of elder abuse. *Clinics in Geriatric Medicine, 30*(4), 743–759. https://doi.org/10.1016/j.cger.2014.08.013

Burston, G. R. (1975). Granny-battering. *British Medical Journal, 3,* 592. https://doi.org/10.1016/j.cger.2014.08.013

Cadmus, E. O., Owoaje, E. T., & Akinyemi, O. O. (2015). Older persons' views and experience of elder abuse in South Western Nigeria: A community-based qualitative survey. *Journal of Aging and Health, 27,* 711–729. https://doi.org/10.1177/0898264314559893

Cohen, M. (2011). Screening tools for the identification of elder abuse. *Journal of Clinical Outcomes Management, 18*(6), 261–270. https://doi.org/10.1111/jocn.13721

DeLiema, M., Gassoumis, Z. D., Homeier, D. C., & Wilber, K. H. (2012). Determining prevalence and correlates of elder abuse using promotores: Low-income immigrant Latinos report high rates of abuse and neglect. *Journal of the American Geriatrics Society, 60*(7), 1333–1339. https://doi.org/10.1111/j.1532-5415.2012.04025.x

Dong, X. (2015). Elder abuse: Systematic review and implications for practice. *Journal of the American Geriatrics Society, 63,* 1214–1238. https://doi.org/10.1111/jgs.13454

Dong, X., Chen, R., & Simon, M. A. (2014). Elder abuse and dementia: A review of the research and health policy. *Health Affairs, 33*(4), 642–649. https://doi.org/10.1377/hlthaff.2013.1261

Dyer, C. B., Connolly, M.-T., & McFeeley, P. (2003). The clinical and medical forensics of elder abuse and neglect. In R. J. Bonnie & R. B. Wallace (Eds.), *Elder mistreatment: Abuse, neglect, and exploitation in an aging America* (pp. 339–381). National Academies Press.

Enguidanos, S., DeLiema, M., Aguilar, I., Lambrinos, J., & Wilber, K. (2014). Multicultural voices: Attitudes of older adults in the United States about elder mistreatment. *Ageing & Society, 34,* 877–903. https://doi.org/10.1017/S0144686X12001389

Eslami, B., Viitasara, E., Macassa, G., Melchiorre, M. G., Lindert, J., Stankunas, M., Torres-Gonzalez, F., Barros, H., Ioannidi-Kapolou, E., & Soares, J. J. F. (2016). The prevalence of lifetime abuse among older adults in seven European countries. *International Journal of Public Health, 61*(8), 891–901. https://doi.org/10.1007/s00038-016-0816-x

Grisso, T., & Appelbaum, P. (1998). *Assessing competence to consent to treatment.* Oxford University Press.

Hall, J. E., Karch, D. L., & Crosby, A. E. (2016). *Elder abuse surveillance: Uniform definitions and recommended core data elements for use in elder abuse surveillance, version 1.0.* National Center for Injury Prevention and Control, Centers for Disease Control and Prevention.

Hamby, S., Smith, A., Mitchell, K., & Turner, H. (2016). Poly-victimization and resilience portfolios: Trends in violence research that can enhance the understanding and prevention of elder abuse. *Journal of Elder Abuse & Neglect, 28*(4–5), 217–234. https://doi.org/10.1080/08946566.2016.1232182

Hernandez-Tejada, M. A., Amstadter, A., Muzzy, W., & Acierno, R. (2013). The National Elder Mistreatment study: Race and ethnicity findings. *Journal of Elder Abuse & Neglect, 25,* 281–293. https://doi.org/10.1080/08946566.2013.770305

Jackson, S. L. (2016). All elder abuse perpetrators are not alike: The heterogeneity of elder abuse perpetrators and implications for intervention. *International Journal of Offender Therapy and Comparative Criminology, 60*(3), 265–285 https://doi.org/10.1177/0306624X14554063

Jackson, S. L. (2018). *Understanding elder abuse: A clinician's guide.* American Psychological Association. https://doi.org/10.1037/0000056-000

Jackson, S. L., & Hafemeister, T. L. (2012). Pure financial exploitation vs. hybrid financial exploitation co-occurring with physical abuse and/or neglect of elderly persons. *Psychology of Violence, 2*(3), 285. https://doi.org/10.1037/a0027273

Kamavarapu, Y. S., Ferriter, M., Morton, S., & Völlm, B. (2017). Institutional abuse – characteristics of victims, perpetrators and organsations: A systematic review. *European Psychiatry, 40,* 45–54. https://doi.org/10.1016/j.eurpsy.2016.07.002

Knight, B. G., Karel, M. J., Hinrichsen, G. A., Qualls, S. H., & Duffy, M. (2009). Pikes Peak model for training in professional geropsychology. *American Psychologist, 64,* 205–214. https://doi.org/10.1037/a0015059

Lachs, M. S., & Pillemer, K. A. (2004). Elder abuse. *Lancet, 364,* 1263–1272. https://doi.org/10.1016/S0140-6736(04)17144-4

Lachs, M. S., & Pillemer, K. A. (2015). Elder abuse. *New England Journal of Medicine, 373*(20), 1947–1956. https://doi.org/10.1056/NEJMra1404688

Lachs, M. S., Williams, C. S., O'Brien, S., & Pillemer, K. A. (2002). Adult protective service use and nursing home placement. *Gerontologist, 42,* 734–739. https://doi.org/10.1093/geront/42.6.734

Laumann, E. O., Leitsch, S. A., & Waite, L. J. (2008). Elder mistreatment in the United States: Prevalence estimates from a nationally representative study. *Journals of Gerontology Series B: Psychological Sciences and Social Sciences, 63*(4), S248-S254. https://doi.org/10.1093/geronb/63.4.S248

Lichtenberg, P. A., Stoltman, J., Ficker, L. J., Iris, M., & Mast, B. (2015). A person-centered approach to financial capacity assessment: Preliminary development of a new rating scale. *Clinical Gerontologist, 38*(1), 49–67. https://doi.org/10.1080/07317115.2014.970318

Marson, D. C., Huthwaite, J. S., & Hebert, K. (2004). Testamentary capacity and undue influence in the elderly: A jurisprudent therapy perspective. *Law & Psychology Review, 28,* 71–96.

McDonald, L., Beaulieu, M., Harbison, J., Hirst, S., Lowenstein, A., Podnieks, E., & Wahl, J. (2012). Institutional abuse of older adults: What we know, what we need to know. *Journal of Elder Abuse & Neglect, 24*(2), 138–160. https://doi.org/10.1080/08946566.2011.646512

McPherson, S., & Koltai, D. (2018). *A practical guide to geriatric neuropsychology.* Oxford University Press.

Montoya, V. (1998). Understanding and combating elder abuse in Hispanic communities. *Journal of Elder Abuse & Neglect, 9*(2), 5–17. https://doi.org/10.1300/J084v09n02_02

Moon, A. (2000). Perceptions of elder abuse among various cultural groups: Similarities and differences. *Generations: Journal of the American Society on Aging, 24,* 75–80.

Moye, J., & Wood, E. (2020). Understanding legal and clinical capacities. In J. Moye (Ed.), *Assessing capacities of older adults: A casebook to guide difficult decisions* (pp. 9–23). American Psychological Association. https://doi.org/10.1037/0000184-000

National Center on Elder Abuse. (2016). Research to practice: Elder abuse screening tools for healthcare professionals. https://ncea.acl.gov/NCEA/media/Publication/Elder-Abuse-Screening-Tools-for-Healthcare-Professionals.pdf

National Research Council. (2003). *Elder mistreatment: Abuse, neglect, and exploitation in an aging America.* National Academies Press.

Neale, A. V., Hwalek, M. A., Scott, R. O., Sengstock, M. C., & Stahl, C. (1991). Validation of the Hwalek-Sengstock elder abuse screening test. *Journal of Applied Gerontology, 10*(4), 406–418. https://doi.org/10.1177/073346489101000403

Patterson, M., & Malley-Morrison, E. (2006). A cognitive-ecological approach to elder abuse in five cultures: Human rights and education. *Educational Gerontology, 32,* 73–82. https://doi.org/10.1080/03601270500338666

Peterson, J. C., Burnes, D. P. R., Caccamise, P. L., Mason, A., Henderson, C. R., Wells, M. T., Berman, J., Cook, A. M., Shukoff, D., Brownell, P., Powell, M., Salamone, A., Pillemer, K. A., & Lachs, M. S. (2014). Financial exploitation of older adults: A population-based prevalence study. *Journal of General Internal Medicine, 29*(12), 1615–1623. https://doi.org/10.1007/s11606-014-2946-2

Pillemer, K., Burnes, D., Riffin, C., & Lachs, M. S. (2016). Elder abuse: Global situation, risk factors, and prevention strategies. *Gerontologist, 56,* S194–S205. https://doi.org/10.1093/geront/gnw004

Pinsker, D. M., Pachana, N. A., Wilson, J., Tilse, C., & Byrne, G. J. (2010). Financial capacity in older adults: A review of clinical assessment approaches and considerations. *Clinical Gerontologist, 33*(4), 332–346. https://doi.org/10.1080/07317115.2010.502107

Quinn, M. J. (2000). Undoing undue influence. *Journal of Elder Abuse & Neglect, 12,* 9–17. https://doi.org/10.1300/J084v12n02_03

Quinn, M. J. (2001). Friendly persuasion, good salesmanship, or undue influence. *Elder Advisor,* 49–56.

Quinn, M. J., Nerenberg, L., Navarro, A., & Wilber, K. H. (2017). Developing an undue influence screening tool for Adult Protective Services. *Journal of Elder Abuse & Neglect, 29,* 157–185. https://doi.org/10.1080/08946566.2017.1314844

Reis, M., & Nahmiash, D. (1995). Validation of the caregiver abuse screen (CASE). *Canadian Journal on Aging/La Revue Canadienne Du Vieillissement, 14*(S2), 45–60. https://doi.org/10.1017/S0714980800005584

Roberto, K. (2016). The complexities of elder abuse. *American Psychologist, 71,* 302–311. https://doi.org/10.1037/a0040259

Saghafi, A., Bahramnezhad, F., Poormollamirza, A., Dadgari, A., & Navab, E. (2019). Examining the ethical challenges in managing elder abuse: a systematic review. *Journal of Medical Ethics and History of Medicine, 12,* 1–18. https://doi.org/10.18502/jmehm.v12i7.1115

Scheiderer, E. M. (2012). Elder abuse: Ethical and related considerations for professionals in psychology. *Ethics & Behavior, 22*(1), 75–87. https://doi.org/10.1080/10508422.2012.638828

Schofield, M. J., & Mishra, G. D. (2003). Validity of self-report screening scale for elder abuse: Women's Health Australia Study. *Gerontologist, 43*(1), 110–120. https://doi.org/10.1093/geront/43.1.110

Spar, J. E., Hankin, M., & Stodden, A. B. (1995). Assessing mental capacity and susceptibility to undue influence. *Behavioral Sciences and the Law, 13,* 391–403. https://doi.org/10.1002/bsl.2370130307

Stiegel, L. A., & Quinn, M. J. (2017, June). *Elder abuse: The impact of undue influence* [Issue brief]. National Center on Law and Elder Rights.

Storey, J. E. (2020). Risk factors for elder abuse and neglect: A review of the literature. *Aggression and Violent Behavior, 50,* 101339. https://doi.org/10.1016/j.avb.2019.101339

Tam, S., & Neysmith, S. (2006). Disrespect and isolation: Elder abuse in Chinese communities. *Canadian Journal on Aging, 25,* 141–151. https://doi.org/10.1353/cja.2006.0043

United Nations, Department of Economic and Social Affairs, Population Division. (2017). *World population ageing* 2017 – *highlights.*

United States Government Accountability Office. (2016, November). *Elder abuse: The extent of abuse by guardians is unknown, but some measures exist to help protect older adults* [Report No. GAO-17-33].

United States Senate Special Committee on Aging. (2019). *Fighting fraud: Senate Aging Committee identified top 10 scams targeting out nation's seniors.*

US Preventative Services Task Force. (2018). Screening for intimate partner violence, elder abuse, and abuse of vulnerable adults: US Preventive Services Task Force final recommendation statement. *JAMA, 320*(16), 1678–1687. https://doi.org/10.1001/jama.2018.14741

Wood, S., & Lichtenberg, P. A. (2017). Financial capacity and financial exploitation of older adults: Research findings, policy recommendations and clinical implications. *Clinical Gerontologist, 40,* 3–13. https://doi.org/10.1080/07317115.2016.1203382

Wood, S., & Liu, P. (2012). Undue influence and financial capacity: A clinical perspective. *Generations: Journal of the American Society on Aging, 36,* 53–58.

World Health Organization. (2018, June). *Fact sheet: Elder abuse.* https://www.who.int/news-room/fact-sheets/detail/elder-abuse

World Health Organization & International Network for the Prevention of Elder Abuse. (2002). *Missing voices: Views of older persons on elder abuse.* World Health Organization.

Yaffe, M. J., Wolfson, C., Lithwick, M., & Weiss, D. (2008). Development and validation of a tool to improve physician identification of elder abuse: The Elder Abuse Suspicion Index (EASI). *Journal of Elder Abuse & Neglect, 20,* 276–300. https://doi.org/10.1080/08946560801973168

Yon, Y., Mikton, C. R., Gassoumis, Z. D., & Wilber, K. H. (2017). Elder abuse prevalence in the community setting: A systematic review and meta-analysis. *Lancet Global Health, 5,* E147–E156. https://doi.org/10.1016/S2214-109X(17)30006-2

Chapter 10

Psychological Interventions Developed Specifically for Use in Palliative Care: A Lifespan Developmental Perspective

Rebecca S. Allen
Julia Kasl-Godley
Candice D. Reel

Authors' Note on the Historical Context of COVID-19

When we first started writing this and the following chapter, on palliative care and bereavement interventions, COVID-19 did not exist. The context for dying and death did not have an overlay of this novel, frightening infectious disease, which has disproportionately impacted people of color and older adults. This disease has laid bare social determinants of health and inequities in our health care system – indeed, of inequalities in society at large. Addressing the mental health sequelae of life and death within the context of COVID-19 has drawn a laser focus on the isolation of sick and dying individuals as well as their loved ones. The need to implement and further refine evidence-based telehealth technologies has never been more acute.

Our focus in these chapters remains living with, and dying from, noncommunicable chronic illnesses, given that these illnesses account for the majority of deaths worldwide. This chapter deals with the universal experience of facing the end of life of our loved ones and issues we each encounter in facing our own death. Specific evidence-based interventions have been developed to address these needs and how they can manifest differently across the adult lifespan. The following chapter focuses on the context of psychopathology concomitant with advanced serious illness and evidence-based interventions that address serious mental health conditions including complicated bereavement.

In both chapters, we want to acknowledge the current context of care with COVID-19 as a new threat and concern for individuals and families. This context includes, but is not limited to, uncertainty, increasing mental health problems, deepening social and racial disparities, and increased need for telehealth and virtual platforms for providing social interaction and clinical services amidst wide disparities in high-speed internet availability and a digital divide in telehealth resources and skills, particularly in rural areas and communities of color.

Introduction

Prior to the onset of COVID-19 in the US, eight of the top 10 leading causes of death were chronic serious illnesses, though the rank order of these causes varied by race and sex (Heron, 2019). Serious illness, defined as "a health condition that carries a high risk of mortality and either negatively impacts a person's daily function or quality of life or excessively strains their caregiver" (Kelley & Bollens-Lund, 2018, p. S8), affects over 12 million US adults (Center to Advance Palliative Care and the National Palliative Care Research Center, 2019). Given that the most common causes of death are from chronic illnesses, individuals and their care partners have, theoretically, enough chronological time to prepare for death. Yet individuals frequently avoid thinking about death, rather than preparing for their future care or discussing plans and wishes for a culturally defined "good death," with loved ones (Bailey et al., 2012; Sörensen et al., 2017; Sörensen & Pinquart, 2001; Zaman et al., 2017). This lack of awareness and engagement with the sureness of our own death may result in discrepancies between the type of care desired and the type of care received (Institute of Medicine, 2015). For psychologists, provision of best practice clinical care during the last phase of life, whenever it occurs in the adult lifespan, must include foundational knowledge of factors that influence individuals' ability to engage in preparation for future care and cope with emergent biopsychosocial, spiritual, and environmental needs.

Palliative care, in contrast to hospice, can be initiated at the time of diagnosis and provided concurrently with other disease-related or even curative treatments at all phases of chronic or advanced serious illness (Kelly & Morrison, 2015). Palliative care aims to improve the quality of life of individuals and their family members through the prevention and relief of suffering by means of early identification and thorough assessment and treatment of pain and other physical, psychosocial, and spiritual problems (World Health Organization [WHO], 2014). Palliative care is associated with reduced symptom burden, improved quality of life, increased individual and family satisfaction with care, longer life expectancy than among similarly ill individuals who do not receive palliative care, and improved bereavement adjustment among family members. Palliative care also is associated with cost savings, achieved through earlier intervention and reductions in emergency department visits, intensive care unit stays, and hospital readmissions (Bickel & Ozanne, 2017; Lustbader et al., 2017; McCarthy et al., 2015; Morrison et al., 2008). Despite the benefits of palliative care and the increasing number of people receiving palliative and hospice care in the US, the percentage receiving care compared with that of those who qualify but do not receive care, remains low (Center to Advance Palliative Care and the National Palliative Care Research Center, 2019). Worldwide, only about 14% of the estimated 40 million people who need palliative care currently receive it, and individuals with greater combinations of low social status identities may experience significant disparities in access to and quality of palliative care (Acquaviva, 2017).

Workforce shortages in palliative care across all disciplines, including psychology, are a significant barrier to palliative care access (National Academies of Sciences, Engineering, and Medicine 2020). Psychologists, however, may play a significant role in the alleviation of psychosocial and behavioral health suffering at the end of life, through offering assessment of needs and delivery of a variety of evidence-based interventions. The range of these roles are described in the American Psychological Association (APA) *Resolution on Palliative Care and End-of-Life Issues and Justification*, a document which examines key issues and suggested recommendations for psychological policy, research, assessment, intervention, and education and training of psychologists in palliative care (APA, 2017). In this and the following chapter, we seek to provide practical information for psychologists and other behavioral health professionals to address the needs of individuals near the end of life, and their care partners. We focus on the role psychologists can play in providing psychological interventions to address clinical issues commonly experienced in palliative care populations. We will use one case example, elaborated across both chapters, to provide a comprehensive clinical context so that readers may consider intervention targets and implementation in palliative and bereavement care cohesively. Though psychologists tend to be underrepresented in palliative care settings, when available, psychological services are well utilized by patients (e.g., Ann-Yi et al., 2018).

We maintain that psychologists working with older adults, particularly with those living with advanced serious illness, can help improve older adults' last phase of life by learning about, promoting, and implementing palliative care psychological interventions, particularly when guided by specific knowledge and skill competencies and informed by lifespan developmental theory. Knowledge of theory is endorsed as an element of competent practice in self-reflective practice guidelines such as the Pikes Peak Geropsychology Knowledge and Skill Assessment Tool (see Appendix 2; Karel et al., 2010) and provides a "road map" or conceptual understanding of clinical issues to address in treatment planning and intervention implementation. We briefly review knowledge and skill competency domains and developmental theory, then discuss goals of care conversations, issues commonly seen in palliative care populations and evidence-based psychological interventions for these issues. We illustrate how one might apply this information and consider multiple intersecting identities, using a hypothetical case example created from an amalgam of our clinical work and woven throughout the chapter. This chapter ends with recommendations for practice change, as well as gaps in science to be addressed to maximize outcomes within the normative context of end of life for diverse patients, families, and health care providers.

Introduction of Clinical Case Example

Mr. R. is a 75-year-old, African-American, retired teacher who lives 2 hrs outside of St. Louis, with his 70-year-old, White male roommate, Mr. M. They have been roommates for nearly 25 years. Mr. R.'s past medical history is significant for chronic obstructive pulmonary disease (COPD), congestive heart failure (CHF), and hepatitis C. Three months ago, he developed abdominal pain and ascites, unexplained weight loss, and jaundice, for which his primary care physician referred him to an outpatient cancer center for evaluation. An abdominal ultrasound and MRI were concerning for hepatocellular cancer. In addition, he recently experienced a COPD exacerbation, characterized by increased breathlessness, wheezing, tightness in his chest, and severe coughing, for which he was hospitalized and intubated, requiring respiratory and speech therapy support. Mr. R. is now recovering at home but has experienced a significant decline in his functional status. He now needs oxygen and can no longer go on his daily walks or visit the local coffee shop on his own. The strain of Mr. R.'s recent health crises has taken a toll on Mr. M. He appears frail, stressed, and is coping with his own health concerns (type 2 diabetes and osteoarthritis). Mr. R. has two older siblings and a 93-year-old mother living in southwest Missouri, near the Arkansas border, all of whom visited Mr. R. after his hospitalization and continue to express concern about his mental state. They are deeply religious (Baptist) and express their desire for him to fight so that he can still receive salvation for his "troubled ways."

Palliative Care Practice Guidelines and Knowledge and Skill Competencies

Psychologists working with older adults living with advanced serious illness will want to be familiar with palliative care practice guidelines as well as palliative care knowledge and skill competency domains. These competencies underlie working with individuals and families during the normative context of death and dying as well as the context of psychopathology and complicated bereavement. The National Coalition for Hospice and Palliative Care's National Consensus Project for Quality Palliative Care (NCP; National Consensus Project for Quality Palliative Care, 2018) outlines clinical practice guidelines covering eight primary domains. These domains are structure and processes of care; ethical and legal aspects of care; physical aspects of care; psychological and psychiatric aspects of care; social aspects of care; spiritual, religious, and existential aspects of care; cultural aspects of care; and care of the patient nearing the end of life.

Although the NCP guidelines are meant for use by all providers working with palliative care populations, psychologists are not explicitly mentioned in the guidelines, albeit they could be seen as being encompassed under "specialist providers." To assist psychologists in thinking about how the guidelines can map onto psychologists' scope of practice, Kasl-Godley and colleagues identified knowledge and skill competencies for psychologists to better address the needs of individuals who receive palliative and hospice care (Kasl-Godley et al., 2014). These competencies are biological aspects of illness and the dying process; psychological, sociocultural, spiritual, and interprofessional factors; normal and abnormal grief and bereavement; communication and facilitation of advance care planning; assessment of common physical and mental health conditions; psychotherapy for patients with chronic, life threatening, or terminal illness; assessment and treatment of families; and interdisciplinary teams, consultation, and professional self-care.

Developmental Theory as a Guide to Palliative Care Interventions

Several theories of adult development inform psychological interventions for individuals nearing the end of life and their care partners. Some theories describe specific psychological activities important to maintaining identity (e.g., reminiscence and life review; Butler, 1963). Others consider shifts in time perception that lead individuals to prioritize meaningful experiences and relationships when time is limited (i.e., socioemotional selectivity theory; Carstensen et al., 1999; Charles, 2010). A particularly relevant theory for conceptualizing issues of focus in psychological interventions provided during the last phase of or near the end of life is Elder's (1998) life course theory and its four core principles of *timing in lives*, *time and place*, *linked lives*, and *agency*. After describing these principles (foundational competency for clinicians), we will illustrate their use (functional competency for clinicians) in the case example.

The principle of *timing in lives* points to differing developmental and clinical issues that may be a focus of psychotherapy, depending on whether death comes at a time that is expected or is "off-time." In other words, clinical targets of intervention for a person near death during middle age – a parent with young children, perhaps – may be quite different from those for a person near death in their 80s or 90s. In psychotherapy with these two individuals, the content of what is meaningful, the targets of anticipated loss, and the definition of effective coping differs. For example, middle-aged parents likely will mourn the loss of sharing in the typical developmental events that will occur in the future lives of their children (e.g., marriage, the birth of grandchildren). They may consider executing ethical wills or creating legacies for their children's future selves (e.g., letters to be opened at specific life events; digital scrapbooks, recipe books, or photo albums). In contrast, an 80-year-old with advanced serious illness may have already spent a great deal of time in life review and legacy making, and may have limited unfinished business, or will want to focus their therapeutic work on issues of forgiveness or gratitude. Notably, what is considered an "on-time" versus an "off-time" death may vary by race or ethnicity, given differences in life expectancy and cause of death driven by disparities.

Any psychotherapy with older adults, and particularly therapy conducted during palliative care or after bereavement, should include consideration of cohort issues, or Elder's principle of *time and place*. This principle pertains to the importance of the historical context of life experiences (time) in support of culturally competent intervention delivery. We use labels for US cohorts as reported by the Pew Research Center (Dimock, 2019) and the Center for Generational Kinetics. For example, the current cohort of older adults (baby boomers and older) in comparison with individuals from Generation X, millennials, or Generation Z individuals, have different attitudes toward psychotherapy, marriage, the choice to rear children, and increased racial and/or ethnic and lesbian, gay, bisexual, transgender, questioning, and other (LGBTQ+) diversity and inclusion.

The current cohort of older adults may be more likely to believe, in comparison with younger generations, that mental health problems are a normal part of aging. This belief may be the result of low mental health literacy (Jorm, 2012) and internalized aging stereotypes (Levy & Leifheit-Limson, 2009). Subsequently, older adults are less likely to report mental health symptoms and seek services than their younger generation counterparts, resulting in delayed diagnosis and treatment of medical and mental health conditions (Cuijpers et al., 2012; Mohlman, 2012). The principle of *place* is seen in the case example in the rural versus urban differences in attitudes toward same-sex couples and disparities in access and care quality. These disparities may increase the need for telehealth and telemedicine delivery.

Implementation of therapeutic interventions near the end of life, of necessity, consider the individual's family and social context. As described in Elder's principle of *linked lives*, social networks and support systems influence an individual's behaviors. These systems include faith communities, family, and fictive kin ("as if" kin or pretend relatives, as in other individuals who assume family-like roles; Fuller et al., 2020; Roberto & Weaver, 2019). Some individuals may be highly interconnected, whereas others may not be, and may possibly be estranged from care partners due to a history of substance use disorder, abusive relationships, or mental health problems. In building and implementing palliative care and bereavement interventions, the principle of linked lives may be critical in goals of care conversations and targeting meaningful activities to reduce existential suffering (e.g., forgiveness, gratitude, legacy).

Finally, every clinician focuses on agency and change as the backbone of therapeutic work, and Elder's principle of *agency* states that an individual practices personal choice in conscious decision making. However, members of ethnic and/or racial groups in the US may feel limited agency, due to disparities in care and evidence-based historical distrust of the medical community. To support agency, clinicians need to work toward therapeutic effectiveness through enacting cultural humility and therapeutic presence (Betancourt et al., 2003; Chochinov et al., 2013). Ultimately, intersecting identities, time, place, agency, and linked lives provide a framework for providing psychotherapeutic interventions near the end of life.

In the case example it can be posited that Mr. R. and Mr. M. may be experiencing a foreshortened sense of future time, and that this changed time perspective may be focusing their attention on meaningful interaction in their own and other relationships, perhaps a clarification of values, and a need to engage in goals of care conversations. Both Mr. R. and Mr. M. are over age 65, and each has chronic illnesses. Hence, timing in lives likely does not play a large role in their situation and does not highlight a particularly useful clinical target. Although Mr. R. and Mr. M. self-identify as "roommates," it may be that they are romantic partners but are not "out" due to the historic time and the rural place in which they have lived and are currently living. Indeed, Mr. R.'s family continue to express concern about his "troubled ways," indicating unspecified family discord that may directly impact the naming of a health care proxy during goals of care discussions. It is possible that Mr. R. possesses intersecting identities related to his cohort and rural location that complicate this experience in life. Moreover, due to their varying race and ethnicity, Mr. R. and Mr. M. bring two different cultural perspectives to the experience of serious, chronic illness, despite their long-term relationship. The principle of place is relevant to our case example of Mr. R., a rural-dwelling, African-American man with limited access to quality care in his own area. In our case example, Mr. R. is now at a point where he may need to more formally document his autonomous wishes regarding care in the context of advanced, serious illness through what may be end-of-life care planning. Mr. R.'s goals of care are in conflict with the beliefs of his family support system. In our case example, Mr. R.'s life is linked both to Mr. M. and to his mother and siblings, representing a potentially conflictual family structure that will impact goals of care conversations as well as management of clinical issues.

Goals of Care Conversations and Advance Care Planning

Understanding what people want for their end of life and in their planning for future care is integral to palliative care and begins with advance care planning or goals of care conversations, and conversations between a health care provider and an ill individual or surrogate for the purpose of determining the individual's values, goals, and preferences for care. Goals of care conversations may involve designation of a *durable power of attorney for health care* to make health care decisions on the individual's behalf if, or when, that individual can no longer do so. Conversations also can include completing advance care directives such as specialized forms that translate the ill individual's preferences with regard to specific treatment decisions into portable medical orders (e.g., Physician Orders for Life-Sustaining Treatment [POLST]). Treatment decisions may include resuscitation, mechanical ventilation, dialysis, artificial nutrition and hydration, antibiotics, hospitalization, chemotherapy, radiation, surgery, or placement or removal of pacemakers or implantable cardioverter defibrillator (ICD). Ideally, goals of care conversations are exploratory and occur in the context of an established relationship, early in the disease process, and repeatedly as illness evolves. When done well, goals of care conversations are associated with improved quality of life, family satisfaction with care, reductions in hospital utilization and aggressiveness of care near the end of life, earlier referral to and increased use of hospice services, greater likelihood of dying in preferred place of death, decreased family conflict, and better adjustment in bereavement (Bernacki & Block, 2014; Brinkman-Stoppelenburg et al., 2014; Detering et al., 2010; Klingler et al., 2016; Wright et al., 2008; Zhang et al., 2009). When goals of care conversations are done poorly, they are pressured, uninformed, transactional, or even adversarial and expect too much from individuals and their care partners too soon. As a result, individuals and families can experience poor quality of life, anxiety, distress, prolongation of the dying process, undesired hospitalizations, and mistrust of the health care system. In situations where the ill individual or care partner or family desires treatment that is deemed by health care providers as inappropriate, clinicians may experience moral distress and be more susceptible to burnout (Piers et al., 2012; St. Ledger et al., 2013).

Psychologists can better facilitate goals of care conversations by being aware of, and addressing, barriers to good goals of care conversations. Barriers commonly fall into three categories, all of which can be more pronounced among diverse communities: patient and family or care partner, clinician, and health care system (Allen et al., 2019; Garrido et al., 2014; Huang et al., 2016; Melhado & Bushy, 2011; Sudore et al., 2010). In terms of patient and family factors, individuals with advanced serious illness may experience feelings of avoidance in addressing the topic of death (Allen et al., 2019; Sörensen et al., 2017; Sörensen & Pinquart, 2001), and such avoidance has been shown to be associated with symptoms of depression 2 years later among primary care patients (Sörensen et al., 2012). Individuals with an advanced serious or terminal illness also may desire to shield or protect family from difficult information, may fear burdening family, or have limited options for surrogate participation. They may wait to initiate conversations because they expect the clinician to start these discussions when appropriate. Individuals and families may share explanatory models of illness (e.g., beliefs about causes of illness and how to treat it; Kleinman, 1978) or cultural and religious beliefs that are different from clinicians which can impact participation (e.g., speaking about death may invoke it, the future is in God's hands, not up to human beings, faith in God's ability to heal, aggressive care can allow time for God to manifest healing). Families may feel guilt over not pursuing life-prolonging treatments or perceive a duty to protect the individual from the health care system by ensuring that the individual receives all treatments available. Families may have difficulty tolerating the thought of the individual dying or desire more time to repair the relationship (Albright et al., 2020; Periyakoil et al., 2016; Sanders et al., 2016).

Clinician barriers often result from inadequate training in goals of care conversations (Back et al., 2019). Clinicians may use vague language that obfuscates understanding of prognosis and treatment choices. Conversations may occur late in an illness trajectory and in pressured contexts due to difficulties with prognostication. Clinicians may miss key stakeholders such as family, fictive kin, or religious or community members by focusing on individual autonomy versus family-centered decision making (Albright et al., 2020). Clinicians may be inattentive to, or reluctant to address, psychosocial-spiritual needs, due to concern that they do not have adequate time to address these needs, discomfort at how to address them, or concern that the conversations may harm individuals and their care partners. Individuals and care partners may encounter health care system barriers, including a default toward high-intensity care and difficulty accessing palliative care services in which goals of care conversations are a central component (Candib, 2002; Carr, 2011; Gerst & Burr, 2008). Often, there is ambiguity about who is responsible for goals of care conversations, as well as how and where these conversations should be documented (Bernacki et al., 2014; Lakin et al., 2016; Sudore & Fried, 2010; Sudore et al., 2017).

In addition to being aware of barriers and helping to address these barriers, psychologists can contribute to good goals of care conversations in other ways. First, psychologists can pay attention to their own biases, beliefs, or assumptions about what the end of life should look like, and to how these beliefs may influence conversations. They should be mindful of health care disparities and individuals' prior experiences with the health care system (Allen et al., 2019; Melhado & Bushy, 2011). When working with individuals in need of having goals of care conversations, psychologists should consider the developmental context (Elder, 1998) and health and mental health literacy, using accessible language and conversation and decision aids such as supplemental written and oral or video materials. Psychologists also can assess factors and values affecting how people make health care decisions. These factors include feeling prepared for, and having a choice with regard to, where and when they die; balancing quality and enjoyment of life with quantity of life; attending to unfinished business or important milestones; needing to maintain autonomy and control; perceiving oneself as a burden; experiencing fears, misunderstanding, and unrelieved physical and psychological symptoms; experiencing family pressure or conflict; and following spiritual and religious beliefs and practices and cultural norms (Lloyd-Williams et al., 2007; Naik et al., 2016).

Resources to Guide Goals of Care Conversations

Psychologists can access many resources to help guide them with goals of care conversations; we will review only a few of them here. See Butler et al. (2014) or Carpenter and McDarby (2018) for a review of tools to support advance care planning. PREPARE for Your Care is an online, evidence-based tool that helps people learn about and prepare for medical decision making (https://prepareforyourcare.org/). It features video stories in English and Spanish, and guides users as they explore their wishes and learn how to discuss them with family, friends, and clinicians. The website also offers written pamphlets and legally binding advance directives (Sudore et al., 2017; Sudore et al., 2018). Vital Talk is an evidence-based program that provides online and in-person communication strategies, tools and video resources (https://www.vitaltalk.org/). The Veterans Administration Life-Sustaining Treatment Decisions initiative outlines standardized practices related to discussing and documenting goals of care conversations, and provides tools and resources to support clinicians and health care facilities (https://www.ethics.va.gov/goalsofcaretraining/team.asp). Ariadre Labs' Serious Illness Conversation Guide program (Bernacki et al., 2015; Lakin et al., 2017) provides clinicians with a guide for asking individuals about their goals, values, and wishes. The guide addresses how to elicit illness understanding and decision-making preferences, share prognostic information according to preferences, understand goals and fears, explore views on trade-offs and impaired function, and discover wishes for family involvement. Use of this guide has resulted in creating more, earlier, better, and more accessible conversations (Paladino et al., 2019) and decreased anxiety and depression in individuals with advanced cancer (Bernacki et al., 2019).

A goals of care conversation with Mr. R. suggested that he was ambivalent about pursuing further diagnostic evaluation or possible treatment for his presumed hepatocellular cancer. He expressed a sense of hopelessness, resignation, and perceived sense of burden and uselessness – at one point indicating that he does not see the point in living any longer. Mr. R. had not completed a health care choices directive although he suggested that he would like Mr. M. to be his durable power for health care. The psychologist from the palliative care team was called in at the request of members of the interprofessional team to meet with Mr. R. and Mr. M. regarding goals of care and future planning. In the midst of this first discussion, the psychologist found that the men were openly discussing their history, the family context and conflict, and sharing in anticipatory grief regarding mutual health decline. Mr. R. openly shared his sadness and anxiety regarding the history of, and current conflict between, his mother and siblings in relation to Mr. M. Additionally, Mr. R. clearly stated a desire for his long-time roommate, Mr. M., to be named his health care proxy rather than his biological relatives who live at a geographic distance and may not share the same values for quality versus quantity of life. Mr. R. and his desired health care proxy, Mr. M., also may share different religious beliefs in comparison with Mr. R.'s mother and siblings, representing yet another potential area of family conflict that may influence goals of care conversations.

Common Issues in the Last Phase of Life and Potential Clinical Targets for Intervention

In addition to the need for timely and clear goals of care conversations, individuals with advanced serious illness and their care partners often need help with a variety of clinical issues. They can encounter a fragmented health care system, experience poorly coordinated care transitions and inattention to practical and social needs. They may experience declining function and high physical symptom burden related to their underlying disease(s) and associated treatment, such as pain, fatigue, appetite and sleep problems, dyspnea, nausea and vomiting, constipation, and cognitive impairment. Individuals may experience psychosocial-spiritual distress including existential suffering; a diminished sense of meaning, purpose, and dignity; adjustment and grief reactions; a crisis of faith; hopelessness, guilt, and a waning will to live; and growing desire for death. They may develop recurrent or recent-onset mental disorders or emergent psychological distress or exacerbation of preexisting psychological symptoms. Individuals also may experience a myriad of changes in their social and physical environment, including changes in roles, status, and lifestyle. They may report interpersonal strain, poor communication, unfinished business, perceived burden, and a sense of isolation or separateness from others. Family systems experience economic burden, and family care partners are at increased risk for psychological distress and physical morbidity and mortality.

In the case example, Mr. R. and Mr. M. had already engaged in goals of care discussions with the psychologist from the palliative care team. At this point, Mr. R. and Mr. M. each might benefit from interventions focused on dignity, legacy, and gratitude to help with anticipatory grief and stress. Mr. R. and his mother and siblings might benefit from interventions focused on forgiveness.

Interventions Developed for Use in Palliative Care to Address Issues of Meaning, Purpose, Self-Worth, and Connection

Several psychological interventions have been developed specifically for use with individuals with advanced illness or with those nearing the end of life, to promote meaning making, a sense of purpose, and self-worth – all targets that have been deemed important to address in any specialized interventions for individuals with advanced disease and their care partners (e.g. Rodin et al., 2020) regardless of the chronological age of the person facing death during adulthood. These interventions include *legacy intervention family enactment* (LIFE; Allen et al., 2008; Allen et al., 2014; Allen et al., 2016), *meaning-centered psychotherapy* (MCP; Breitbart, 2016; Breitbart et al., 2010; Masterson et al., 2018), and *dignity therapy* (Chochinov, 2012; Chochinov et al., 2005). Both of the identity maintenance theories that focus on limited time perspective (e.g., socioemotional selectivity theory; Carstensen et al., 1999) and several principles of Elder's life course theory (agency, linked lives, and time and place) help inform therapeutic targets for these intervention approaches.

Legacy Intervention Family Enactment

LIFE integrates reminiscence and creative activity as mechanisms to address practice targets near the end of life for seriously ill individuals and at least one care partner. LIFE involves dyads and can be delivered by master's degree–prepared mental health professionals (Allen et al., 2008) or trained community health advisors, peer mentors, or retired senior volunteers (Allen et al., 2014, 2016). LIFE utilizes the individual's perspective of limited time left to live, to promote engagement in meaning-based coping which leads the seriously ill individual and care partner to sustained coping and the experience of positive emotions. This strengths-based intervention may be considered a simplified version of dignity therapy delivered across three sessions and best implemented with the involvement of a care partner in addition to the person facing death. The first session involves a series of questions addressed to each individual in the care dyad and, based on these responses, the identification of one time period in the seriously ill person's life to be represented in a specific legacy activity. The second and third sessions involve engagement in creating the legacy and reviewing present-moment awareness of this process of creativity and life review dyadically. LIFE addresses the mediating influence of social and activity engagement in the intervention process on outcomes for all participants (patients, care partners, and volunteers). This format makes the intervention accessible to practitioners with any training background, or to lay community health advisors and peer mentors.

For seriously ill individuals, LIFE is associated with decreased symptom distress (breathing difficulties, pain), fewer emotional symptoms, less emotional symptom "bother," less of a sense of being abandoned by one's God, increased existential meaning, and more experienced forgiveness. Among care partners, LIFE has shown reduced caregiving stress and more existential meaning (Allen, 2009; Allen et al., 2008, 2014, 2016; unpublished treatment manual available at request from rsallen@ua.edu or on the website at https://rsallen.people.ua.edu/). LIFE has shown efficacy among non-Hispanic White and African-American community-dwelling dyads and across disease contexts.

Meaning-Centered Psychotherapy

MCP is designed to help individuals sustain or enhance a sense of meaning, peace, and purpose in their lives even as they approach the end of life, and has most frequently been used within the illness context of cancer. MCP uses a combination of didactics, discussion, and experiential exercises, and participants are assigned readings and homework tailored to specific meaning-centered themes (Breitbart, 2016; Breitbart & Poppito, 2014a, 2014b). Sessions 1–3 entail sharing of the individual's cancer story, the impact of cancer on identity, and reviewing sources of meaning and legacy. Sessions 4–6 involve identifying attitudinal, creative, and experiential sources of meaning, respectively. Session 7 closes with the individual's reflections on therapy and hopes for the future. Though initially developed for individuals with advanced cancer, MCP has been used in other illness contexts (Masterson et al., 2018). MCP initially was provided in group format and subsequently, it has been adapted for individual treatment (IMCP; Breitbart et al., 2018) as well as for care partners (MCP-C) both in-person (Applebaum et al., 2015) and in web-based formats (Applebaum et al., 2017). It has been abbreviated for individuals close to the end of life (Rosenfeld et al., 2017) and has been modified to place greater emphasis on cultivating compassion and self-compassion (Gil et al., 2018). MCP also has been adapted to a variety of cultural contexts (see Ryu et al., 2018; Leng et al., 2019).

MCP is made readily accessible through the publication of treatment manuals (Breitbart & Poppito, 2014a, 2014b) as well as through training opportunities. It is associated with improved spiritual well-being and sense of meaning; improved quality of life; reduced desire for hastened death; and decreased depression, hopelessness, and physical symptom burden (Breitbart et al., 2010, 2012, 2015, 2018; Rosenfeld et al., 2017), and decreased anxiety and anxious preoccupation (Ryu et al., 2018). An enhanced sense of meaning and peace has been shown to mediate the decrease in psychological distress (Rosenfeld et al., 2018).

Dignity Therapy

Dignity therapy is the best-known and most international intervention developed for use in palliative care. It is based on an empirical, dignity-conserving model developed by

Chochinov (Chochinov, 2002; Johnston et al., 2015) informed by reports by individuals with end-stage cancer describing their beliefs and experiences with dignity. The model is divided into three primary domains that address physical (illness-related concerns), existential and/or spiritual (dignity-conserving repertoire), and social (social dignity inventory) considerations, each bearing on the person's sense of dignity. The first domain regards concerns that result from the illness and threaten to, or actually do, impinge on the individual's sense of dignity.

The second domain consists of beliefs (dignity-conserving perspectives) and behaviors (dignity-conserving practices) that promote dignity. Dignity-conserving perspectives include beliefs related to continuity of self, role preservation, generativity and legacy, autonomy and control, maintenance of pride and hope, acceptance, and resilience or fighting spirit. Dignity-conserving practices consist of living in the moment, maintaining normalcy, and seeking spiritual comfort.

The third domain is a social dignity inventory which describes the quality of interactions with others that enhance or detract from the individual's sense of dignity.

Dignity therapy seeks to promote individuals' desire to go on living in the face of impending death by helping them identify and share meaningful, important aspects of their lives, their hopes and wishes for their loved ones, life values, and future goals. It does so by asking specific questions meant to elicit some aspect of personhood, provide opportunities for affirmation, or help reconnect the person with elements of themselves that were or still remain meaningful and valued. Conversations are recorded, transcribed, edited, and eventually compiled into a document that is then bequeathed to an identified loved one. Questions include: "What do I need to know about you as a person to take the best care of you that I can?" "Tell me a little about your life history, particularly the parts that you either remember most, or think are the most important. When did you feel most alive?" "Are there specific things that you would want your family to know about you, and are there particular things you would want them to remember?" "What are the most important roles you have played in life (family roles, vocational roles, community service roles, etc.)? Why were they so important to you, and what do you think you accomplished in those roles?" "What are your most important accomplishments, and what do you feel most proud of?" "Are there particular things that you feel still need to be said to your loved ones, or things that you would want to take the time to say once again?" "What are your hopes and dreams for your loved ones?" "What have you learned about life that you would want to pass along to others? What advice or words of guidance would you wish to pass along to your (son, daughter, husband, wife, parents, others)?" and "Are there words or perhaps even instructions you would like to offer your family to help prepare them for the future?"

Dignity therapy is readily accessible in a book by Chochinov, outlining the intervention (Chochinov, 2012). It has shown efficacy across disease contexts, and for both individuals with advanced serious illness and their care partners. Dignity therapy is associated with decreased depressive and anxiety symptoms (Julião et al., 2013; Julião et al., 2017); increased quality of life and increased sense of dignity, purpose, meaning, and will to live; perceived positive change in how ill individuals' families see and appreciate them (Houmann et al., 2014; Chochinov et al., 2012, 2011, 2005); and improved bereavement adjustment among care partners (McClement et al., 2007). International randomized controlled trials have demonstrated efficacy across racial and ethnic and cultural contexts (Anable et al., 2018), as well as considerations of ways to make the intervention more culturally congruent (e.g., Li et al., 2014). In addition, it has been modified to better meet the dual needs of care partners and ill individuals (Mowll et al., 2015) and to promote meaningful conversation between individuals with advanced serious illness and their family members (Guo et al., 2018).

In the case of Mr. R., he and Mr. M. participated in a dignity therapy intervention with the psychologist from the palliative care team to create a legacy that addressed their life together, values, and wishes for other members of the family. Across the course of the intervention, both Mr. R. and Mr. M. reported increased meaning and more positive affect, including feelings of gratitude and decreased symptoms of depression. In the case example, Mr. R. expressed feeling hopeless, useless, fear of being a burden on Mr. M., and an indication that he might desire a hastened death. Both Mr. R. and Mr. M. worked with the psychologist from the palliative care team to clarify goals of care and participate in dignity therapy. Through the process of this work, Mr. R.'s feelings of hopelessness and uselessness lessened. The stress and feelings of being overwhelmed previously reported by Mr. M. also diminished. Although tension still existed between Mr. R.'s mother, siblings, and Mr. M., the documentation of Mr. R.'s goals of care and everyone's involvement (either in person or via telephone delivery) in gratitude and values-based, meaning-focused interventions decreased the tension significantly. Prior to Mr. R.'s death, he told the psychologist on the palliative care team, "I finally feel some sense of peace."

Conclusions and Implications

In this chapter, we used the case example of Mr. R. and Mr. M. to illustrate how theories of adult development that involve identity maintenance strategies and life course principles (Elder's concepts of agency, linked lives, time and place, and timing in lives) may inform psychologists' choice of practice targets and use of specific therapeutic approaches when working with individuals with advanced serious illness and their care partners. Using Elder's theory, it was noted that goals of care conversations and meaning-centered interventions may have nuanced intervention targets for individuals with serious illness during their 40s or 50s, in comparison with those facing death during their 80s or 90s.

One of the most important take-aways for psychologists and other practitioners based on the information in this chapter concerns a knowledge of how to evaluate practice competencies in psychosocial palliative care. Useful tools include the Pikes Peak Geropsychology Knowledge and Skill Assessment Tool (see Appendix 2; Karel et al., 2010) and Kasl-Godley and colleagues' (2014) knowledge and skill competencies for psychologists to better address the needs of individuals who receive palliative and hospice care. Both of these guidelines emphasize the importance of having awareness of one's own foundational competencies, including knowledge of the biological aspects of illness and the dying process; lifecourse developmental theory; and the psychological, sociocultural, spiritual, and interprofessional context of care. Moreover, accurate awareness and assessment of one's functional competencies in conducting goals of care conversations and meaning-based interventions is key to high-quality clinical practice (Hinrichsen et al., 2018). We strongly recommend that interested practitioners acquire a detailed working knowledge of these guidelines and engage in serial self-assessment of foundational and functional competencies in providing psychosocial palliative care.

One area of critical future clinical and research development is greater use of an intersectional lens to facilitate cultural competency and address the needs of diverse individuals and care partners at the end of life. The case example presented in this chapter illustrated various needs, including how to approach goals of care conversations within the context of family conflict (Albright et al., 2020) and address issues of meaning, purpose, self-worth, and forgiveness during existentially oriented and couples-based intervention. Intersecting identities interact simultaneously and dynamically to influence one's life experiences (Bauer, 2014; Bowleg, 2012; Earnshaw et al., 2018), including choice of, access to, and outcomes of palliative care. A vastly understudied aspect of intersectionality is the influence of aging (chronological changes within individuals across time) or cohort (Elder's historical time and place). Psychologists must be aware of intersecting identities within individuals and systems to provide culturally informed and therapeutically effective care throughout the illness trajectory, from goals of care conversations through to psychosocial interventions near the end of life. Knowledge of specific skill competencies identified by Kasl-Godley and colleagues (2014), in tandem with the ability to understand foundational lifespan theory, will assist psychologists in identifying practice targets for intervention (goals of care conversations vs. meaning and existential needs) and choosing specific evidence-based strategies to facilitate change.

In summary, we wish to emphasize the following future practice and research targets: (1) shoring up the evidence base of promising treatments; (2) greater inclusion of developmental and intersectionality theories to inform choice of treatment across diverse cultures and illness contexts; (3) adaptation of evidence-based interventions to telehealth platforms, and (4) focused translation of effective intervention into everyday clinical practice. For readers interested in reading first person accounts of living a meaningful life in the context of advanced serious illness, learning more about specific interventions used in palliative care, or personal accounts of working in these settings, we have listed several suggested readings.

Suggested Resources on a Lifespan Devleopmental Perspective of Palliative Care

Allen, R. S., Carpenter, B. D., & Eichorst, M. K. (Eds). (2018). *Perspectives on behavioural interventions in palliative and end-of-life care. Aging and mental health research series.* Routledge; Taylor & Francis Group. ISBN: 978-0-4|57-9152-6.

Breitbart, W. S. (Ed.). (2016). *Meaning-centered psychotherapy in the cancer setting: Finding meaning and hope in the face of suffering.* Oxford University Press.

Byock, I. (2014). *The four things that matter most: A book about living.* Simon and Schuster.

Byock, I., & Byock, A. (1997). *Dying well: The prospect for growth at the end of life* (p. 299). Riverhead Books.

Chochinov, H. M. (2012). *Dignity therapy: Final words for final days.* Oxford University Press.

Kalanithi, P. (2016). *When breath becomes air.* Random House.

Qualls, S. H., & Kasl-Godley, J. E. (2010). *End-of-life issues, grief, and bereavement: What clinicians need to know* (Vol. 6). John Wiley & Sons.

Wilson, K. G., & Murrell, A. R. (2004). Values work in Acceptance and Commitment Therapy: Setting a Course for Behavioral Treatment. In S. C. Hayes, V. M. Follette, & M. Linehan (Eds.), *Mindfulness & Acceptance: Expanding the cognitive-behavioral tradition* (pp. 120–151). Guilford Press.

References

Acquaviva, K. D. (2017). *LGBTQ-inclusive hospice and palliative care.* Harrington Park Press. https://doi.org/10.17312/harringtonparkpress/2017.03lgbtqihpc

Albright, A., Hilgeman, M. M., & Allen, R. S. (2020). Addressing family conflicts when assessing capacities. In J. Moye (Ed.), *Assessing capacities of older adults: A casebook to guide difficult decisions* (pp. 299–325). American Psychological Association. https://doi.org/10.1037/0000184-013

Allen, R. S. (2009). The Legacy Project intervention to enhance meaningful family interactions: Case examples. *Clinical Gerontologist, 32*(2), 164–176. https://doi.org/10.1080/07317110802677005

Allen, R. S., Azuero, C. B., Csikai, E. L., Parmelee, P. A., Shin, H. J., Kvale, E., Durkin, D. W., & Burgio, L. D. (2016). "It was very rewarding for me...": senior volunteers' experiences with implementing a reminiscence and creative activity intervention. *Gerontologist, 56*(2), 357–367. https://doi.org/10.1093/geront/gnu167

Allen, R. S., Harris, G. M., Burgio, L. D., Azuero, C. B., Miller, L. A., Shin, H., Eichorst, M. K., Csikai, E. L., DeCoster, J., Dunn, L. L., Kvale, E. A., & Parmelee, P. (2014). Can senior volunteers deliver reminiscence and creative activity interventions? Results of the Legacy Intervention Family Enactment (LIFE) randomized controlled trial. *Journal of Pain and Symptom Management, 48*(4), 590–601. https://doi.org/10.1016/j.jpainsymman.2013.11.012

Allen, R. S., Hilgeman, M. M., Ege, M. A., Shuster, J. L., & Burgio, L. D. (2008). Legacy activities as interventions approaching the end of life. *Journal of Palliative Medicine, 11*(7), 1029–1038. https://doi.org/10.1089/jpm.2007.0294

Allen, R. S., Oliver, J. S., Eichorst, M. K., Mieskowski, L., Payne-Foster, P., & Sörensen, S. (2019). Preparation and planning for future care in the Deep South: Adapting a validated tool for cultural sensitivity. *Gerontologist, 59*(6), e643–e652. https://doi.org/10.1093/geront/gny102

American Psychological Association. (2017). *Resolution on assisted dying and justification.* http://www.apa.org/about/policy/assisted-dying-resolution.aspx.

Anable, G., Chochinov, H. M., McClement, S., & Thompson, G. (2018). Dignity therapy. In R. S. Allen, B. D. Carpenter, & M. K. Eichorst (Eds.). *Perspectives on behavioural interventions in palliative and end-of-life care* (pp. 12–47). Routledge. https://doi.org/10.4324/9781315212265-5

Ann-Yi, R. E., & Block, S. D. (2014). Communication about serious illness care goals: a review and synthesis of best practices. *JAMA internal medicine, 174*(12), 1994–2003.

Applebaum, A. J., Buda, K. L., Schofield, E., Faberov, M., Teitelbaum, N. D., Evans, K., Cowens-Alvarado, R., & Cannady, R. S. (2017). Exploring the cancer caregiver's journey through web-based meaning-centered psychotherapy. *Psycho-Oncology, 27,* 847–856. https://doi.org/10.1002/pon.4583

Applebaum, A. J., Kulikowski, J. R., & Breitbart, W. (2015). Meaning-centered psychotherapy for cancer caregivers (MCP-C): Rationale and overview. *Palliative and Support Care, 13*(6), 1631–1641. https://doi.org/10.1017/S1478951515000450

Back, A. L., Fromme, E. K., & Meier, D. E. (2019). Training clinicians with communication skills needed to match medical treatments to patient values. *Journal of the American Geriatrics Society, 67*(S2), S435–S441. https://doi.org/10.1111/jgs.15709

Bailey, F. A., Allen, R. S., Williams, B. R., Goode, P. S., Granstaff, S., Redden, D. T., & Burgio, K. L. (2012). Do-Not-Resuscitate orders in the last days of life. *Journal of Palliative Medicine, 15*(7), 751–759. https://doi.org/10.1089/jpm.2011.0321

Bauer, G. R. (2014). Incorporating intersectionality theory into population health research methodology: Challenges and the potential to advance health equity. *Social Science & Medicine, 110,* 10–17. https://doi.org/10.1016/j.socscimed.2014.03.022

Bernacki, R. E., & Block, S. D. (2014). Communication about serious illness care goals: A review and synthesis of best practices. *JAMA Internal Medicine, 174*(12), 1994–2003. https://doi.org/10.1001/jamainternmed.2014.5271

Bernacki, R., Hutchings, M., Vick, J., Smith, G., Paladino, J., Lipsitz, S., Gawande, A. A., & Block, S. D. (2015). Development of the Serious Illness Care Program: A randomised controlled trial of a palliative care communication intervention. *BMJ Open, 5*(10), Article e009032. https://doi.org/10.1136/bmjopen-2015-009032

Bernacki, R., Paladino, J., Neville, B. A., Hutchings, M., Kavanagh, J., Geese, O. P., Lakin, J., Sanders, J. J., Miller, K., Lipsitz, S., Gawande, A. A., & Block, S. (2019). Effect of the Serious Illness Care Program in outpatient oncology: a cluster randomized clinical trial. *JAMA Internal Medicine, 179*(6), 751–759. https://doi.org/10.1001/jamainternmed.2019.0077

Betancourt, J. R., Green, A. R., Carrillo, J. E., & Owusu Ananeh-Firempong, I. I. (2003). Defining cultural competence: A practical framework for addressing racial/ethnic disparities in health and health care. *Public Health Reports, 118,* 293–302. https://doi.org/10.1016/S0033-3549(04)50253-4

Bickel, K., & Ozanne, E. (2017). Importance of costs and cost effectiveness of palliative care. *Journal of Oncology Practice, 13*(5), 287–289. https://doi.org/10.1200/JOP.2016.019943

Bowleg, L. (2012). The problem with the phrase women and minorities: Intersectionality – an important theoretical framework for public health. *American Journal of Public Health, 102,* 1267–1273. https://doi.org/10.2105/AJPH.2012.300750

Breitbart, W. S. (Ed.). (2016). *Meaning-centered psychotherapy in the cancer setting: Finding meaning and hope in the face of suffering.* Oxford University Press.

Breitbart, W., Pessin, H., Rosenfeld, B., Applebaum, A. J., Lichtenthal, W. G., Li, Y., Saracino, R. M., Marziliano, A. M., Masterson, M., Tobias, K., & Fenn, N. (2018). Individual meaning-centered psychotherapy for the treatment of psychological and existential distress: a randomized controlled trial in patients with advanced cancer. *Cancer, 124*(15), 3231–3239.

Breitbart, W. S., & Poppito, S. R. (2014a). *Individual meaning-centered psychotherapy for patients with advanced cancer: A treatment manual.* Oxford University Press. https://doi.org/10.1093/med/9780199837243.001.0001

Breitbart, W. S., & Poppito, S. R. (2014b). *Meaning-centered group psychotherapy for patients with advanced cancer: A treatment manual.* Oxford University Press. https://doi.org/10.1093/med/9780199837243.001.0001

Breitbart, W., Poppito, S., Rosenfeld, B., Vickers, A. J., Li, Y., Abbey, J., Olden, M., Pessin, H., Lichtenthal, W., Sjoberg, D., & Cassileth, B. R. (2012). Pilot randomized controlled trial of individual meaning-centered psychotherapy for patients with advanced cancer. *Journal of Clinical Oncology, 30*(12), 1304–1309. https://doi.org/10.1200/JCO.2011.36.2517

Breitbart, W., Rosenfeld, B., Gibson, C., Pessin, H., Poppito, S., Nelson, C., Tomarken, A., Timm, A. K., Berg, A., Jacobson, C., Sorger, B., Abbey, J., & Olden, M. (2010). Meaning-centered group psychotherapy for patients with advanced cancer: A pilot randomized controlled trial. *Psycho-Oncology, 19*(1), 21–28. https://doi.org/10.1002/pon.1556

Breitbart, W., Rosenfeld, B., Pessin, H., Applebaum, A., Kulikowski, J., & Lichtenthal, W. G. (2015). Meaning-centered group psychotherapy: An effective intervention for improving psychological well-being in patients with advanced cancer. *Journal of Clinical Oncology, 33*(7), 749–754. https://doi.org/10.1200/JCO.2014.57.2198

Brinkman-Stoppelenburg, A., Rietjens, J. A. C., & van der Heide, A. (2014). The effects of advance care planning on end-of-life care: a systematic review. *Palliative Medicine, 28*(8), 1000–1025. https://doi.org/10.1177/0269216314526272

Butler, R. N. (1963). The life review: An interpretation of reminiscence in the aged. *Psychiatry, 26*(1), 65–76. https://doi.org/10.1080/00332747.1963.11023339

Butler, M., Ratner, E., McCreedy, E., Shippee, N., & Kane, R. L. (2014). Decision aids for advance care planning: an overview of the state of the science. *Annals of Internal Medicine, 161,* 408–418. https://doi.org/10.7326/M14-0644

Candib, L. M. (2002). Truth telling and advance planning at end of life: problems with autonomy in a multicultural world. *Families, Systems & Health, 20*(3), 213–228. https://doi.org/10.1037/h0089471

Carpenter, B. D., & McDarby, M. (2018). Interventions to enhance communication and decision-making in the context of serious illness. In R. S. Allen, B. D. Carpenter, & M. K. Eichorst (Eds.), *Perspectives on behavioural interventions in palliative and end-of-life care* (pp. 12–47). Routledge.

Carr, D. (2011). Racial differences in end-of-life planning: Why don't Blacks and Latinos prepare for the inevitable? *Omega, 63*(1), 1–20. https://doi.org/10.2190/OM.63.1.a

Carstensen, L. L., Isaacowitz, D. M., & Charles, S. T. (1999). Taking time seriously: A theory of socioemotional selectivity. *American Psychologist, 54*(3), 165. https://doi.org/10.1037/0003-066X.54.3.165

Center to Advance Palliative Care & the National Palliative Care Research Center. (2019). *America's care of serious illness: A state-by-state report card on access to palliative care in our nation's hospitals.*

Charles, S. T. (2010). Strength and vulnerability integration: A model of emotional well-being across adulthood. *Psychological Bulletin, 136*(6), 1068. https://doi.org/10.1037/a0021232

Chochinov, H. M. (2002). Dignity-conserving care – a new model for palliative care: helping the patient feel valued. *JAMA, 287*(17), 2253–2260. https://doi.org/10.1001/jama.287.17.2253

Chochinov, H. M. (2012). *Dignity therapy: Final words for final days.* Oxford University Press.

Chochinov, H. M., Cann, B., Cullihall, K., Kristjanson, L., Harlos, M., McClement, S. E., Hack, T. F., & Hassard, T. (2012). Dignity therapy: A feasibility study of elders in long-term care. *Palliative and Supportive Care, 10*(1), 3–15. https://doi.org/10.1017/S1478951511000538

Chochinov, H. M., Hack, T., Hassard, T., Kristjanson, L. J., McClement, S., & Harlos, M. (2005). Dignity therapy: a novel psychotherapeutic intervention for patients near the end of life. *Journal of Clinical Oncology, 23*(24), 5520–5525. https://doi.org/10.1200/JCO.2005.08.391

Chochinov, H. M., Kristjanson, L. J., Breitbart, W., McClement, S., Hack, T. F., Hassard, T., & Harlos, M. (2011). Effect of dignity therapy on distress and end-of-life experience in terminally ill patients: A randomised controlled trial. *Lancet Oncology, 12*(8), 753–762. https://doi.org/10.1016/S1470-2045(11)70153-X

Chochinov, H. M., McClement, S. E., Hack, T. F., McKeen, N. A., Rach, A. M., Gagnon, P., Sinclair, S., & Taylor-Brown, J. (2013). Health care provider communication: An empirical model of therapeutic effectiveness. *Cancer, 119*(9), 1706–1713. https://doi.org/10.1002/cncr.27949

Cuijpers, P., Reynolds, C. F., Donker, T., Li, J., Andersson, G., & Beekman, A. (2012). Personalized treatment of adult depression: medication, psychotherapy, or both? A systematic review. *Depression and Anxiety, 29*(10) , 855–864. https://doi.org/10.1002/da.21985

Detering, K. M., Hancock, A. D., Reade, M. C., & Silvester, W. (2010). The impact of advance care planning on end of life care in elderly patients: Randomised controlled trial. *BMJ, 340,* 1345. https://doi.org/10.1136/bmj.c1345

Dimock, M. (2019, January 17). *Defining generations: Where millennials end and Generation Z begins.* Pew Research Center.

Earnshaw, V. A., Rosenthal, L., Gilstad-Hayden, K., Carroll-Scott, A., Kershaw, T. S., Santilli, A., & Ickovics, J. R. (2018). Intersectional experiences of discrimination in a low-resource urban community: An exploratory latent class analysis. *Journal of Community & Applied Social Psychology, 28,* 80–93. https://doi.org/10.1002/casp.2342

Elder, G. H., Jr. (1998). The life course as developmental theory. *Child Development, 69*(1), 1–12. https://doi.org/10.1111/j.1467-8624.1998.tb06128.x

Fuller, H. R., Ajrouch, K. J., & Antonucci, T. C. (2020). The convoy model and later-life family relationships. *Journal of Family Theory & Review, 12*(2), 126–146.

Garrido, M. M., Harrington, S. T., Prigerson, H. G. (2014). End-of-life treatment preferences: A key to reducing ethnic/racial disparities in advance care planning. *Cancer, 120*(24), 3981–3986. https://doi.org/10.1002/cncr.28970

Gerst, K., & Burr, J. A. (2008). Planning for end-of-life care: Black-White differences in the completion of advance directives. *Research on Aging, 30*(4), 428–449. https://doi.org/10.1177/0164027508316618

Gil, F., Fraguell, C., Benito, L., Casellas-Grau, & Limonero, J. T. (2018). Meaning-centered psychotherapy integrated with elements of compassion: A pilot study to assess feasibility and utility. *Palliative and Supportive Care, 6*(6), 643–647. https://doi.org/10.1017/S1478951518000548

Guo, Q., Chochinov, H. M., McClement, S., Thompson, G., & Hack T. (2018). Development and evaluation of the Dignity Talk question framework for palliative patients and their families: A mixed-methods study. *Palliative Medicine, 32*(1), 195–205. https://doi.org/10.1177/0269216317734696

Heron, M. (2019). Deaths: Leading causes for 2017. *National Vital Statistics Reports*, 68(6). National Center for Health Statistics.

Hinrichsen, G. A., Emery-Tiburcio, E. E., Gooblar, J., & Molinari, V. A. (2018). Building foundational knowledge competencies in professional geropsychology: Council of Professional Geropsychology Training Programs (Co PGTP) recommendations. *Clinical Psychology: Science and Practice, 25*(2), Article e12236. https://doi.org/10.1111/cpsp.12236

Houmann, L. J., Chochinov, H. M., Kristjanson, L. J., Petersen, M. A., & Groenvold, M. (2014). A prospective evaluation of dignity therapy in advanced cancer patients admitted to palliative care. *Palliative Medicine, 28*(5), 448–458. https://doi.org/10.1177/0269216313514883

Huang, C. H. S., Crowther, M., Allen, R. S., DeCoster, J., Kim, G., Azuero, C., Ang, X., & Kvale, E. (2016). A pilot feasibility intervention to increase advance care planning among African Americans in the Deep South. *Journal of Palliative Medicine, 19*(2), 164–173. https://doi.org/10.1089/jpm.2015.0334

Institute of Medicine. (2015). *Dying in America: Improving quality and honoring individual preferences near the end of life.*

Johnston, B., Larkin, P., Connolly, M., Barry, C., Narayanasamy, M., Östlund, U., & McIlfatrick, S. (2015). Dignity-conserving care in palliative care settings: An integrative review. *Journal of Clinical Nursing, 24*(13–14), 1743–1772. https://doi.org/10.1111/jocn.12791

Jorm, A. F. (2012). Mental health literacy: Empowering the community to take action for better mental health. *American Psychologist, 67*(3), 231–243. https://doi.org/10.1037/a0025957

Julião, M., Barbosa, A., Oliveira, F., Nunes, B., Carneiro, A. V. (2013). Efficacy of dignity therapy for depression and anxiety in terminally ill patients: Early results of a randomized controlled trial. *Palliative and Supportive Care, 11*(6), 481–489. https://doi.org/10.1017/S1478951512000892

Julião, M., Oliveira, F., Nunes, B., Carneiro, A. V., & Barbosa, A. (2017). Effect of dignity therapy on end-of-life psychological distress in terminally ill Portuguese patients: A randomized controlled trial. *Palliative & Supportive Care, 15*(6), 628–637. https://doi.org/10.1017/S1478951516001140

Karel, M. J., Emery, E. E., Molinari, V., & CoPGTP Task Force on the Assessment of Geropsychology Competencies. (2010). Development of a tool to evaluate geropsychology knowledge and skill competencies. *International Psychogeriatrics, 22*(6), 886–896. https://doi.org/10.1017/S1041610209991736

Kasl-Godley, J. E., King, D. A., & Quill, T. E. (2014). Opportunities for psychologists in palliative care: Working with patients and families across the disease continuum. *American Psychologist, 69*(4), 364. https://doi.org/10.1037/a0036735

Kelley, A. S., & Bollens-Lund, E. (2018). Identifying the population with serious illness: The "denominator" challenge. *Journal of Palliative Medicine, 21*(S2), S7–S16. https://doi.org/10.1089/jpm.2017.0548

Kelly, A. S., & Morrison, R. S. (2015). Palliative care for the seriously ill. *New England Journal of Medicine, 373*(8), 747–755. https://doi.org/10.1056/NEJMra1404684

Kleinman, A. (1978). Concepts and a model for the comparison of medical systems as cultural systems. *Social Science and Medicine, 12*(2-B), 85–93. https://doi.org/10.1016/0160-7987(78)90014-5

Klingler, C., in der Schmitten, J., & Marckmann, G. (2016). Does facilitated advance care planning reduce the costs of care near the end of life? Systematic review and ethical considerations. *Palliative Medicine, 30*(5), 423–433. https://doi.org/10.1177/0269216315601346

Lakin, J. R., Block, S. D., Billings, J. A. Koritsanszky, L. A., Cunningham, R., Wichmann, L., Harvey, D., Lamey, J., & Bernacki, R. E. (2016). Improving communication about serious illness in primary care: A review. *JAMA Internal Medicine, 176*(9), 1380–1387. https://doi.org/10.1001/jamainternmed.2016.3212

Lakin, J. R., Koritsanszky, L. A., Cunningham, R., Maloney, F. L., Neal, B. J., Paladino, J., Palmore, M. C., Vogeli, C., Ferris, T. G., Block, S. G., Gawande, A. A., & Bernacki, R. E. (2017). A systematic intervention to improve serious illness communication in primary care. *Health Affairs, 36*(7), 1258–1264. https://doi.org/10.1377/hlthaff.2017.0219

Leng, J., Lui, F., Huang, X. Breitbart, W., & Gany, F. (2019). Patient perspectives on adapting meaning-centered psychotherapy in advanced cancer for the Chinese immigrant population. *Supportive Care in Cancer, 27*, 3431–3438. https://doi.org/10.1007/s00520-019-4638-2

Levy, B. R., & Leifheit-Limson, E. (2009). The stereotype-matching effect: greater influence on functioning when age stereotypes correspond to outcomes. *Psychology and Aging, 24*(1), 230. https://doi.org/10.1037/a0014563

Li, H. C., Richardson, A., Speck, P., & Armes, J. (2014). Conceptualizations of dignity at the end of life: Exploring theoretical and cultural congruence with dignity therapy. *Journal of Advanced Nursing, 70*(12), 2920–2931. https://doi.org/10.1111/jan.12455

Lloyd-Williams, M., Kennedy, V., Sixsmith, A., & Sixsmith, J. (2007). The end of life: A qualitative study of perceptions of people over the age of 80 on issues surrounding death and dying. *Journal of Pain and Symptom Management, 34*(1), 60–66. https://doi.org/10.1016/j.jpainsymman.2006.09.028

Lustbader, D., Mitchell, M., Romano, C., Lukoski, E., Chang, A., Mittelberger, J., Scherr, T., Cooper, D. (2017). The impact of a home-based palliative care program in an accountable care organization. *Journal of Palliative Medicine, 20*(1), 23–28. https://doi.org/10.1089/jpm.2016.0265

Masterson, M., Rosenfeld, B., & Breitbart, W. (2018). Meaning-centered psychotherapy for cancer patients with advanced and terminal illness. In R. S. Allen, B. D. Carpenter, & M. K. Eichorst (Eds.), *Perspectives on behavioural interventions in palliative and end-of-life care* (pp. 80–102). Routledge.

McCarthy, I. M., Robinson, C., Huq, S., Philastre, M., & Fine, R. L. (2015). Cost savings from palliative care teams and guidance for a financially viable palliative care program. *Health Services Research, 50*(1), 217–236. https://doi.org/10.1111/1475-6773.12203

McClement, S., Chochinov, H. M., Hack, T., Hassard, T., Kristjanson, L. J., & Harlos, M. (2007). Dignity therapy: Family member perspectives. *Journal of Palliative Medicine, 10*(5),1076–1082. https://doi.org/10.1089/jpm.2007.0002

Melhado, L., & Bushy, A. (2011). Exploring uncertainty in advance care planning in African Americans: Does low health literacy influence decision making preference at end of life. *American Journal of Hospice and Palliative Care, 28,* 495–500. https://doi.org/10.1177/1049909110398005

Mohlman, J. (2012). A community based survey of older adults' preferences for treatment of anxiety. *Psychology and Aging, 27*(4), 1182–1190. https://doi.org/10.1037/a0023126

Morrison, R. S., Penrod, J. D., Cassel, J. B., Caust-Ellenbogen, M., Litke, A., Spragens, L., Meier, D. E.; for the Palliative Care Leadership Centers' Outcomes Group. (2008). Cost savings associated with US hospital palliative care consultation programs. *Archives of Internal Medicine, 168*(16), 1783–1790. https://doi.org/10.1001/archinte.168.16.1783

Mowll, J., Lobb, E. A., Lane, L., Lacey, J., Chochinov, H. M. Kelly, B., Agar, M., Links, M., & Kearsley, J. H. (2015). A preliminary study to develop an intervention to facilitate communication between couples in advanced cancer. *Palliative and Supportive Care, 13*(5), 1381–1390. https://doi.org/10.1017/S1478951514001333

Naik, A. D., Martin, L. A., Moye, J., & Karel, M. J. (2016). Health values and treatment goals of older, multimorbid adults facing life-threatening illness. *Journal of the American Geriatrics Society, 64,* 625–631. https://doi.org/10.1111/jgs.14027

National Academies of Sciences, Engineering, and Medicine. (2020). *Building the workforce we need for people with serious illness: Proceedings of a workshop.* National Academies Press. https://doi.org/10.17226/25789

National Consensus Project for Quality Palliative Care. (2018). *Clinical practice guidelines for quality palliative care* (4th ed.). National Coalition for Hospice and Palliative Care. https://www.nationalcoalitionhpc.org/ncp

Paladino, J., Bernacki, R., Neville, B. A., Kavanagh, J., Miranda, S. P., Palmor, M., Lakin, J., Desai, M., Lamas, D., Sander, J. J., Gass, J., Henrich, N., Lipsitz, S., Fromme, E., Gawande, A. A., & Block, S. D. (2019). Evaluating an intervention to improve communication between oncology clinicians and patients with life-limiting cancer: A cluster randomized clinical trial of the Serious Illness Care Program. *JAMA Oncology, 5*(6), 801–809.

Periyakoil, V. S., Neri, E., & Kraemer, H. (2016). Patient-reported barriers to high-quality, end-of-life care: A multiethnic, multilingual, mixed methods study. *Journal of Palliative Medicine, 19*(4), 373–379. https://doi.org/10.1089/jpm.2015.0403

Piers, R. D., Van den Eynde, M., Steeman, E., Vlerick, P., Benoit, D. D., & Van Den Noortgate, N. J. (2012). End-of-life care of the geriatric patient and nurses' moral distress. *Journal of the American Medical Directors Association, 13*(1), 80-e7. https://doi.org/10.1016/j.jamda.2010.12.014

Roberto, K. A., & Weaver, R. H. (2019). Late-life families. In B. H. Fiese, M. Celano, K. Deater-Deckard, E. N. Jouriles, & M. A. Whisman (Eds.), *APA handbook of contemporary family psychology: Foundations, methods, and contemporary issues across the lifespan* (Vol. 1, pp. xxvi–815). American Psychological Association. https://doi.org/10.1037/0000099-035

Rodin, G., An, E., Shnall, J., & Malfitano, C. (2020). Psychological interventions for patients with advanced disease: Implications for oncology and palliative care. *Journal of Clinical Oncology, 38*(9), 885–904. https://doi.org/10.1200/JCO.19.00058

Rosenfeld, B., Cham, H., Pessin, H., & Breitbart, W. (2018). Why is meaning-centered group psychotherapy (MCGP) effective? Enhanced sense of meaning as the mechanism of change for advanced cancer patients. *Psycho-Oncology, 27*(2), 654–660. https://doi.org/10.1002/pon.4578

Rosenfeld, B., Saracino, R., Tobias, K., Masterson, M., Pessin, H., Applebaum, A., Brescia, R., & Breitbart, W. (2017). Adapting meaning-centered psychotherapy for the palliative care setting: Results of a pilot study. *Palliative Medicine, 31*(2), 140–146. https://doi.org/10.1177/0269216316651570

Ryu, J. S., Choi, S. W., Yun, S. S., Koo, B. H., Choi, I. S., Kim, S. J., Park, J. S., Seok, J. H., & Yoon, D. S. (2018). Preliminary findings on the effectiveness of meaning-centered psychotherapy in patients with pancreatobiliary cancer. *Yonsei Medical Journal, 59*(9), 1107–1114. https://doi.org/10.3349/ymj.2018.59.9.1107

Sanders, J. J., Robinson, M. T., & Block, S. D. (2016). Factors impacting advance care planning among African Americans: Results of a systematic integrated review. *Journal of Palliative Medicine, 19*(2), 202–227. https://doi.org/10.1089/jpm.2015.0325

Sörensen, S., Chapman, B. J., Duberstein, P. R. Pinquart, M., & Lyness, J. M. (2017). Assessing future care preparation in late life: Two short measures. *Psychological Assessment, 29*(12), 1480–1495. https://doi.org/10.1037/pas0000446

Sörensen, S., Mak, W., Chapman, B., Duberstein, P. R., & Lyness, J. M. (2012). The relationship of preparation for future care to depression and anxiety in older primary care patients at 2-year follow-up. *The American Journal of Geriatric Psychiatry, 20*(10), 887–894.

Sörensen, S., & Pinquart, M. (2001). Developing a measure of older adults' preparation for future care needs. *International Journal of Aging and Human Development, 53*(2), 137–165. https://doi.org/10.2190/1R0D-30TC-F4K1-F0DW

St. Ledger, U., Begley, A., Reid, J., Prior, L., McAuley, D., & Blackwood, B. (2013). Moral distress in end-of-life care in the intensive care unit. *Journal of Advanced Nursing, 69*(8), 1869–1880. https://doi.org/10.1111/jan.12053

Sudore, R. L., Boscardin, J., Feuz, M. A., McMahan, R. D., Katen, M. T., & Barnes, D. E. (2017). Effect of the PREPARE website vs an easy-to-read advance directive on advance care planning documentation and engagement among veterans: A randomized clinical trial. *JAMA Internal Medicine, 177*(8), 1102–1109. https://doi.org/10.1001/jamainternmed.2017.1607

Sudore, R. L., & Fried, T. R. (2010). Redefining the "planning" in advance care planning: preparing for end-of-life decision making. *Annals of Internal Medicine, 153*(4), 256–261. https://doi.org/10.7326/0003-4819-153-4-201008170-00008

Sudore, R. L., Lum, H. D., You, J. J., Hanson, L. C., Meier, D. E., Pantilat, S. Z., Matlock, D. D., Rietjenz, J. A. C., Korfage, I. J., Ritchie, C. S., Kutner, J. S., Teno, J. M., Thomas, J., McMahon, R. D., & Heyland, D. K. (2017). Defining advance care planning for adults: A consensus definition from a multidisciplinary Delphi panel. *Journal of Pain and Symptom Management, 53*(5), 821–832. https://doi.org/10.1016/j.jpainsymman.2016.12.250

Sudore, R. L., Schillinger, D., Katen, M. T., Shi, Y., Boscardin, W. J., Osua, S., & Barnes, D. E. (2018). Engaging diverse English-and Spanish-speaking older adults in advance care planning: the PREPARE randomized clinical trial. *JAMA Internal Medicine, 178*(12), 1616–1625. https://doi.org/10.1001/jamainternmed.2018.4657

Sudore, R. L., Schillinger, D., Knight, S. J., & Fried, T. R. (2010). Uncertainty about advance care planning treatment preferences among diverse older adults. *Journal of Health Communication, 15*(S2), 159–171. https://doi.org/10.1080/10810730.2010.499982

World Health Organization. (2014). *Strengthening of palliative care as a component of comprehensive care throughout the life course.* Sixty-seventh World Health Assembly.

Wright, A. A., Zhang, B., Ray, A., Mack, J. W., Trice, E., Balboni, T., Mitchell, S. L., Jackson, V. A., Block, S. D., Maciejewski, P. K., & Prigerson, H. G. (2008). Associations between end-of-life discussions, patient mental health, medical care near death, and caregiver bereavement adjustment. *JAMA, 300*(14), 1665–1673.

Zaman, S., Inbadas, H., Whitelaw, A., & Clark, D. (2017). Common or multiple futures for end of life care around the world? Ideas from the 'waiting room of history.' *Social Science & Medicine, 172*, 72–79. https://doi.org/10.1016/j.socscimed.2016.11.012

Zhang, B., Wright, A. A., Huskamp, H. A., Maciejewski, M. L., Earle, C. C., Block, S. D., Maciejewski, P. K., & Prigerson, H. G. (2009). Health care costs in the last week of life: associations with end-of-life conversations. *Archives of Internal Medicine, 169*(5), 480–488. https://doi.org/10.1001/archinternmed.2008.587

Chapter 11

Psychological Palliative Care and Bereavement Interventions: Psychopathology and Family Contexts

Julia Kasl-Godley
Rebecca S. Allen

Authors' Note on the Historical Context of COVID-19

As we stated in the last chapter, when we first started writing the chapters on palliative care and bereavement interventions, COVID-19 did not exist. This disease has laid bare social determinants of health and inequities in our health care system and has further challenged the ways that we care for sick and dying individuals who may be isolated from loved ones in the days preceding death. Moreover, the context of COVID-19 has highlighted the needs of families during bereavement, particularly because culturally relevant rituals before and after a loved one's death have been interrupted due to social distancing guidelines.

This chapter focusses on dying from noncommunicable chronic illnesses, which historically account for the majority of deaths worldwide. Nevertheless, we also want to acknowledge the current COVID-19 context of care. This context includes, but is not limited to, increasing mental health and substance use problems and the impact of social isolation on bereavement.

Introduction

Before COVID-19, noncommunicable diseases, predominantly cancer, cardiovascular disease, chronic respiratory diseases, and diabetes, accounted for nearly three quarters of the estimated 57 million annual deaths worldwide, and approximately 60% of these deaths occurred in adults 70 years and older (Bennett et al., 2018). Over 12 million US adults (Center to Advance Palliative Care and the National Palliative Care Research Center, 2019) live with serious illness, defined as "a health condition that carries a high risk of mortality and either negatively impacts a person's daily function or quality of life or excessively strains their caregiver" (Kelley & Bollens-Lund, 2018, p. S8). In the context of chronic illness, individuals and their care partners have the opportunity, if they so choose, to prepare for death. However, many individuals avoid preparing for future care needs (Sörensen et al., 2017), resulting in difficulty coping with emergent psychosocial-spiritual and environmental needs (Institute of Medicine, 2015) and care partners who are at risk for complications in bereavement.

Palliative care is defined by the World Health Organization as meeting the physical, psychological, and religious and spiritual needs of individuals and their care partners, typically through collaborative efforts of interprofessional teams. Palliative care may be initiated at the time of diagnosis and provided concurrently with other disease-related or even curative treatments at all phases of chronic or advanced serious illness (Kelly & Morrison, 2015). Unfortunately, the percentage of patients receiving care compared with those who qualify for but do not receive care remains low (Center to Advance Palliative Care and the National Palliative Care Research Center, 2019).

In this chapter, which builds upon Chapter 10, we discuss psychological interventions to address serious mental health conditions that may arise concomitant with advanced serious illness and palliative care. We highlight *acceptance and commitment therapy* (ACT) as a particularly useful evidence-based intervention to alleviate suffering across a variety of illness contexts and mental health conditions. The mental health and coping among individuals receiving palliative care impact their care partners and can increase risk for complications in bereavement; therefore, effective interventions for complicated bereavement also are reviewed. To illustrate how one might apply this information, we refocus and expand the hypothetical case example created in the last chapter from an amalgam of our clinical work. This chapter ends with a summary of skill competencies and suggested targets for scientific and clinical work.

Case Example Continued and Expanded

In the case example, Mr. R. was a 75-year-old, African-American, retired teacher who lived 2 hrs outside of St. Louis, with Mr. M., his 70-year-old, White male roommate of 25 years. Mr. R. expressed feeling hopeless, useless, and fearful of being a burden on Mr. M., an indication that he might have a desire for hastened death. Both Mr. R. and Mr. M. worked with the psychologist from the palliative care team to clarify goals of care and participate in dignity therapy. Through the process of this work, Mr. R.'s feelings of hopelessness and uselessness lessened. The stress and feelings of being overwhelmed previously reported by Mr. M. also diminished. Although tension still existed between Mr. R.'s mother, siblings, and Mr. M., the documentation of Mr. R.'s goals of care and everyone's involvement (either in person or via telephone delivery) in values-based, meaning-centered interventions decreased the tension significantly. Prior to Mr. R.'s death, he told the psychologist on the palliative care team, "I finally feel some sense of peace."

After Mr. R.'s death, and beginning with making funeral arrangements, however, tensions among Mr. M. and Mr. R.'s mother (Mrs. R., aged 93) and two older siblings (Mr. N., aged 76, and Ms. J., aged 77) intensified. The deeply religious R. family wanted Mr. R. to be buried in the family plot in southwest Missouri. The agreed-upon plan prior to his death, however, had been for him to be cremated and for his ashes to be split between Mr. M. and Mrs. R.. Moreover, Mr. N. and Ms. J. were now discussing contesting Mr. Bill R.'s will and estate. They argued their brother "was not of sound mind" when the goals of care and advance planning documentation was executed and that his portion of the 23-acre property he owned with Mr. M. outside St. Louis should now be transferred to Mrs. R. Once again the stress associated with this conflict was exacerbating symptoms of Mr. M.'s health conditions (type 2 diabetes and osteoarthritis). The palliative care psychologist suggested that Mr. M. consult with an elder law attorney about these ongoing issues with Mr. R.'s family.

Acceptance and Commitment Therapy in Palliative Care

Though not developed specifically for individuals with advanced serious illness, ACT is an excellent theoretical fit. ACT is a third-generation cognitive behavior therapy (CBT) that seeks to promote psychological flexibility, or the ability to fully contact the present moment and persist in value-based behavior, through a number of acceptance and mindfulness, as well as commitment and behavior change, processes. ACT maintains that primary pain is inevitable, whereas suffering is not. Suffering is directly connected to individuals' relationship with their thoughts and feelings. Individuals suffer when they try to get rid of painful experiences (e.g., anxiety, sadness, negative thoughts, bad memories, chronic pain), often through attempting to avoid or control these experiences. Suffering also can arise from a lack of clarity regarding one's values or a diminished ability to live in accordance with one's values. Values are chosen life directions, not a destination, and provide a sense of meaning or purpose and motivation to face life's obstacles. The goal is for individuals to embrace and accept their psychological experience, while living life in accordance with their values.

Compared with individuals without disease, individuals living with advanced cancer show greater experiential avoidance, greater psychological inflexibility, and reduced ability to act in accordance with their values (Mosher et al., 2017; Serfaty et al., 2019). Values commonly expressed among terminally ill individuals include family, pleasure, caring, a sense of accomplishment, true friendship, and rich experience (Hack et al., 2010). Among individuals living with cancer, ACT is associated with lower depression, anxiety, and psychological distress; greater psychological flexibility; improved acceptance and mindfulness skills; improved quality of life (QOL; Feros et al., 2013; Mohabbat-Bahar et al., 2015); and decreased interference of physical symptoms in their daily life (Mosher et al., 2018). Among people living with pain, a symptom commonly experienced in chronic and advanced serious illnesses, individual, group-based, and internet-delivered ACT is associated with increased psychological flexibility (McCracken & Gutiérrez-Martínez, 2011), lower depression and pain-related anxiety (Buhrman et al., 2013; Wetherell et al., 2011), less physical disability, higher pain acceptance, lower pain intensity (McCracken & Jones, 2012; Vowles & McCracken, 2008), and lower pain interference in daily life (Trompetter et al., 2015), with gains being maintained at 3 months (McCracken et al., 2013) and for as long as 3 years (Vowles et al., 2011). Given the efficacy of ACT within the context of advanced cancer and painful conditions, this treatment approach offers guidance across a broad range of psychopathology.

Specific Mental Disorders, Psychiatric Symptoms, and Their Treatment in Palliative Care

Some of the most commonly experienced mental disorders among individuals living with advanced serious illness are major depression, anxiety disorders, posttraumatic stress disorder (PTSD), and substance use. In discussing psychological interventions for these disorders in the context of palliative care, we assume working knowledge of their treatment in older adults, covered elsewhere in this book (i.e., see Chapter 3 for a discussion of treatment of depression in older adults and Chapter 5 for a discussion of treatment of anxiety and PTSD in late life). In this chapter, we focus on specific adaptations of psychological interventions for use within the context of psychopathology in palliative care populations.

Major Depressive Disorder

Between 5% and 50% of individuals living with advanced serious illness experience major depressive disorder (Akizuki et al., 2016; Mitchell et al., 2011), though prevalence varies by setting (Walker et al., 2013), disease type (Walker, Hansen, Martin, Symeonides, Ramessu et al., 2014), and assessment method and classification criteria (Janberidizee et al., 2014). Risk factors include complications of disease and treatment, high symptom burden (controlling for disease, treatment status, and prognosis; Grotmol et al., 2019), functional dependence, loss of control and autonomy, diminished purpose and meaning, pain, previous history of depression, perception of oneself as a burden, poor support, and concurrent stressors (e.g., financial strain; King et al., 2005; Wilson et al., 2009). The incidence of suicide among individuals with cancer, particularly those with lung, stomach, and head and neck cancers, is twice that of the general US population, with the risk highest in the first 5 years after diagnosis (Misono et al., 2008). In addition, physical illness and functional disability are more likely to be associated with suicidal ideation and behaviors when they threaten independence, QOL, sense of purpose and usefulness, value, dignity and pleasure (Fässberg et al., 2016). Depression is an independent predictor of poor adherence to disease-modifying therapies and survival in advanced cancer, and of rehospitalization and death from heart failure (Freedland et al., 2016).

Use of psychological interventions for major depression in individuals with advanced serious illness should be informed by an understanding of risk factors and an evidence base with palliative care patients. Outcome research supports a variety of interventions including dignity therapy, meaning-centered psychotherapy, ACT, depression care for people with cancer (DCPC), and managing cancer and living meaningfully (CALM). DCPC is a collaborative care intervention for depression in individuals with advanced cancer, combining antidepressants, problem-solving therapy, behavioral activation, and care coordination among the primary care physician, psychiatrist, and oncologist (Walker & Sharpe, 2009). Two randomized controlled trials (RCTs) comparing DCPC with usual care in individuals with major depression with either good or poor cancer prognosis found that DCPC resulted in significantly reduced depressive symptoms and improved QOL (Sharpe et al., 2014; Walker, Hansen, Martin, Symeonides, Gourley et al., 2014). Of note, a recent large-scale RCT of manualized, 12-session CBT in treating depression in advanced cancer did not achieve clinical benefit, leading the study authors to recommend use of a more integrated care model such as DCPC (Serfaty et al., 2019). The benefit of CBT alone for depression in advanced illness (as opposed to anxiety, which is reviewed in the following section) is equivocal.

CALM (Hales et al., 2015) is a brief, semistructured, evidence-based intervention broadly rooted in attachment theory and relational theory, and designed to help individuals with advanced cancer manage their disease, broaden their perspective beyond living with illness to other possibilities for living, remain engaged in life, and attend to relationships and personal identity. It consists of three to six individual sessions, each lasting 45–60 minutes, delivered over 3 to 6 months. Sessions are structured around four empirically derived domains found to be important to this population: (1) symptom management and communication with health care providers; (2) changes in self and relations with close others; (3) sense of meaning and purpose; and (4) thinking of the future, hope, and mortality. Individuals' primary care partners are also offered the opportunity to participate. CALM resulted in reduced depression and anxiety and increased psychological growth (Nissim et al., 2012; Lo et al., 2014, 2019; Rodin et al., 2018). Please see Wilson et al. (2009) for an overview of assessment and treatment of depression at the end of life.

Anxiety Disorders

Between 2% and 30% (mean 10%) of individuals living with advanced serious illness have anxiety disorders (Kadan-Lottick et al., 2005; Miovic & Block, 2007), with 8–18% prevalence rates among individuals with advanced cancer (Spencer et al., 2010; Stark et al., 2002; Wilson et al., 2007). Risk factors include younger age, being female, underlying disease (pneumonia, pulmonary embolism, lung cancer, pleural effusion, chronic obstructive pulmonary disease) and associated physical symptoms (pain, dyspnea, nausea, fatigue), with risk increasing with increased physical symptom burden (Hofmann et al., 2017). Medications (e.g., adverse or paradoxical reactions to corticosteroids or stimulants), conditioned responses to medical treatment (radiation and/or chemotherapy), history of an anxiety disorder (generalized anxiety disorder, obsessive-compulsive disorder, or panic disorder), substance use, and anxiety in the care partner also increase risk (Bambauer et al., 2006; Hendriksen et al., 2015). The last risk factor argues for inclusion of the care partner in treatment. In addition, fears of living with a life-limiting illness, time constraints for attending to unresolved issues, and rumination about the future or concerns about the past increase the risk for anxiety disorders. Of note, individuals may be less likely to endorse the word "anxiety" rather than words such as "worry," "feeling tense," or "scared" (Zweers et al., 2019).

As is the case with depression, choice of psychological intervention for anxiety should be informed by the presence of risk factors and the nature of the anxiety and fears. Outcome research on the treatment of anxiety in palliative care populations shows support for dignity therapy, meaning-centered psychotherapy, ACT, CBT, and mindfulness-based interventions. Greer and colleagues (2010, 2012) piloted a modified CBT intervention for anxiety among individuals with terminal cancer, the goals of which were to provide information, promote control, engender good symptom management, and build on existing coping strategies. The intervention included psychoeducation and goal setting, relaxation training, coping strategies for cancer-related fears using cognitive therapy, and activity planning and pacing. In comparison with a waitlist control group, individuals receiving the modified CBT intervention demonstrated significant reductions in anxiety, which is consistent with prior research (Moorey et al., 2009).

Mindfulness-based stress reduction (MBSR) and mindfulness-based cognitive therapy (MBCT) have been used effectively with palliative care populations. Men with advanced prostate cancer in MBCT showed reduced anxiety, improved mindfulness skills, and reductions in avoidance and fear of cancer recurrence (Chambers et al., 2012). Peer learning in a group format appeared to contribute to the effectiveness of this intervention. A systematic review of the efficacy of MBCT or MBSR for individuals with cancer found reduced anxiety, stress (Shennan et al., 2011), and depressive symptoms, and improvements in mindfulness skills (Piet et al., 2012) though the studies were not specific to advanced serious illness or end of life. Please see Roth & Massie (2009) for an overview of assessment and treatment of anxiety at the end of life and Sage et al. (2008) for practical strategies and worksheets that could be used in treating anxiety in palliative care populations.

Posttraumatic Stress Disorder

Diagnosis of a life-limiting or terminal illness, particularly cancer, in combination with the challenges of medical treatment, may increase risk for PTSD or lead to persistence of PTSD (Gold et al., 2012). Most of what we know about PTSD in advanced illness comes from individuals diagnosed with cancer. Prevalence rates of PTSD in people with cancer typically range from 2% to 15%, depending on cancer site, assessment method, and time since diagnosis (Abbey et al., 2015; Kangas et al., 2005; Esser et al., 2019). In addition, individuals with non-cancer related PTSD are thought to be more vulnerable to an exacerbation of preexisting PTSD symptoms or to disease-related PTSD when diagnosed with a life-limiting illness (Wachen et al., 2014). For example, among newly diagnosed individuals with cancer, up to one third of individuals who were diagnosed with PTSD at the time of diagnosis had persistent or worsening PTSD 4 years later (Chan et al., 2018). Individuals at a more advanced stage of disease at the time of diagnosis were at greater risk (Abbey et al., 2015). Elevated dissociative reactions and acute emotional distress within the initial months following cancer diagnosis have been found to predict development of PTSD at 3 months posttreatment (Kangas et al., 2005).

Other factors that may increase risk or worsen symptoms, include fear of death, type of cancer and treatment, preexisting mental disorder, personal medical care, lack of privacy/control, and naturally occurring life review (Cordova et al., 2017; French-Rosas et al., 2011; Swartzman et al., 2017). Younger, female individuals may be at greatest risk, as are those with a higher number of physical and psychological symptoms (Nipp et al., 2018). In addition, pain interference or the disruption of activity or functioning because of pain or fear of pain, has been found to be associated with PTSD symptoms. Daily awareness of pain interference may act as a reminder of cancer-related trauma. However, pain anxiety and pain catastrophizing appear to mediate the relationship between pain interference and PTSD symptoms (Roth et al., 2013). Of note is that care partners may show the same degree of PTSD as individuals living with cancer (Swartzman et al., 2017), arguing for inclusion of care partners in psychological interventions.

Though the evidence base is not well-established for treatment of PTSD in advanced illness (i.e., Dimitrov et al., 2019), grounding strategies, mindfulness exercises, general coping skills, modified Eye Movement Desensitization and Reprocessing (EMDR) Therapy, CBT, and ACT may be appropriate. One study found that CBT with components of imaginal and in vivo exposure was more effective than supportive therapy in reducing PTSD symptoms in individuals with head and neck cancer (Kangas et al., 2013). Traditional trauma-focused psychotherapeutic interventions used to treat PTSD, including cognitive processing therapy (CPT) and prolonged exposure (PE), may require careful considerations in palliative care populations. These considerations include whether the individual wishes or is able to emotionally and cognitively process trauma, the likelihood of increased short-term distress, or time constraints. One promising intervention model that addresses these factors but has yet to be evaluated empirically is a stepwise psychosocial palliative care model (Feldman et al., 2014). Please see Glick et al. (2018) for a broader discussion of these issues.

Substance Use Disorders

Among individuals living with cancer, including those admitted to palliative care units or seen through outpatient palliative care services, the prevalence of substance use disorders ranges from 15% to 40% (Braiteh et al., 2007; Dev et al., 2011; Parsons et al., 2008). Substance use disorders can exacerbate suffering, decrease QOL, complicate management of symptoms, and distress family care partners (Krashin et al., 2012; Passik & Theobald, 2000). Individuals actively using can be difficult to engage in treatment. Individuals with addiction histories may be at increased risk of relapse when prescribed pain medication. Therefore, risk or fear of relapse should be acknowledged and nonpharmacological interventions, such as mindfulness-based relapse prevention, offered (Bowen et al., 2010).

The context of substance use disorders or fear of opioid misuse can complicate pain management. Cancer pain is undertreated in the US and Europe, with a third of patients not receiving pain medication proportional to their pain intensity (e.g., Greco et al., 2014), especially among US minorities (Fisch et al., 2012). Concern for substance use disorders, particularly opioid addiction and opioid misuse (i.e., the taking of pain medication in any way not prescribed, whether intentionally or inadvertently, and whether or not harm results) contributes to inadequate pain management. However, even individuals with clear risk factors for misuse or abuse may legitimately have moderate to severe pain. Clinicians must consider reasons for misuse, including poor pain control and pseudoaddiction (when patients have inadequate pain control and seek greater pain relief). Pain specialists, addiction specialists, oncologists, palliative care providers, psychologists, and behavioral health professionals can work collaboratively to explore fears of unmanaged pain and issues of misuse or addiction. High-risk individuals should be monitored for unusual behavior, provided education on safe opioid use, and have their emotional needs addressed (Kwon et al., 2015). Opioid risk management strategies can be implemented, including pain monitoring tools (urine drug testing, pill counts, pain intensity assessments), treatment agreements, periodic pain assessments, and abuse-deterrent formulations and packaging (Pergolizzi et al., 2016).

Care Partners of Individuals With Advanced Serious Illness or at End of Life

Between a quarter and a third of care partners of individuals living with advanced serious illness experience moderate to severe depression and anxiety (Oliver et al., 2017) and between 3.5% and 8.0% experience a mental disorder (Vanderwerker et al., 2005). Care partner mental health is often interdependent with that of the person for whom they are caring, such that addressing mental health and coping in the person living with advanced serious illness will also benefit the care partner. For example, depression and anxiety in the care partner is related to the care recipient's understanding of the severity of their disease (prognosis) and coping efforts (Nipp et al., 2016). Unfinished business with the care recipient, which can complicate meaning making and legacy-building activities, also contributes to depression and grief in the care partner (Yamashita et al., 2017). Ira Byock's four things (Byock, 2014) – forgive me, I forgive you, thank you, and I love you – can assist families in the completion of emotional unfinished business. Byock argues that these messages of gratitude and forgiveness must be shared before saying goodbye. Despite these significant impacts on care partners, care partners underutilize mental health and bereavement services, although this use increases significantly when providers discuss mental health concerns predeath (Lichtenthal et al., 2011).

> In the case example, Mr. R., Mr. M., and members of Mr. R.'s family engaged in gratitude and values-based, meaning-centered interventions via dignity therapy (described in Chapter 10). However, after Mr. R.'s death, tensions escalated between Mr. M., Mr. R.'s mother (Mrs. R.), and the older siblings. Specifically, Mrs. R. shared with the palliative care psychologist that she and her other children forgave Mr. R. prior to his death, but instead held resentment against Mr. M. for the "troubled ways" of his shared life with Mr. R. At the urging of her son Mr. N., Mrs. R. attempted to intervene with the funeral home director and stop the cremation of Mr. R.'s remains so that he could be buried in the family plot. This caused Mr. N. renewed stress and consternation, feelings of depression and anxiety, and an exacerbation of his osteoarthritis (OA) pain, as well as decreased adherence to his dietary regimen and monitoring of his blood sugar to manage his type 2 diabetes.

Factors Affecting Bereavement in Care Partners

As illustrated in the case example, family dysfunction commonly occurs among palliative care populations and is related to psychosocial distress in the seriously ill individual and care partners (Schuler et al., 2017) as well as to care partner adjustment to bereavement. Family focused grief therapy (FFGT; Kissane & Bloch, 2002) was developed to help families experiencing a high degree of conflict and dysfunction better cope with, and adapt to, illness-related changes in the family and promote adaptation in bereavement. The goal is to improve overall family functioning by strengthening cohesiveness, conflict resolution, and open expression of illness-related concerns. Therapy occurs in five stages: assessment, agreement regarding concerns or issues to address in treatment, active treatment, consolidation, and termination. The timing and frequency of sessions is adapted to the needs of the family and particulars of the illness. Typically, sessions occur for 90 minutes every other week or monthly. This approach is described in detail in Kissane and Bloch (2002) and is thereby easily accessible. Considerations of family and cultural norms such as family hierarchy; loyalty and tradition; expectations about caregiving; intergenerational tension; gender-determined roles; and the role of emotions, faith, and religion are important to address when working with diverse families (del Gaudio et al., 2012; Mondia et al., 2012). FFGT is associated with reduced distress and depression (Kissane et al., 2006) and reduced complicated grief symptom severity (Kissane et al., 2016).

Although grief and anticipatory grief are common experiences among individuals living with advanced serious illness and their care partners, due to space limitations, we focus here on bereavement in the care partners. In general, most people adapt to bereavement, with nearly one half to two thirds being resilient (Bonanno et al., 2004; Nielsen et al., 2019;

Ott et al., 2007). However, a sizable minority of individuals experience a persistent and pervasive grief response characterized by longing for, or preoccupation with, the deceased, difficulty accepting the death, separation distress, feeling that one has lost a part of oneself, inability to experience positive affect, and difficulty engaging in activities. These complications in grief, known commonly as prolonged grief disorder (PGD) or persistent complex bereavement disorder (PCBD), are distinct from other mental disorders (Boelen et al., 2010), though associated with an increase in major depression, anxiety, PTSD, suicidal ideation, negative health behaviors (e.g., alcohol, tobacco use), functional impairment, and poor physical health (Simon et al., 2007; Zhang et al., 2006).

PGD or PCBD affect between approximately 3–23% of bereaved individuals, with rates of 25% in bereaved older adults (Newson et al., 2011). Prevalence varies as a function of relationship to the deceased, cause of death, income, education, age, assessment instrument, and diagnostic criteria used in the study (*Diagnostic and Statistical Manual of Mental Disorders*, 5th edition [DSM-5] vs. *International Classification of Diseases,* 11th edition [ICD-11]). For example, when comparing the DSM-5 persistent complex bereavement disorder with the ICD-11 prolonged grief disorder criteria, prevalence was found to be 8% and 19%, respectively (Boelen et al., 2019). Among care partners of individuals receiving hospice and palliative care, the rate of complicated grief ranged from 10% to 20% (e.g., Nanni et al., 2014). Individuals with intersecting identities may be at particularly high risk given that they often experience additional stressors that impact bereavement. For example, lesbian, gay, bisexual, transgender, questioning, and other (LGBTQ+) bereaved individuals reported failure to acknowledge their relationship to the deceased and additional legal and financial stressors that shaped their bereavement experience (Bristowe et al., 2016). This finding could have had implications for the case example, wherein the relationship between Mr. R. and Mr. M. seemed to remain ambiguous and ill-defined to his family members.

Early identification of factors that put care partners at risk for complications in bereavement is critical. Yet, risk assessment strategies are often imprecise or inconsistently implemented (Ghesquiere et al., 2015). Hospice and palliative care providers have been found to be no better than chance at identifying those care partners at risk for future complications in bereavement, yet most hospice and palliative care services in the US do not use standardized risk assessment tools that could improve identification (Breen et al., 2014).

Psychologists can assist with risk assessment and management by assessing and addressing factors that put individuals at risk for complicated grief. Risk factors include poor physical health, concurrent stressful life events, psychological vulnerabilities, particular interpersonal factors, and nature of the dying experiences and death (Allen et al., 2013; Lobb et al., 2010; Hebert et al., 2009; Tomarken et al., 2008; Schulz et al., 2006). These risk factors can be clinical targets for intervention. Psychological vulnerabilities include experiential avoidance, intolerance of uncertainty, rumination, cognitive misappraisals, low self-efficacy, depression, and preloss grief (Boelen, 2010; Eisma, Schut et al., 2015; Eisma & Stroebe, 2017; Nielsen et al., 2017; Shear, 2010). Interpersonal factors include quality of the relationship with the seriously ill individual, degree to which individuals define themselves by their relationship with the seriously ill individual, attachment style, family conflict, absence of other caregivers, low satisfaction with or unavailable social support, perceived burden, separation anxiety, and exposure to trauma including previous deaths (Mancini et al., 2009; Nanni et al., 2014). Factors related to the death of the seriously ill individual include lack of preparation or forewarning of death, nonacceptance of the death, the nature and circumstances of the death, quality of the caregiving and dying experience, dissatisfaction with palliative or end-of-life care, decisional conflict and regret, perceived distress of the patient, and unresolved family issues (Holland et al., 2013; Lovell et al., 2015; Miyajima et al., 2014).

In addition to attempting to minimize and manage risk factors prior to the care recipient's death, psychologists also can promote protective factors. They can help care partners build their perceived self-efficacy and agency and emotion regulation skills. They can work with core schema and cultivate core beliefs that one can learn and grow from both positive and negative life experiences, that one is worthy even in the absence of the loved one. Psychologists can help care partners make sense of loss or find compensatory benefit and identify purpose. They also can assist in mobilizing social support (Bonanno, 2004; Neimeyer et al., 2006; Ong et al., 2004).

Bereavement Interventions for Care Partners

Psychologists and behavioral health professionals also can advocate for and provide bereavement interventions. Although bereavement services are an integral part of hospice and palliative care, services often are limited (Barry et al., 2012), and interventions typically are not theoretically driven or evidence-based, in part because the evidence base is not well-established or is equivocal (Breen et al., 2014; She & Prigerson, 2018). A national survey of US hospices (National Hospice Survey) found that just 27% provided comprehensive bereavement services, defined as ongoing discussion of family preferences for care, ongoing screening for depression and complicated grief, and provision of at least 8 of 10 specific bereavement services. These services include telephone calls to the bereaved, a card sent at the time of death or anniversary of death, educational information on grief, home visits, staff and/or volunteer attendance at funerals, memorial ceremonies, support groups or workshops, predeath planning, individual therapy, and group therapy. The survey also found that only 55% of hospices provided both screening for complicated grief and depression as well as access to bereavement therapy (Ghesquiere et al., 2015). Data were not collected on the type of screens used to identify complicated grief, or on the type of therapy provided to care partners or by whom it was provided.

The type of therapy offered is often limited by availability of providers who have familiarity with, and comfort providing, psychotherapy for complicated grief. Psychotherapy interventions for complicated grief that are supported by outcome data include, though are not limited to: (1) complicated grief treatment (Shear, 2015; Shear et al., 2014, 2016); (2) CBT and CBT with exposure (Boelen et al., 2011; Boelen et al., 2007; Boelen et al., 2006; Bryant et al., 2014, 2019; Eisma, Boelen et al., 2015; Wagner & Maercker, 2007; Wagner et al., 2006); (3) prolonged grief-specific CBT (PG-CBT; Rosner et al., 2011, 2014, 2015, 2018); (4) metacognitive grief therapy for prolonged grief (Wenn, O'Connor, Kane et al., 2019; Wenn, O'Connor, Breen et al., 2019; Wenn et al., 2015); and (5) constructivist grief therapy/narrative-based (Neimeyer et al., 2008, 2010; Neimeyer, 2001). Collectively, these approaches target cognitive processes, avoidance, emotion regulation, meaning making, and skills development.

Complicated Grief Treatment

Complicated grief treatment (CGT; Shear, 2015) is an evidence-based, 16-session, manualized treatment informed by the dual process model (Stroebe & Schut, 2010), which maintains that bereaved people cope with loss dialectically, attending to the dual processes of loss-oriented coping and restoration-oriented coping. When engaged in loss-oriented coping, individuals are consumed by the pain of grief and negative emotions triggered by the death. They struggle with redefining their attachment relationship with the deceased and temporarily deny or distract themselves from the demands of the world that have been changed by the death. When using restoration-orientated coping, bereaved individuals are engaged in activities that help them adapt to the myriad changes resulting from the death, such as learning new skills, assuming new roles, and forming new relationships, as well as distancing from the pain of grief. The goal of CGT is to help bereaved individuals move from primarily loss-oriented coping toward primarily restoration-orientated coping, and to reduce the intensity of grief, facilitate enjoyment of fond memories of the deceased, and support reengagement in daily activities and relationships. Sessions include (1) psychoeducation about the model of complicated grief and treatment strategies, (2) retelling the story of the death with a focus on revising troubling thinking regarding the circumstances or consequences of the death such as blaming oneself or believing life has no meaning without the deceased, (3) confronting situations that are avoided because of the death, (4) engaging with memories and pictures of the deceased, and (5) imagining conversations with the deceased. A supportive person usually attends the third session. The entire treatment manual, which includes outcome data, is available for purchase online (https://complicatedgrief.columbia.edu/professionals/manual-tools/).

In RCTs, CGT resulted in reductions in negative thoughts about the future, avoidance of situations or emotions connected to the loss, and reductions in anxiety and complicated grief symptoms (Glickman et al., 2017; Shear et al., 2005; Supiano & Luptak, 2014). Cognitive reappraisal and self-compassion are central mediators in these outcomes (Glickman et al., 2017).

CBT With Exposure for Complicated Grief

CBT with exposure for complicated grief (CBT for CG) is based on the assumption that to address complicated grief symptoms, an intervention needs to target negative cognitions and avoidance behaviors (Boelen et al., 2006). CBT for CG is a manualized, evidence-based therapy consisting of 6 sessions of cognitive restructuring and 6 sessions of exposure therapy (Boelen et al., 2007). Through cognitive restructuring, cognitions central to the bereaved individuals' problems are targeted, including attributions of meaning of the death, and differentiation of letting-go from forgetting the deceased. Through exposure, individuals gradually increase confrontation with the reality of the loss. They tell the story of the death and write down internal (memories, thoughts) and external (places, people) grief-eliciting stimuli that they tend to avoid. These grief-eliciting stimuli are hierarchically organized and subsequently confronted through flooding and graduated exposure. Reductions in complicated grief through CBT for CG were associated with changes in negative cognitions about life (e.g., my life is meaningless since my partner died) and catastrophic misinterpretations of grief reactions (e.g., if I express my feelings, I will go crazy) (Boelen et al., 2011).

Byrant and colleagues (2014, 2019) evaluated CBT for CG, with and without exposure. Treatment consisted of 10 weekly, 2-hr group CBT sessions and four individual exposure therapy sessions versus 10 weekly, 2-hr group CBT sessions and four individual sessions in which participants discussed whatever they wished. Individuals were taught skills to manage avoidance, rumination, and common maladaptive, grief-related appraisals. They were helped to facilitate positive memories of the deceased by sharing positive experiences as well as unresolved issues. They also identified future goals, steps to achieve these goals, and relapse prevention strategies for high-risk times (e.g., anniversaries). In the exposure condition, individuals were asked to think about the death of the person, attending to their emotional, cognitive, sensory, and somatic reactions. CBT+exposure compared with CBT alone was associated with greater reductions in grief and depressive symptoms and increased psychological and social functioning. Grief symptom reduction persisted at 6-month follow-up.

Prolonged Grief–Specific CBT

PG-CBT is an integrative, though predominantly CBT, approach that combines psychoeducation, exposure, cognitive restructuring, and homework with solution-focused, experiential and systemic strategies. PG-CBT consists of 20 individual sessions (plus four optional sessions). Sessions include psychoeducation on how symptoms are maintained, exposure to grief-related avoidance, cognitive restructuring of grief-related thoughts, relaxation skills, integration of the death and maintaining a healthy attachment to the deceased, and future goals. PG-CBT resulted in a reduction of grief symptoms and an increase in personal growth (Bartl et al., 2017).

Metacognitive Grief Therapy

MCGT (Wenn et al., 2015) was developed as a modified version of metacognitive therapy for anxiety and depression which targets metacognitive beliefs guiding maladaptive coping strategies – such as, worry, rumination and fixation of attention on perceived threat, which in turn allows for metacognitive flexibility. This intervention is provided in a group format, 2 hrs weekly for 6 weeks. Sessions review the metacognitive model of grief; the association between metacognitions, emotions, and behavior; and specific strategies including cognitive restructuring, detached mindfulness, attention training, rumination and worry postponement, and relapse prevention. An RCT demonstrated reductions in prolonged grief, depression, anxiety, stress, and rumination, and increased QOL, effects that were maintained at 3- and 6-month follow-ups (Wenn et al., 2019).

Constructivist/Narrative-Based Interventions

Constructive/narrative-based interventions confront and integrate the bereavement-related loss into life stories while consolidating memories of the relationship and reconstructing a changed sense of oneself. Either loss is written into existing narratives or new narratives are created. The task is to reorganize the individual's self-narrative to accommodate a changed life, and to recreate or reconstruct meaning. The various processes of meaning reconstruction (sense making, benefit finding, progressive identity change) have been found to mitigate the impact of interpersonal factors and characteristics of the dying process and death, on risk for complicated bereavement (Neimeyer et al., 2006).

Narrative strategies that promote meaning making regarding loss can mitigate complications in bereavement (Shear et al., 2005). High meaning making predicts better grief outcomes. The ability to find some form of benefit or silver lining, to experience a progressive rather than regressive transformation of one's identity, and to make sense of loss in personal, practical, existential and spiritual ways, predicts positive outcomes (Holland et al., 2006). Bereaved individuals who are able to make sense of loss in personally meaningful ways experience fewer symptoms of complicated grief (Neimeyer et al., 2006).

> Mr. M. began experiencing an exacerbation of his OA pain symptoms as well as anxiety, depression, and helplessness, after the death of Mr. R., due to his conflict with Mrs. R., and N. and Ms. J. over Mr. R.'s burial and estate. He also felt unmoored in his life and struggled with finding meaning and purpose now that the reality of life without Mr. R. was taking hold. In addition to working with the elder law attorney referred by the palliative care psychologist, Mr. M. began narrative-based grief therapy with the psychologist. This approach was chosen due to the previous success experienced to some degree by all family members with dignity therapy prior to Mr. R.'s death. The psychologist self-defined as an ACT practitioner and noted in a self-assessment of her skill competencies that a narrative-based grief therapy approach would match her skill set. The psychologist worked with Mr. M. to redefine his narrative to include his long-term romantic partnership with Mr. R. and to accept that, in large part, it was unlikely that his relationship with Mr. R.'s mother and siblings would change meaningfully. She also worked with Mr. M. using mindfulness and CBT principles to help him actively choose behavioral goals to resolve the conflict about the burial while relinquishing control to the elder law attorney regarding Mr. R.'s contested estate will and the disposition of their shared property. At the end of treatment, Mr. M. expressed relief and confidence that he could face the challenges of the family system with a sense of well-being and peace.

Conclusions and Implications

In this chapter, we expanded upon the case example of Mr. R. and Mr. M. to delve more deeply into issues that may affect care partners and family members after bereavement. We reviewed evidence-based interventions for serious mental health conditions that may arise concomitant to living with advanced serious illness, including depression, anxiety, PTSD, and substance use disorder. We explored effective interventions for complicated bereavement and the factors that put care partners at risk for mental health disorders and complicated bereavement. The current chapter also provided information regarding ACT as one psychotherapy approach particularly well-suited to treat psychological issues commonly seen in palliative care.

As in Chapter 10, we advocate for clinician self-assessment of skill and further training needs using the Pikes Peak Geropsychology Knowledge and Skill Assessment Tool (see Appendix 2; Karel et al., 2010) and Kasl-Godley and colleagues' (2014) description of knowledge and skill competencies for psychologists working in palliative care and hospice. The specific competencies covered in this chapter include foundational and functional knowledge of psychotherapy for individuals with concomitant chronic, life-threatening or terminal illness, and significant psychopathology as well as normal and abnormal grief and bereavement.

Expansion of the case example in this chapter highlighted family conflicts that may arise after bereavement and illustrated diversity and inclusion issues that may be more prevalent in earlier-born and specific age cohorts. Such conflict may be predicated upon claims of incapacity as the individual nearing death loses functionality. These capacity issues are beyond the scope of this chapter, but interested readers may wish to explore Carpenter and Merz (2020) regarding capacity to discuss medical aid in dying during goals of care conversations, Albright and colleagues (2020) regarding addressing family conflicts, and Chapter 7 of this book on determining basic decisional capacity.

Finally, we wish to emphasize the need to expand the evidence base of promising psychological treatments and translate these treatments into everyday clinical practice. One way this might be done is through the use of telehealth technology. Increasing the availability of evidence-based palliative and bereavement care interventions to telehealth platforms must be the focus of current and future research. The COVID-19 pandemic has brought into stark focus issues of death and dying, as well as mental health and social isolation. Bereavement within the context of COVID-19 poses many complex challenges, as families must rely upon telehealth platforms and the availability of health care staff to support saying final goodbyes with loved ones. Future efforts to support psychologists outside of Veterans Administration settings in providing palliative and bereavement care will likely rely upon current efforts such as the Psychology Interjurisdictional Compact (PSYPACT; https://www.asppb.net/general/custom.asp?page=psypact) in support of national licensure for telehealth delivery. The future of psychologists as part of integrated behavioral health teams in palliative and hospice care is poised to expand exponentially as telehealth delivery becomes a form of standard clinical practice.

Suggested Resources on Palliative Care, Psychopathology and Family Contexts

Allen, R. S., Carpenter, B. D., & Eichorst, M. K. (Eds). (2018). *Perspectives on palliative and end-of-life care: Disease, social and cultural context.* Aging and mental health research series. Routledge. ISBN: 978-1-138-59381-7 https://doi.org/10.4324/9780429489259

Byock, I., & Byock, A. (1997). *Dying well: The prospect for growth at the end of life* (p. 299). Riverhead Books.

Hayes, S. C., Strosahl, K. D., & Wilson, K. G. (2011). *Acceptance and commitment therapy: The process and practice of mindful change.* Guilford Press.

Moye, J. E. (2020). *Assessing capacities of older adults: A casebook to guide difficult decisions.* American Psychological Association. https://doi.org/10.1037/0000184-000

Qualls, S. H., & Kasl-Godley, J. E. (2010). *End-of-life issues, grief, and bereavement: What clinicians need to know* (Vol. 6). John Wiley & Sons.

Wilson, K. G., & Murrell, A. R. (2004). Values work in acceptance and commitment therapy: Setting a course for behavioral treatment. In S. C. Hayes, V. M. Follette, & M. Linehan, (Eds.), *Mindfulness & Acceptance: Expanding the cognitive-behavioral tradition* (pp. 120–151). Guilford Press.

References

Abbey, G., Thompson, S. B. N., Hickish, T., & Heathcote, D. (2015). A meta-analysis of prevalence rates and moderating factors for cancer-related post-traumatic stress disorder. *Psycho-Oncology, 24,* 371–381. https://doi.org/10.1002/pon.3654

Akizuki, N., Shimizu, K., Asai, M., Nakano, T., Okusaka, T., Shimada, K., Inoguchi, H., Inagaki, M., Fujimori, M., Akechi, T., & Uchitomi, Y. (2016). Prevalence and predictive factors of depression and anxiety in patients with pancreatic cancer: A longitudinal study. *Japanese Journal of Clinical Oncology, 46*(1), 71–77. https://doi.org/10.1093/jjco/hyv169

Albright, A., Hilgeman, M. M., & Allen, R. S. (2020). Addressing family conflicts when assessing capacities. In J. Moye (Ed.), *Assessing capacities of older adults: A casebook to guide difficult decisions.* American Psychological Association.

Allen, J. Y., Haley, W. E., Small, B. J., Schonwetter, R. S., & McMillan, S. C. (2013). Bereavement among hospice caregivers of cancer patients one year following loss: Predictors of grief, complicated grief, and symptoms of depression. *Journal of Palliative Medicine, 16*(7), 745–751 https://doi.org/10.1089/jpm.2012.0450

Bambauer, K Z., Zhang, B., Maciejewski, P. K., Sahay, N., Pirl, W. F., Block, S. D., & Prigerson, H. G. (2006). Mutuality and specificity of mental disorders in advanced cancer patients and caregivers. *Social Psychiatry and Psychiatric Epidemiology, 41,* 819–824. https://doi.org/10.1007/s00127-006-0103-x

Barry, C. L., Carlson, M. D., Thompson, J. W., Schlesinger, M., McCorkle, R., Kasl, S. V., & Bradley, E. H. (2012). Caring for grieving family members: Results from a national hospice survey. *Medical Care, 50*(7), 578–584. https://doi.org/10.1097/MLR.0b013e318248661d

Bartl, H., Hagl, M., Kotoucova, M., Pfoh, G., & Rosner, R. (2017). Does prolonged grief treatment foster posttraumatic growth? Secondary results from a treatment study with long-term follow-up and mediation analysis. *Psychology and Psychotherapy: Theory, Research and Practice, 91,* 27–41 https://doi.org/10.1111/papt.12140

Bennett, J. E., Stevens, G. A, Mathers, C. D., Bonita, R., Rehm, J., Kruk, M. E., Riley, L. M., Dian, K., Kengne, A. P., Chalkidou, K., Beagley, J., Kishore, S. P., Chen, W., Saxena, S., Bettcher, D. W., Grove, J. T., Beaglehole, R., & Ezzati, M. (2018). NCD Countdown 2030: Worldwide trends in non-communicable disease mortality and progress towards sustainable development goal target. *Lancet, 392*(10152), 1072–1088.

Boelen, P. (2010). Intolerance of uncertainty and emotional distress following the death of a loved one. *Anxiety, Stress & Coping, 23*(4), 471–478. https://doi.org/10.1080/10615800903494135

Boelen, P. A., de Keijser, J., van den Hout, M. A., & van den Bout, J. (2007). Treatment of complicated grief: A comparison between cognitive-behavioral therapy and supportive counseling. *Journal of Consulting and Clinical Psychology,75*(2), 277–284. https://doi.org/10.1037/0022-006X.75.2.277

Boelen, P. A., de Keijser, J., van den Hout, M. A., & van den Bout, J. (2011). Factors associated with outcome of cognitive-behavioral therapy for complicated grief: A preliminary study. *Clinical Psychology and Psychotherapy, 18*(4), 284–291. https://doi.org/10.1002/cpp.720

Boelen, P. A., Lenferink, L. I. M., & Smid, G. E. (2019). Further evaluation of the factor structure, prevalence, and concurrent validity of DSM-5 criteria for Persistent Complex Bereavement Disorder and ICD-11 criteria for Prolonged Grief Disorder. *Psychiatry Research, 273,* 206–210. https://doi.org/10.1016/j.psychres.2019.01.006

Boelen, P. A., van den Hout, M. A., & van den Bout, J. (2006). A cognitive-behavioral conceptualization of complicated grief. *Clinical Psychology: Science & Practice, 13,* 109–128. https://doi.org/10.1111/j.1468-2850.2006.00013.x

Boelen, P. A., van de Schoot, R., van den Hout, M. A., de Keijser, J., & van den Bout, J. (2010). Prolonged Grief Disorder, depression, and posttraumatic stress disorder are distinguishable syndromes. *Journal of Affective Disorders, 125*(1–3), 374–378. https://doi.org/10.1016/j.jad.2010.01.076

Bonanno, G. A. (2004). Loss, trauma, and human resilience: Have we underestimated the human capacity to thrive after extremely aversive events? *American Psychologist, 59*(1), 20–28. https://doi.org/10.1037/0003-066X.59.1.20

Bonanno, G. A., Wortman, C. B., & Nesse, R. M. (2004). Prospective patterns of resilience and maladjustment during widowhood. *Psychology and Aging, 19*(2), 260. https://doi.org/10.1037/0882-7974.19.2.260

Bowen, S., Chawla, N., Marlatt, G. A., & Parks, G. A. (2010). *Mindfulness-based relapse prevention.* Guilford Press.

Braiteh, F., El Osta, B., Palmer, J. L., Reddy, S. K., & Bruera, E. (2007). Characteristics, findings, and outcomes of palliative care inpatient consultations at a comprehensive cancer center. *Journal of Palliative Medicine, 10*(4), 948–955. https://doi.org/10.1089/jpm.2006.0257

Breen, L. J., Aoun, S. M., O'Connor, M., & Rumbold, B. (2014). Bridging the gaps in palliative care bereavement suppAn international perspective. *Death Studies, 38*(1–5), 54–61. https://doi.org/10.1080/07481187.2012.725451

Bristowe, K., Marshall, S., & Harding, R. (2016). The bereavement experiences of lesbian, gay, bisexual and/or trans* people who have lost a partner: A systematic review, thematic synthesis and modelling of the literature. *Palliative Medicine, 30*(8), 730–744. https://doi.org/10.1177/0269216316634601

Bryant, R. A, Kenny L., Joscelyne, A., Rawson, N., Maccallum, F., Cahill, C., Hopwood, S., Aderka, I., & Nickerson, A. (2014). Treating prolonged grief disorder: A randomized clinical trial. *JAMA Psychiatry, 71*(12), 1332–1339. https://doi.org/10.1001/jamapsychiatry.2014.1600

Bryant, R. A., Kenny, L., Joscelyne, A., Rawson, N., Maccallum, F., Cahill, C., & Hopwood, S. (2019). Predictors of treatment response for cognitive behaviour therapy for prolonged grief disorder. *European Journal of Psychotraumatology, 8*(6), 1556551. https://doi.org/10.1080/20008198.2018.1556551

Buhrman, M., Skoglund, A.,, Husell, J., Bergström, K., Gordh, T., Hursti, T., Bendelin, N., Furmark, T., & Andersson, G. (2013). Guided internet-delivered acceptance and commitment therapy for chronic pain patients: A randomized controlled trial. *Behavior Research and Therapy, 51,* 307–315. https://doi.org/10.1016/j.brat.2013.02.010

Byock, I. (2014). *The four things that matter most: A book about living.* Simon and Schuster.

Carpenter, B. D., & Merz, C. C. (2020). Assessment of capacity in medical aid in dying. In J. Moye (Ed.), *Assessing capacities of older adults: A casebook to guide difficult decisions* (p. 243–267). American Psychological Association.

Center to Advance Palliative Care & the National Palliative Care Research Center. (2019). *America's care of serious illness: A state-by-state report card on access to palliative care in our nation's hospitals.*

Chambers, S. K., Foley, E., Galt, E., Ferguson, M., & Clutton, S. (2012). Mindfulness groups for men with advanced prostate cancer: A pilot study to assess feasibility and effectiveness and the role of peer support. *Supportive Care in Cancer, 20*(6), 1183–1192. https://doi.org/10.1007/s00520-011-1195-8

Chan, C. M. H., Ng, C. G., Taib, N. A., Wee, L. H., Krupat, E., & Meyer, F. (2018). Course and predictors of post-traumatic stress disorder in a cohort of psychologically distressed patients with cancer: A 4-year follow-up study. *Cancer, 124,* 406–416. https://doi.org/10.1002/cncr.30980

Cordova, M. J., Riba, M. B., & Spiegel, D. (2017). Post-traumatic stress disorder and cancer. *Lancet Psychiatry, 4*(4), 330–338. https://doi.org/10.1016/S2215-0366(17)30014-7

del Gaudio, F., Hichenberg, S., Eisenberg, M., Kerr, E., Zaider, T. I., & Kissane, D. W. (2012). Latino values in the context of palliative care: illustrative cases from the Family Focused Grief Therapy trial. *American Journal of Hospice & Palliative Medicine, 30*(3), 271–278. https://doi.org/10.1177/1049909112448926

Dev, R., Parsons, H. A., Palla, S., Palmer, J. L., Del Fabbro, E., & Bruera, E. (2011). Undocumented alcoholism and its correlation with tobacco and illegal drug use in advanced cancer patients. *Cancer, 117,* 4551–4556. https://doi.org/10.1002/cncr.26082

Dimitrov, L., Moschopoulou, E., & Korszun, A. (2019). Interventions for the treatment of cancer-related traumatic stress symptoms: A systematic review of the literature. *Psycho-Oncology, 28,* 970–979. https://doi.org/10.1002/pon.5055

Eisma, M. C., Boelen, P. A., van den Bout, J., Stroebe, W., Schut, H. A. W., Lancee, J., & Stroebe, M. S. (2015). Internet-based exposure and behavioral activation for complicated grief and rumination: A randomized controlled trial. *Behavior Therapy, 46*(6), 729–748. https://doi.org/10.1016/j.beth.2015.05.007

Eisma, M. C., Schut, H. A., Stroebe, M. S., Boelen, P. A., van den Bout, J., & Stroebe, W. (2015). Adaptive and maladaptive rumination after loss: A three-wave longitudinal study. *British Journal of Clinical Psychology, 54*(2), 163–180. https://doi.org/10.1111/bjc.12067

Eisma, M. C., & Stroebe, M. S. (2017). Rumination following bereavement: An overview. *Bereavement Care, 36*(2), 58–64. https://doi.org/10.1080/02682621.2017.1349291

Esser, P., Glaesmer, H., Faller, H., Koch, U., Harter, M., Schulz, H., Wegscheider, K., Weis, J., & Mehnert, A. (2019). Postraumatic stress disorder among cancer patients – findings from a large and representative interview-based study in Germany. *Psycho-Oncology, 28,* 1278–1285. https://doi.org/10.1002/pon.5079

Fässberg, M. M., Cheung, G., Canetto, S. S., Erlangsend, A., Lapierre, S., Lindner, R., Draper, B., Gallo, J. J., Wong, C., Wu, J., Duberstein, P., & Wærn, M. (2016). A systematic review of physical illness, functional disability, and suicidal behaviour among older adults. *Aging & Mental Health, 20*(2), 166–194.

Feldman, D. B., Sorocco, K. H., & Bratkovich, K. L. (2014). Treatment of posttraumatic stress disorder at the end-of-life: Application of the stepwise psychosocial palliative care model. *Palliative and Supportive Care, 12,* 233–243. https://doi.org/10.1017/S1478951513000370

Feros, D. L., Lane, L., Ciarrochi, J., & Blackledge, J. T. (2013). Acceptance and commitment therapy (ACT) for improving the lives of cancer patients: A preliminary study. *Psycho-Oncology, 22,* 459–464.

Fisch, M. J., Lee, J. W., Weiss, M., Wagner, L. I., Chang, V. T., Cella, D., Manola, J. B., Minasian, L. M., McCaskill-Stevens, W., Mendoza, T. R., & Cleeland, C. S. (2012). Prospective, observational study of pain and analgesic prescribing in medical oncology outpatients with breast, colorectal, lung, or prostate cancer. *Journal of Clinical Oncology, 30*(16), 1980–1988.

Freedland, K. E., Carney, R. M., Rich, M. W., Steinmeyer, B. C., Skala, J. A., & Dávila-Román, V. G. (2016). Depression and multiple rehospitalizations in patients with heart failure. *Clinics of Cardiology, 39*(5), 257–262. https://doi.org/10.1002/clc.22520

French-Rosas, L. N., Moye, J., & Naik, A. D. (2011). Improving the recognition and treatment of cancer-related posttraumatic stress disorder. *Journal of Psychiatric Practice, 17*(4), 270–276. https://doi.org/10.1097/01.pra.0000400264.30043.ae

Ghesquiere, A. R., Aldridge, M. D., Johnson-Hürzeler, R., Kaplan, D., Bruce, M. L., & Bradley, E. (2015). Hospice services for complicated grief and depression: results from a national survey. *Journal of the American Geriatrics Society, 63*(10), 2173–2180. https://doi.org/10.1111/jgs.13656

Glick, D. M., Cook, J. M., Moye, J., & Kaiser, A. P. (2018). Assessment and treatment considerations for post traumatic stress disorder at end of life. *American Journal of Hospice and Palliative Care, 35*(8), 1133–1139. https://doi.org/10.1177/1049909118756656

Glickman, K., Shear, M. K., & Wall, M. M. (2017). Mediators of outcome in complicated grief treatment. *Journal of Clinical Psychology, 73*(7), 817–828. https://doi.org/10.1002/jclp.22384

Gold, J. I., Douglas, M. K., Thomas, M. L., Elliott, J. E., Rao, S. M., & Miaskowski, C. (2012). The relationship between posttraumatic stress disorder, mood states, functional status, and quality of life in oncology outpatients. *Journal of Pain and Symptom Management, 44*(4), 20–531. https://doi.org/10.1016/j.jpainsymman.2011.10.014

Greco, M. T., Roberto, A., Corli, O., Deandrea, S., Bandieri, E., Cavuto, S., & Apolone, G. (2014). Quality of cancer pain management: An update of a systematic review of undertreatement of patients with cancer. *Journal of Clinical Oncology, 32*(36), 4149–4154. https://doi.org/10.1200/JCO.2014.56.0383

Greer, J. A., Park, E. R., Prigerson, H. G., & Safren, S. A. (2010). Tailoring cognitive-behavioral therapy to treat anxiety comorbid with advanced cancer. *Journal of Cognitive Psychotherapy, 24,* 294–313. https://doi.org/10.1891/0889-8391.24.4.294

Greer, J. A., Traeger, L., Bemis, H., Solis, J., Hendriksen, E. S., Park, E. R., Pirl, W. F., Temel, J. S., Prigerson, H. G., & Safren, S. A. (2012). A pilot randomized controlled trial of brief cognitive-behavioral therapy for anxiety in patients with terminal cancer. *Oncologist, 17,* 1337–1345. https://doi.org/10.1634/theoncologist.2012-0041

Grotmol, K. S., Lie, H. C., Loge, J. H., Aass, N., Haugen, D. Stone, P. C., Kaasa, S., Hjermstad, M. J.; on behalf of the European Palliative Care Research Collaborative (EPCRC). (2019). Patients with advanced cancer and depression report a significantly higher symptom burden than non-depressed patients. *Palliative and Supportive Care, 17,* 143–149.

Hack, T. F., McClement, S. E., Chochinov, H. M., Cann, B. J., Hassard, T. H., Kristjanson, L. J., & Harlos, M. (2010). Learning from dying patients during their final days: life reflections gleaned from dignity therapy. *Palliative Medicine, 24*(7), 715–723. https://doi.org/10.1177/0269216310373164

Hales, S., Lo, C., & Rodin, G. (2015). *Managing cancer and living meaningfully (CALM). Treatment manual: An individual psychotherapy for patients with advanced cancer.* Princess Margaret Cancer Centre, University Health Network.

Hendriksen, E., Williams, E., Sporn, N., Greer, J., DeGrange, A., & Koopman, C. (2015). Worried together: A qualitative study of shared anxiety in patients with metastatic non-small cell lung cancer and their family caregivers. *Supportive Care in Cancer, 23*(4), 1035-1041. https://doi.org/10.1007/s00520-014-2431-9

Hebert, R. S., Schulz, R., Copeland, V. C., & Arnold, R. M. (2009). Preparing family caregivers for death and bereavement: Insights from caregivers of terminally ill patients. *Journal of Pain and Symptom Management, 37*(1), 3–12. https://doi.org/10.1016/j.jpainsymman.2007.12.010

Hofmann, S., Hess, S., Klein, C., Lindena, G., Radbruch, L., & Ostgathe, C. (2017). Patients in palliative care – Development of a predictive model for anxiety using routine data. *PLoS ONE, 12*(8). https:/doi.org/10.1371/journal.pone.0179415

Holland, J. M., Currier, J. M., & Neimeyer, R. A. (2006). Meaning reconstruction in the first two years of bereavement: The role of sense-making and benefit-finding. *Omega, 53*(3), 175–191. https://doi.org/10.2190/FKM2-YJTY-F9VV-9XWY

Holland, J. M., Futterman, A., Thompson, L. W., Moran, C., & Gallagher-Thompson, D. (2013). Difficulties accepting the loss of a spouse: A precursor for intensified grieving among widowed older adults. *Death Studies, 37*(2),126–144. https://doi.org/10.1080/07481187.2011.617489

Institute of Medicine. (2015). *Dying in America: Improving quality and honoring individual preferences near the end of life*. The National Academies Press.

Janberidizee, E., Hjermstad, M. J., Haugen, D. F., Haugen, D. F., Sigurdardottir, K. R., Løhre, E. T., Lie, H. C., Loge, J. H., Kaasa, S., Knudsen, K. & EURO IMPACT. (2014). How are patient populations characterized in studies investigating depression in advanced cancer? Results from a systematic literature review. *Journal of Pain and Symptom Management, 48*(4), 678–698.

Kadan-Lottick, N. S., Vanderwerker, L. C., Block, S. D., Zhang, B., & Prigerson, H. G. (2005). Psychiatric disorders and mental health service use in patients with advanced cancer: A report from the coping with cancer study. *Cancer, 104*(12), 2872–2881. https://doi.org/10.1002/cncr.21532

Kangas, M., Henry, J. L., & Bryant, R. A. (2005). Predictors of posttraumatic stress disorder following cancer. *Health Psychology, 24*(6), 579–585. https://doi.org/10.1037/0278-6133.24.6.579

Kangas, M., Milross, C., Taylor, A., & Bryant, R. A. (2013). A pilot randomized controlled trial of a brief early intervention for reducing posttraumatic stress disorder, anxiety and depressive symptoms in newly diagnosed head and neck cancer patients. *Psycho-Oncology, 22*(7), 1665–1673. https://doi.org/10.1002/pon.3208

Karel, M. J., Emery, E. E., Molinari, V., & CoPGTP Task Force on the Assessment of Geropsychology Competencies. (2010). Development of a tool to evaluate geropsychology knowledge and skill competencies. *International Psychogeriatrics, 22*(6), 886–896. https://doi.org/10.1017/S1041610209991736

Kasl-Godley, J. E., King, D. A., & Quill, T. E. (2014). Opportunities for psychologists in palliative care: Working with patients and families across the disease continuum. *American Psychologist, 69*(4), 364. https://doi.org/10.1037/a0036735

Kelley, A. S., & Bollens-Lund, E. (2018). Identifying the population with serious illness: The "denominator" challenge. *Journal of Palliative Medicine, 21*(S2), S7–S16. https://doi.org/10.1089/jpm.2017.0548

Kelly, A. S., & Morrison, R. S. (2015). Palliative care for the seriously ill. *New England Journal of Medicine, 373*(8), 747–755. https://doi.org/10.1056/NEJMra1404684

King, D. A., Heisel, M. J., & Lyness, J. M. (2005). Assessment and psychological treatment of depression in older adults with terminal or life-threatening illness. *Clinical Psychology: Science and Practice, 12*(3), 339–353. https://doi.org/10.1093/clipsy.bpi029

Kissane, D. W., & Bloch, S. (2002). *Family focused grief therapy: A model of family-centred care during palliative care and bereavement (facing death)*. Open University Press.

Kissane, D. W., McKenzie, M., Bloch, S., Moskowitz, C., McKenzie, D. P., & O'Neill, I. (2006). Family focused grief therapy: A randomized, controlled trial in palliative care and bereavement. *American Journal of Psychiatry, 163*(7), 1208–1218. https://doi.org/10.1176/ajp.2006.163.7.1208

Kissane, D. W., Zaider, T. I., Li, Y., Hichenberg, S., Schuler, T., Lederberg, M., Lavelle, L., Loeb, R., & del Gaudio, F. (2016). Randomized controlled trial of family therapy in advanced cancer continued into bereavement. *Journal of Clinical Oncology, 34*(16), 1921–1927. https://doi.org/10.1200/JCO.2015.63.0582

Krashin, D., Murinova, N., & Ballantyne, J. (2012). Management of pain with comorbid substance abuse. *Current Psychiatry Reports, 14*(5), 462–468. https://doi.org/10.1007/s11920-012-0298-3

Kwon, J. H., Hui, D., & Bruera, E. (2015). A pilot study to define chemical coping in cancer patients using the Delphi method. *Journal of Palliative Medicine, 18*(8), 703–706. https://doi.org/10.1089/jpm.2014.0446

Lichtenthal, W. G., Nilsson, M., Kissane, D. W., Breitbart, W., Kacel, E., Jones, E. C., & Prigerson, H. C. (2011). Underutilization of mental health services among bereaved caregivers with prolonged grief disorder. *Psychiatric Services, 62*(10), 1225–1229. https://doi.org/10.1176/ps.62.10.pss6210_1225

Lo, C., Hales, S., Jung, J., Chiu, A., Panday, T., Malfitano, C., Jung, J., Rydall, A., Li, M., Nissim, R., Zimmermann, C., & Rodin, G. (2019). Managing cancer and living meaningfully (CALM): Randomised feasibility trial in patients with advanced cancer. *BMJ Supportive & Palliative Care, 9*(2), 209–218.

Lo, C., Hales, S., Jung, J., Chiu, A., Panday, T., Rydall, A., Nissim, R., Malfitano, C., Petricone-Westwood, D., Zimmermann, C., & Rodin, G. (2014). Managing Cancer and Living Meaningfully (CALM): Phase 2 trial of a brief individual psychotherapy for patients with advanced cancer. *Palliative Medicine, 28*(3), 234–242. https://doi.org/10.1177/0269216313507757

Lobb, E. A., Kristjanson, L. J., Aoun, S. M., Monterosso, L., Halkett, G. K. B., & Davies, A. (2010). Predictors of complicated grief: A systematic review of empirical studies. *Death Studies, 34*(8), 673–698. https://doi.org/10.1080/07481187.2010.496686

Lovell, G. P., Smith, T., & Kannis-Dymand, L. (2015). Surrogate end-of-life care decision makers' postbereavement grief and guilt responses. *Death Studies, 39*(10), 647–653. https://doi.org/10.1080/07481187.2015.1047062

Mancini, A. D., Robinaugh, D., Shear, K., & Bonanno, G. A. (2009). Does attachment avoidance help people cope with loss? The moderating effects of relationship quality. *Journal of Clinical Psychology, 65*(10), 1127–1136. https://doi.org/10.1002/jclp.20601

McCracken, L. M., & Gutiérrez-Martínez, O. (2011). Processes of change in psychological flexibility in an interdisciplinary group-based treatment for chronic pain based on acceptance and commitment therapy. *Behavior Research and Therapy, 49*(4), 267–274. https://doi.org/10.1016/j.brat.2011.02.004

McCracken, L. M., & Jones, R. (2012). Treatment for chronic pain for adults in the seventh and eighth decades of life: A preliminary study of acceptance and commitment therapy (ACT). *Pain Medicine, 13*(7), 861–867. https://doi.org/10.1111/j.1526-4637.2012.01407.x

McCracken, L. M., Sato, A., & Taylor, G. J. (2013). A trial of a brief group-based form of acceptance and commitment therapy (ACT) for chronic pain in general practice: Pilot outcome and process results. *Journal of Pain, 14*(11), 1398–1406. https://doi.org/10.1016/j.jpain.2013.06.011

Miovic, M., & Block, S. (2007). Psychiatric disorders in advanced cancer. *Cancer, 110*(8), 1665–1676. https://doi.org/10.1002/cncr.22980

Misono, S., Weiss, N. S., Fann, J. R., Redman, M., & Yueh, B. (2008). Incidence of suicide in persons with cancer. *Journal of Clinical Oncology, 26*(29), 4731–4738. https://doi.org/10.1200/JCO.2007.13.8941

Mitchell, A. J., Chan, M., Bhatti, H., Halton, M., Grassi, L., Johansen, C., & Meader, N. (2011). Prevalence of depression, anxiety, and adjustment disorder in oncological, haematological, and palliative- care settings: A meta-analysis of 94 interview-based studies. *Lancet Oncology, 12*(2), 160–174. https://doi.org/10.1016/S1470-2045(11)70002-X

Miyajima, K., Fujisawa, D., Yoshimura, K., Ito, M., Nakajima, S., Shirahase, J., Mimuru, M., & Miyashita, M. (2014). Association between quality of end-of-life care and possible complicated grief among bereaved family members. *Journal of Palliative Medicine, 17*(9),1025–1031. https://doi.org/10.1089/jpm.2013.0552

Mohabbat-Bahar, S., Maleki-Rizi, F., Akbari, M. E., & Moradi-Joo, M. (2015). Effectiveness of group training based on Acceptance and Commitment Therapy on anxiety and depression of women with breast cancer. *Iranian Journal of Cancer Prevention, 8*(2), 71–76.

Mondia, S., Hichenberg, S., Kerr, E., Eisenberg, M., & Kissane, D. W. (2012). The impact of Asian American value systems on palliative care: Illustrative cases from the family-focused grief therapy trial. *American Journal of Hospice & Palliative Medicine, 29*(6), 443–448. https://doi.org/10.1177/1049909111426281

Moorey, S., Cort, E., Kapari, M., Monroe, B., Hansford, P., Mannix, K., Henderson, M., Fisher, L., & Hotopf, M. (2009). A cluster randomized controlled trial of cognitive behavior therapy for common mental disorders in patients with advanced cancer. *Psychological Medicine, 39,* 713—723. https://doi.org/10.1017/S0033291708004169

Mosher, C. E., Secinti, E., Li, R., Hirsh, A. T., Bricker, J., Miller, K. D., Schneider, B., Storniolo, A. M., Mina, L., Newton, E. V., Champion, V. L., Johns, S. A. (2018). Acceptance and commitment therapy for symptom interference in metastatic breast cancer patients: A pilot randomized trial. *Support Care Cancer, 26*(6), 1993–2004.

Mosher, C. E., Tometich, D. B., Hirsh, A., Rand, K. L., Johns, S. A., Matthias, M. S., Outcalt, S. D., Bricker, J., Schneider, B. Mina, L., Storniolo, A. M., Newton, E., & Miller, K. (2017). Symptom experiences in metastatic breast cancer patients: Relationships to activity engagement, value-based living, and psychological inflexibility. *Psycho-Oncology, 26*(11), 1944–1951.

Nanni, M. G., Biancosino, B., & Grassi, L. (2014). Pre-loss symptoms related to risk of complicated grief in caregivers of terminally ill cancer patients. *Journal of Affective Disorders, 160,* 87–91. https://doi.org/10.1016/j.jad.2013.12.023

Neimeyer, R. A. (2001). The language of loss: grief therapy as a process of meaning reconstruction. In R. A. Neimeyer (Ed.), *Meaning reconstruction & the experience of loss* (pp. 261–268). American Psychological Association. https://doi.org/10.1037/10397-014

Neimeyer, R. A., Baldwin, S. A., & Gillies, J. (2006). Continuing bonds and reconstructing meaning: Mitigating complications in bereavement. *Death studies, 30*(8),715–738. https://doi.org/10.1080/07481180600848322

Neimeyer, R. A., Burke, L. A., MacKay, M. M., & van Dyke Stringer, J. G. (2010). Grief therapy and the reconstruction of meaning: From principles to practice. *Journal of Contemporary Psychotherapy, 40,* 73–83. https://doi.org/10.1007/s10879-009-9135-3

Neimeyer, R. A., Holland, J. M., Currier, J. M., & Mehta, T. (2008) Meaning reconstruction in later life: Toward a cognitive-constructivist approach to grief therapy. In D. Gallagher-Thompson, A. M. Steffen, & L. W. Thompson (Eds), *Handbook of behavioral and cognitive therapies with older adults* (pp. 264–277). Springer. https://doi.org/10.1007/978-0-387-72007-4_17

Newson, R. S., Boelen, P. A., Hek, K., Hofman, A., & Tiemeier, H. (2011). The prevalence and characteristics of complicated grief in older adults. *Journal of Affective Disorders, 132,* 231–238. https://doi.org/10.1016/j.jad.2011.02.021

Nielsen, M. K., Carlsen, A. H, Neergaard, M. A., Bidstrup, P. E., & Guldin, M. (2019). Looking beyond the mean in grief trajectories: A prospective, population-based cohort study. *Social Science & Medicine, 232,* 460–469. https://doi.org/10.1016/j.socscimed.2018.10.007

Nielsen, M. K., Neergaard, M. A., Jensen, A. B., Vedsted, P., Bro, F., & Guldin, M. B. (2017). Preloss grief in family caregivers during end-of-life cancer care: A nationwide population-based cohort study. *Psycho-Oncology, 26*(12), 2048–2056. https://doi.org/10.1002/pon.4416

Nipp, R. D., El-Jawahri, A., D'Arpino, S. M., Chan, A., Fuh, C., Johnson, P. C., Lage, D. E., Wong, R. L., Pirl, W. F., Traeger, L., Cashavelly, B. J., Jackson, V. A., Ryan, D. P., Hochberg, E. P., Temel, J. S., & Greer, J. A. (2018). Symptoms of posttraumatic stress disorder among hospitalized patients with cancer. *Cancer, 124,* 3445–3453. https://doi.org/10.1002/cncr.31576

Nipp, R. D., El-Jawahri, A., Fishbein, J. N., Gallagher, E. R., Stagl, J. M., Parke, E. R., Jackson, V. A., Pirl, W. F., Greer, J. A., & Temel, J. S. (2016). Factors associated with depression and anxiety symptoms in family caregivers of patients with incurable cancer. *Annals of Oncology, 27,* 1607–1612. https://doi.org/10.1093/annonc/mdw205

Nissim, R., Freeman, E., Lo, C., Zimmermann, C., Gagliese, L., Rydall, A., Hales, S., & Rodin, G. (2012). Managing Cancer and Living Meaningfully (CALM): A qualitative study of a brief individual psychotherapy for individuals with advanced cancer. *Palliative Medicine, 26*(5), 713–721. https://doi.org/10.1177/0269216311425096

Oliver, D. P., Washington, K., Smith, J., Uraizee, A., & Demiris, G. (2017). The prevalence and risks for depression and anxiety in hospice caregivers. *Journal of Palliative Medicine, 20*(4), 366–371. https://doi.org/10.1089/jpm.2016.0372

Ong, A. D., Bergeman, C. S., & Bisconti, T. L. (2004). The role of daily positive emotions during conjugal bereavement. *Journal of Gerontology B: Psychological Sciences & Social Sciences, 59*(4), P168–P176.

Ott, C. H., Lueger, R. J., Kelber, S. T., & Prigerson, H. G. (2007). Spousal bereavement in older adults: Common, resilient, and chronic grief with defining characteristics. *Journal of Nervous and Mental Disease, 195*(4), 332–341. https://doi.org/10.1097/01.nmd.0000243890.93992.1e

Parsons, H. A., Delgado-Guay, M. O., Osta, B. E., Chacko, R., Poulter, V., Palme, L., & Bruera, E. (2008). Alcoholism screening in patients with advanced cancer: Impact on symptom burden and opioid use. *Journal of Palliative Medicine, 11*(7), 964–968. https://doi.org/10.1089/jpm.2008.0037

Passik, S. D., & Theobald, D. E. (2000). Managing addiction in advanced cancer patients: Why bother? *Journal of Pain and Symptom Management, 19,* 229–234. https://doi.org/10.1016/S0885-3924(00)00109-3

Pergolizzi, J. V., Zampogna, G., Taylor, R., Gonima, E., Posada, J., & Raffa, R. B. (2016). A guide for pain management in low and middle income communities: Managing the risk of opioid abuse in patients with cancer pain. *Frontiers in Pharmacology, 7*(42), 1–9. https://doi.org/10.3389/fphar.2016.00042

Piet, J., Wurtzen, H., & Zachariae, R. (2012). The effect of mindfulness-based therapy on symptoms of anxiety and depression in adult cancer patients and survivors: A systematic review and meta-analysis. *Journal of Consulting and Clinical Psychology, 80*(6), 1007–1020. https://doi.org/10.1037/a0028329

Rodin, G., Lo, C., Rydall, A., Shnall, J., Malfitano, C., Chiu, A., Panday, T., Watt, S., An, E., Nissim, R., Li, M., Zimmermann, C., & Hales, S. (2018). Managing Cancer and Living Meaningfully (CALM): A randomized controlled trial of a psychological intervention for patients with advanced cancer. *Journal of Clinical Oncology, 36*(23), 2422–2432. https://doi.org/10.1200/JCO.2017.77.1097

Rosner, R., Bartl, H., Pfoh, G., Kotoučová, M., & Hagl, M. (2015). Efficacy of an integrative CBT for prolonged grief disorder: A long-term follow-up. *Journal of Affective Disorders, 183,* 106–112. https://doi.org/10.1016/j.jad.2015.04.051

Rosner, R., Pfoh, G., & Kotoučová, M. (2011). Treatment of complicated grief. *European Journal of Psychotraumatology, 2*(1). https://doi.org/10.3402/ejpt.v2i0.7995

Rosner, R., Pfoh, G., Kotoučová, M., & Hagl, M. (2014). Efficacy of an outpatient treatment for prolonged grief disorder: A randomized controlled clinical trial. *Journal of Affective Disorders, 167,* 56–63. https://doi.org/10.1016/j.jad.2014.05.035

Rosner, R., Rimane, E., Vogel, A., Rau, J., & Hagl, M. (2018). Treating prolonged grief disorder with prolonged grief-specific cognitive behavioral therapy: Study protocol for a randomized controlled trial. *Trials, 19,* 241. https://doi.org/10.1186/s13063-018-2618-3

Roth, A. J., & Massie, M. J. (2009). Anxiety in palliative care. In H. M. Chochinov & W. Breitbart (Eds.), *Handbook of psychiatry in palliative medicine* (2nd ed., pp. 69–80). Oxford University Press.

Roth, M. L., St. Cyr, K., Harle, I., & Katz, J. D. (2013). Relationship between pain and post-traumatic stress symptoms in palliative care. *Journal of Pain and Symptom Management, 46*(2), 182–191. https://doi.org/10.1016/j.jpainsymman.2012.07.015

Sage, N., Sowden, M., Chorlton, E., & Edeleanu, A. (2008). *CBT for chronic illness and palliative care: A workbook and toolkit*. John Wiley & Sons.

Schuler, T. A., Zaider, T. I., Li, Y., Masterson, M., McDonnell, G. A., Hichenberg, S. Loeb, R., Kissane, D. W. (2017). Perceived family functioning predicts baseline psychosocial characteristics in U.S. participants of a Family Focused Grief Therapy trial. *Journal of Pain and Symptom Management, 54*(1), 126–131.

Schulz, R., Boerner, K., Shear, K., Zhang, S., & Gitlin, L. N. (2006). Predictors of complicated grief among dementia caregivers: A prospective study of bereavement. *American Journal of Geriatric Psychiatry, 14*(8), 650–658. https://doi.org/10.1097/01.JGP.0000203178.44894.db

Serfaty, M., King, M., Nazareth, I., Moorey, S., Aspden, T., Tookman, A., Mannix, K., Gola, A., Davis, S., Wood, J., & Jones, L. (2019). Manualised cognitive-behavioral therapy in treatment depression in advanced cancer: The CanTalk RCT. *Health Technology Assessment, 23*(19). https://doi.org/10.3310/hta23190

Sharpe, M., Walker, J., Hansen, C. H., Martin, P., Symeonides, S., Gourley, C., Wall, L., Weller, D., & Murray, G., for the SMaRT Oncology-2 Team. (2014). Integrated collaborative care for comorbid major depression in patients with cancer (SMaRT Oncology-2): A multicenter randomised controlled effectiveness trial. *Lancet, 384*, 1099–1108.

She, W. J., & Prigerson, H. G. (2018). "Caregrieving" in palliative care: Opportunities to improve bereavement services. *Palliative Medicine, 32*(11), 1635–1636. https://doi.org/10.1177/0269216318780587

Shear, M. K. (2010). Exploring the role of experiential avoidance from the perspective of attachment theory and the dual process model. *Omega, 61*(4), 357–369. https://doi.org/10.2190/OM.61.4.f

Shear, M. K. (2015). *Complicated grief treatment manual*. Columbia Center for Complicated Grief. htps://complicatedgrief.columbia.edu/professionals/manual-tools/

Shear, M. K., Frank, E., Houck, P. R., & Reynolds, C. F. (2005). Treatment of complicated grief: A randomized controlled trial. *JAMA, 293*(21), 2601–2608. https://doi.org/10.1001/jama.293.21.2601

Shear, M. K., Reynolds, C. F., 3rd, Simon, N. M., Zisook, S., Wang, Y., Mauro, C., Duan, N., Lebowitz, B., & Skritskaya, N. (2016). Optimizing treatment of complicated grief: A randomized clinical trial. *JAMA Psychiatry, 73*(7), 685–694. https://doi.org/10.1001/jamapsychiatry.2016.0892

Shear, M. K., Wang, Y., Skritskaya, N., Duan, N., Mauro, C., & Ghesquiere, A. (2014). Treatment of complicated grief in elderly persons: A randomized clinical trial. *JAMA Psychiatry, 71*(11), 1287–1295. https://doi.org/10.1001/jamapsychiatry.2014.1242

Shennan, C., Payne, S., & Fenlon, D. (2011). What is the evidence for the use of mindfulness-based interventions in cancer care? A review. *Psycho-Oncology, 20*(7), 681–697. https://doi.org/10.1002/pon.1819

Simon, N. M., Shear, K. M., Thompson, E. H., Zalta, A. K., Perlman, C., Reynolds, C. F., Frank, E., Melhem, N. M., & Silowash, R. (2007). The prevalence and correlates of psychiatric comorbidity in individuals with complicated grief. *Comprehensive Psychiatry, 48*(5), 395–399. https://doi.org/10.1016/j.comppsych.2007.05.002

Sörensen, S., Chapman, B. J., Duberstein, P. R. Pinquart, M., & Lyness, J. M. (2017). Assessing future care preparation in late life: Two short measures. *Psychological Assessment, 29*(12), 1480–1495. https://doi.org/10.1037/pas0000446

Spencer, R., Nilsson, M., Wright, A., Pirl, W., & Prigerson, H. (2010). Anxiety disorders in advanced cancer patients: Correlates and predictors of end-of-life outcomes. *Cancer, 116*, 1810–1819. https://doi.org/10.1002/cncr.24954

Stark, D., Kiely, M., Smith, A., Velikova, G., House, A., & Selby, P. (2002). Anxiety disorders in cancer patients: Their nature, associations, and relation to quality of life. *Journal of Clinical Oncology, 20*(14), 3137–3148. https://doi.org/10.1200/JCO.2002.08.549

Stroebe, M., & Schut, H. (2010). The dual process model of coping with bereavement: A decade on. *OMEGA-Journal of Death and Dying, 61*(4), 273–289. https://doi.org/10.2190/OM.61.4.b

Supiano, K. P., & Luptak, M. (2014). Complicated grief in older adults: A randomized controlled trial of complicated grief group therapy. *Gerontologist, 54*(5), 840–856. https://doi.org/10.1093/geront/gnt076

Swartzman, S., Booth, J. N., Munro, A., & Sani, F. (2017). Posttraumatic stress disorder after cancer diagnosis in adults: A meta-analysis. *Depression and Anxiety, 34,* 327–339. https://doi.org/10.1002/da.22542

Tomarken, A., Holland, J., Schachter, S., Vanderwerker, L., Zuckerman, E., Nelson, C., Coups, E., Ramirez, P. M., & Prigerson, H. (2008). Factors of complicated grief pre-death in caregivers of cancer patients. *Psycho-Oncology, 17*(2), 105–111. https://doi.org/10.1002/pon.1188

Trompetter, H. R., Bohlmeijer, E. T., Veehof, M. M., & Schreurs, K. M. G. (2015). Internet-based guided self-help intervention for chronic pain based on Acceptance and Commitment Therapy: A randomized controlled trial. *Journal of Behavioral Medicine, 38,* 66–80. https://doi.org/10.1007/s10865-014-9579-0

Vanderwerker, L. C., Laff, R. E., Kadan-Lottick, N. S., McColl, S., & Prigerson, H. G. (2005). Psychiatric disorders and mental health service use among caregivers of advanced cancer patients. *Journal of Clinical Oncology, 23*(28), 6899–6907. https://doi.org/10.1200/JCO.2005.01.370

Vowles, K. E., & McCracken, L. M. (2008). Acceptance and values-based action in chronic pain: A study of treatment effectiveness and process. *Journal of Consulting and Clinical Psychology, 76*(3), 397–407. https://doi.org/10.1037/0022-006X.76.3.397

Vowles, K. E., McCracken, L. M., & O'Brien, J. Z. (2011). Acceptance and values-based action in chronic pain: A three-year follow-up analysis of treatment effectiveness and process. *Behavior Research and Therapy, 49,* 748-755. https://doi.org/10.1016/j.brat.2011.08.002

Wachen, J. S., Patidar, S. M., Mulligan, E. A., Naik, A. D., & Moye, J. (2014). Cancer-related PTSD symptoms in a veteran sample: Association with age, combat PTSD, and quality of life. *Psycho-Oncology, 23,* 921–927. https://doi.org/10.1002/pon.3494

Wagner, B., Knaevelsrud, C., & Maercker, A. (2006). Internet-based cognitive-behavioral therapy for complicated grief: A randomized controlled trial. *Death Studies, 30,* 429–453. https://doi.org/10.1080/07481180600614385

Wagner, B., & Maercker, A. (2007). A 1.5 year follow-up of an internet-based intervention for complicated grief. *Journal of Traumatic Stress, 20*(4), 625–629.

Walker, J., Hansen, C. H., Martin, P., Sawhney, A., Thekkumpurath, P., Beale, C., Symeonides, S., Wall, L., Murray, G., & Sharpe, M. (2013). Prevalence of depression in adults with cancer: A systematic review. *Annals of Oncology, 24,* 895–900. https://doi.org/10.1093/annonc/mds575

Walker, J., Hansen, C. H., Martin, P., Symeonides, S., Gourley, C., Wall, L. Weller, D., Murray, G, & Sharpe, M.; for the SMaRT Oncology-3 Team. (2014). Integrated collaborative care for major depression comorbid with poor prognosis cancer (SMaRT Oncology-3): A multicenter randomised controlled trial in patients with lung cancer. *Lancet, 15,* 1168–1176.

Walker, J., Hansen, C. H., Martin, P., Symeonides, S., Ramessur, R., Murray, G., & Sharpe, M. (2014). Prevalence, associations, and adequacy of treatment of major depression in patients with cancer: A cross-sectional analysis of routinely collected clinical data. *Lancet Psychiatry, 1,* 343–350. https://doi.org/10.1016/S2215-0366(14)70313-X

Walker, J., & Sharpe, M. (2009). Depression care for people with cancer: A collaborative care intervention. *General Hospital Psychiatry, 31,* 436–441. https://doi.org/10.1016/j.genhosppsych.2009.05.010

Wenn, J., O'Connor, M., Breen, L. J., Kane, R. T., & Rees, C. S. (2015). Efficacy of metacognitive therapy for prolonged grief disorder: protocol for a randomised controlled trial. *BMJ Open, 5,* Article e007221. https://doi.org/10.1136/bmjopen-2014-007221

Wenn, J., O'Connor, M., Breen, L. J., & Rees, C. S. (2019). Exploratory study of metacognitive beliefs about coping processes in prolonged grief symptomatology. *Death Studies, 43*(3), 143–153 https://doi.org/10.1080/07481187.2018.1440032

Wenn, J. A., O'Connor, M., Kane, R. T., Rees, C. S., & Breen, L. J. (2019). A pilot randomized controlled trial of metacognitive therapy for prolonged grief. *BMJ Open*, 9(1). Article e021409. https://doi.org/10.1136/bmjopen-2017-021409

Wetherell, J. L., Afari, N., Rutledge, T., Sorrell, J. T., Stoddard, J. A., Petkus, A. J., Solomon, B. C., Lehman, D. H., Liu, L., Lang, A. J., & Atkinson, J. H. (2011). A randomized, controlled trial of acceptance and commitment therapy and cognitive-behavioral therapy for chronic pain. *Pain, 152*(9), 2098–2107. https://doi.org/10.1016/j.pain.2011.05.016

Wilson, K. G., Chochinov, H. M., Skirko, M. G., Allard, P., Chary, S., Gagnon, P. R., Macmillan, K., De Luca, M., O'Shea, F., Kuhl, D., Fainsinger, R. L., & Clinch, J. J. (2007). Depression and anxiety disorders in palliative cancer care. *Journal of Symptom Management, 33*(2), 118–129. https://doi.org/10.1016/j.jpainsymman.2006.07.016

Wilson, K. G., Lander, M., & Chochinov, H. M. (2009). Diagnosis and management of depression in palliative care. In H. M. Chochinov & W. Breitbart (Eds.), *Handbook of psychiatry in palliative medicine* (2nd ed., pp. 39–68). Oxford University Press.

Yamashita, R., Arao, J., Takao, A., Masutani, E., Morita, T., Shima, Y., Kizawa, Y., Tsuneto, S., Aoyama, M., & Miyashita, M. (2017). Unfinished business in families of terminally ill with cancer patients. *Journal of Pain and Symptom Management, 54*(6), 861–869. https://doi.org/10.1016/j.jpainsymman.2017.04.013

Zhang, B., El-Jawahri, A., & Prigerson, H. G. (2006). Update on bereavement research: evidence-based guidelines for the diagnosis and treatment of complicated bereavement. *Journal of Palliative Medicine, 9*(5), 1188–1203. https://doi.org/10.1089/jpm.2006.9.1188

Zweers, D., de Graeff, A., Duijn, J., de Graaf, E., Witteveen, P. O., & Teunissen, S. C. C. M. (2019). Patients' needs regarding anxiety management in palliative cancer care: A qualitative study in a hospice setting. *American Journal of Hospice and Palliative Medicine, 36*(11), 947–954. https://doi.org/10.1177/1049909119846844

Appendix

Pikes Peak Geropsychology Competencies: Attitude, Knowledge, and Skill Competencies for Practice in Professional Geropsychology

I. Attitudes

1. Psychologists are encouraged to work with older adults within their scope of competence, and to seek consultation or make appropriate referrals when indicated. (G1; *Note.* G1–G19 refer to the guidelines published in "Guidelines for Psychological Practice With Older Adults, by the American Psychological Association, 2004, *American Psychologist*, *59*, 236–260.)
2. Psychologists are encouraged to recognize how their attitudes and beliefs about aging and about older individuals may be relevant to their assessment and treatment of older adults, and to seek consultation or further education about these issues when indicated. (G2)
3. Psychologists are encouraged to expand their awareness of how individual diversity in all of its manifestations (including sex, age, cohort, ethnicity, language, religion, socioeconomic status, sexual orientation, gender identity, disability status, and urban or rural residence) interacts with attitudes and beliefs about aging, to utilize this awareness to inform their assessment and treatment of older adults, and to seek consultation or further education when indicated.
4. Psychologists are encouraged to increase their knowledge, understanding, and skills with respect to working with older adults, through continuing education, training, supervision, and consultation. (G20)

II. Knowledge Base

A. Knowledge: General Knowledge About Adult Development, Aging, and the Older Adult Population

1. Theoretical models and research methodologies for understanding the processes of aging, including the life-span developmental perspective, conceptions of positive or successful aging, and methodological issues in conducting or evaluating research on aging. (G3)
2. Demographics of aging, including where to obtain current knowledge on changes in population dynamics.
3. Normal or "usual" aging, including:
   - Biological and health-related aspects of aging and mind-body interactions. (G6–adapted)
   - Psychology of aging, including normative continuity and change in the domains of sensory processes, cognition, personality, and emotions.
   - Social dynamics of the aging process, including issues such as work and retirement, friendships, roles, and family relationships. (G4)

4. Awareness of diversity in the aging process, particularly how sociocultural factors such as sex, age, cohort, ethnicity, language, religion, socioeconomic status, sexual orientation, gender identity, disability status, and urban or rural residence may influence the experience and expression of health and of psychological problems in later life, and how this knowledge may inform the assessment and treatment of older adults. (G5)

B. Knowledge: Foundations of Clinical Practice With Older Adults

1. The neuroscience of aging, its applications to changes in cognition, and its implications for clinical interventions with older adults. (G7–adapted)
2. Knowledge of the salience of functional changes in later adulthood, including resulting problems in daily living. (G8)
3. Awareness of the concept of person–environment interaction and the implications of this concept for adaptation in late life. (G8)
4. Psychopathology in middle and later adulthood, including differences in the prevalence, etiology, presentation, associated features, comorbidities, and course of mental disorders in older adults, as well as the health-related consequences of treated and untreated psychological disorders in late life. (G9)
5. Knowledge of common medical illnesses in late life.

C. Knowledge: Foundations of Assessment of Older Adults (G10 and G11, Expanded)

1. Theory and research informing psychological assessment of older adults, including the broad array of assessment domains, methods, and instruments which are psychometrically suitable for assessing older adults.
2. Issues in the limits of using assessment instruments created for younger persons with older adults without adequate standardization.
3. Knowledge of contextual issues in the assessment of older adults, including the system or environment in which the elder functions, and the impact on assessment process and outcomes.

D. Knowledge: Foundations of Intervention, Consultation, and Other Service Provision

1. Theory, research, and practice of various methods of intervention with older adults, including current research evidence about their efficacy and effectiveness as applied to diverse groups within the older adult population. (G13, G14)
2. Health, illness, and pharmacology as related to assessment and treatment of late-life mental health problems, including awareness of medical and/or medication factors which may affect treatment outcomes (e.g., illness, medication side effects, polypharmacy).
3. Issues pertaining to the provision of services in the specific settings in which older adults typically live or seek treatment. (G15)
4. Knowledge of aging services in the local community (e.g., day care, transportation, residential) and how to refer clients to these services.

5. Prevention and health promotion services, and their relevance for middle-aged and older adults at risk for mental disorders. (G16)
6. Awareness of the broad array of potential clients (e.g., family members, other caregivers, health care professionals, and organizations) for psychological consultation and intervention, and appropriate intervention strategies in these contexts. (G17)
7. Models and methods of interdisciplinary collaboration, including an understanding of the varied components, roles, and contexts of interdisciplinary treatment of late-life mental disorders. (G18)
8. Knowledge of ethical and legal standards related to psychological intervention with older adults and care systems, with particular attention to aging-specific issues of informed consent, confidentiality, substitute or end-of-life decision making and potential conflicts of interest, capacity and/or competency, and elder abuse and neglect.

III. Skill Competencies

A. Skills: Professional Geropsychology Functioning (Foundational Competencies)

1. Understand and apply ethical and legal standards, with particular attention to aging-specific issues, such as informed consent, confidentiality, capacity/competency, end-of-life decision making, and elder abuse and neglect.
2. Understand cultural and individual diversity as relevant to assessment, intervention, and consultation, and apply to practice with diverse older adults.
3. Address complex biopsychosocial issues among many older adults by collaborating with other disciplines in multidisciplinary and interdisciplinary teams.
4. Practice self-reflection, self-assessment (e.g., self-awareness of ageist assumptions/biases; recognition of boundaries of competence and when/how to refer elsewhere)
5. Relate effectively and empathically with older adults clients, families, and other stakeholders in a range of professional roles and settings (e.g., senior center, hospital, long-term care).
6. Apply scientific knowledge to geropsychology practice and policy advocacy.
7. Practice appropriate documentation, billing, and reimbursement procedures for geropsychological services, in compliance with state and federal laws and regulations (especially regarding Medicare and Medicaid services), including assessment and documentation of medical necessity.
8. Advocate for clients' needs and provide case management for needed services.

B. Skills: Assessment (G11 and G12, Adapted)

1. Conduct clinical assessment leading to *Diagnostic and Statistical Manual of Mental Disorders* (DSM) diagnoses and other clinically relevant problems, formulation of treatment plans, and specifically, differential diagnosis (common problems and issues include, but are not limited to, depression, anxiety, grief, delirium, and dementia; and medication and physical disorders and their effects on functioning).
2. Use psychometrically sound screening instruments for cognition, psychopathology, and personality to inform treatment planning.

3. Refer for neuropsychological, neurological, psychiatric, medical, or other evaluations as indicated.
4. Use cognitive assessments and/or neuropsychological reports to clarify clinical issues and inform treatment planning (some geropsychologists have also been trained as neuropsychologists, and would thus be able to conduct neuropsychological evaluations within their scope of competence).
5. Evaluate decision-making and functional capacities (e.g., for managing finances, independent living, driving, and making health care decisions).
6. Assess risk (e.g., suicidality, self-neglect, elder abuse).
7. Adapt instruments and tailor assessments to accommodate older adults' specific characteristics and contexts.
8. Communicate assessment results to various stakeholders with relevant, practical, and clearly understandable recommendations, with appropriate consideration for confidentiality issues.

C. Skills: Intervention

1. Apply individual, group, and family interventions to older adults using appropriate modifications to accommodate distinctive biopsychosocial functioning of older adults and distinct therapeutic relationship characteristics.
2. Use available evidence-based treatments for older adults.
3. Develop psychotherapeutic interventions based on empirical literature, theory, and clinical judgment when insufficient efficacy research is available on older adults.
4. Be proficient in using commonly employed late-life interventions such as those focusing on life review, grief, end-of-life care, and caregiving.
5. Use interventions to enhance health of diverse older persons (e.g., chronic health problems, healthy aging, and cognitive fitness).
6. Demonstrate ability to intervene in settings where older adults and their family members are often seen (e.g., health services, housing, and community programs) with a range of strategies, including those targeted at the individual, family, environment, and system.

D. Skills: Consultation and Training

1. Advise families, professionals, programs, health care facilities, legal systems, and other agencies and organizations that serve older adults.
2. Provide training on geropsychological issues (e.g., inhouse services and workshops, in community settings, to different disciplines).
3. Participate in interprofessional teams that serve older adults.
4. Communicate psychological conceptualizations to medical and other professionals in concise and useful manner.
5. Implement strategies for systems analysis and change in organizations and facilities that serve older adults.
6. Design and participate in different models of aging services delivery (e.g., integration).
7. Collaborate and coordinate with other agencies and professionals that serve older adults.
8. Recognize and negotiate multiple roles in older adult consultation settings.

E. Skills: Delivery of Services in Different Settings

Delivery of services in two or more different settings, including:
1. Outpatient mental health services.
2. Outpatient primary care and medical settings.
3. Inpatient medical service.
4. Inpatient psychiatric service.
5. Long-term care settings, including nursing homes, assisted living facilities, home care, and day programs.
6. Rehabilitation settings.
7. Hospice.
8. Community-based programs.
9. Forensic settings.
10. Home delivered psychological services.
11. Research settings.

Pikes Peak Geropsychology Knowledge and Skill Assessment Tool

Purpose

This evaluation tool is for learners who are working to develop knowledge and skills for providing optimal care to older adults, their families, and related care systems. Psychology trainees, their supervisors, and practicing psychologists may use this tool to evaluate progress in developing geropsychology competencies, and to help define ongoing learning goals and training needs.

Pikes Peak Competencies

The competencies for professional geropsychology practice are aspirational, rather than required of any particular psychologist. Even the most accomplished geropsychologist will have relative strengths and weaknesses across the spectrum of competencies for geropsychology. The Pikes Peak Model for Geropsychology Training (Knight et al., 2009), and created the Council of Professional Geropsychology Training Programs (CoPGTP). CoPGTP developed this competency evaluation tool for learners and supervisors to have a measure by which to gauge competence in serving older adults. For the purposes of this evaluation tool, each Pikes Peak geropsychology knowledge and skill competency is specified by behaviorally descriptive items, and can be rated along a continuum from novice to expert. Some redundancy is inherent in this measure. The intent is to evaluate both the learner's knowledge base and skill set, separately for the same domains, as the awareness of information and ability or experience in applying it may differ.

Geropsychology Practice

Geropsychologists provide assessment, intervention, consultation, and other professional services across a wide range of medical, mental health, residential, community, and other care settings, with a population of demographically and socioculturally diverse older adults. The Pikes Peak competencies are applicable across varied geriatric care settings and populations. It is recognized also that each work area or training setting may call for the development of particular competencies, not all of which may be addressed in this document. Both the APA Guidelines for Psychological Practice with Older Adults (APA, 2004) and the Pikes Peak model highlight core attitudes for practice with older adults. Although this tool does not evaluate attitudes explicitly, the knowledge and skill competencies reflect core geropsychology practice attitudes, including recognition of scope of competence, self-awareness of attitudes and beliefs about aging and older adults, appreciation of diversity among older adults, and commitment to continuing education.

Using the Competency Evaluation Tool

This tool is intended to be used both by supervisors to assess trainees and by psychologists to assess their own knowledge and skills. Supervisors in geropsychology training programs may choose to evaluate the domains relevant to the goals of their program. Evaluation should include the learner's perspective (self-assessment), observation of the learner's work (e.g., direct observation, audiotape, videotape, cotherapy), as well as regular supervision involving case discussion. Psychologists and trainees conducting self-assessments can use the tool to evaluate their training and supervision needs in each area. The tool can also gauge a learner's progress over time.

The learner can be rated on each Pikes Peak knowledge domain and skill competency as novice (N), intermediate (I), advanced (A), proficient (P), or expert (E), as described below. Each Pikes Peak competency (highlighted in light gray in the chart below) is delineated by several specifiers (indicated by letters "a.," "b.," "c.," etc. in the chart). The specifiers are designed to help define the knowledge domain or skill competency and do not need to be rated separately. However, the specifiers can be rated individually if that level of assessment is desired.

Rating Scale Anchors

This rating scale assumes that professional competence is developed over time, as learners develop knowledge and skills with ongoing education, training, and supervision. The anchors, then, reflect developmental levels of competence, from novice through expert. The scale is adapted from previous efforts, as summarized by Hatcher and Lassiter (2007). Because the scale reflects development of competence, the same scale can be used at different levels of training. For example, graduate practica students would be expected to perform at novice through advanced levels, while postdoctoral fellows in geropsychology would be expected to perform from intermediate to expert levels. Development of knowledge and skills may differ significantly across domains, depending upon previous training experiences.

To illustrate use of the scale, we provide a brief case example and a description of how an individual at each level might approach the case.

Case example

A 78-year-old Irish-American man is referred to the mental health clinic by his primary care physician because his daughter-in-law complained that, in recent months, he has become depressed and forgetful and is no longer involved in his hobbies. He has several chronic medical problems including mild diabetes and hypertension. His Korean-American wife of 52 years is angry that he is not completing his household chores. His three adult children have varied levels of involvement in his life, with one daughter and one son living nearby. He comes to the clinic for an initial evaluation.

Novice (N): Possesses entry-level skills; needs intensive supervision.

Novices have limited knowledge and understanding of case conceptualization and intervention skills, and the processes and techniques of implementing them. Novices do not yet recognize consistent patterns of behavior relevant for diagnosis and care planning and do not differentiate well between important and unimportant details.

In this case example: The novice learner is able to identify salient symptoms, but does not appreciate possible contributions of medical, neurological, and family system factors to the older adult's presentation, and does not know how to formulate differential diagnosis questions.

Intermediate (I): Has a background of some exposure and experience; ongoing supervision is needed.

Experience has been gained through practice, supervision, and instruction. The intermediate learner is able to recognize important recurring issues and select appropriate strategies. Generalization of skills is limited and support is needed to guide performance.

In this case example: The intermediate learner recognizes multiple possible contributions to the older adult's presentation, is able to collect history from the patient (and his daughter-in-law, with his permission), administer depression and cognitive screening tools, and consult with supervisor to discuss possible implications and to plan further evaluation. Learner may not appreciate complex, late-life family and cultural systems issues affecting patient's coping.

Advanced (A): Has solid experience, handles typical situations well; requires supervision for unusual or complex situations.

Knowledge of the competency domain is more integrated, including application of appropriate research literature. The advanced learner is more fluent in the ability to recognize patterns and select appropriate strategies to guide diagnosis and treatment.

> In this case example: The advanced learner is able to integrate multiple sources of information (e.g., behavioral observation, cognitive testing data, medical records, collateral reports) and complex history (medical, psychiatric, family, occupational, and cultural context) to rule out possibility of early dementia plus depression, and make recommendations to the primary care provider and family about further assessment and treatment options. Learner consults with supervisor about local resources for older adults, and how best to handle issues around wife's difficulty in coping with patient's changes, related marital conflict, family dynamics, culture, and treatment planning.

Proficient (P): Functions autonomously, knows limits of ability; seeks supervision or consultation as needed.

Proficiency is demonstrated in perceiving situations as wholes and not only summations of parts, including an appreciation of longer-term implications of current situation. The psychologist has a perspective on which of the many existing attributes and aspects in the present situation are important ones, and has developed a nuanced understanding of the clinical situation.

> In this case example: The proficient learner is able to integrate information, as above, collaborate with family and medical (e.g., psychiatrist, neurologist) and social service providers for ongoing assessment and intervention for the patient and family (e.g., psychoeducation, couple's therapy, and exploration of community support options). Learner functions as a full member of an interdisciplinary team to address the biopsychosocial needs of the client and his family, and is able to assume a leadership role.

Expert (E): Serves as resource or advisor to others, is recognized as having expertise

With a significant background of experience, the geropsychologist is able to focus in on the essentials of the problem quickly and efficiently. Analytical problem solving is used to consider unfamiliar situations, or when initial impressions are not borne out.

> In this case example: An expert learner is frequently contacted by other psychologists in their community to provide advice regarding care of older adults with dementia. Learner is able to use the above case as a teaching example for the need to provide a thorough biopsychosocial assessment in geriatric care, to implement an interdisciplinary team plan, and to be knowledgeable about geriatric resources in the community.

I. General knowledge about adult development, aging, and the older adult population	
A. The psychologist/trainee has *knowledge* of:	
1. Models of aging	**N I A P E**
a. Development as a life-long process encompassing early to late life, and encompassing both gains and losses over the lifespan	
b. Different theories of late-life development and adaptation	
c. Biopsychosocial perspective for understanding an individual's physical and psychological development within the sociocultural context	
d. Concept of, and variables associated with, positive or successful aging	
e. Relevant research on adult development and aging, including methodological considerations in cross-sectional and longitudinal research.	
2. Demographics	**N I A P E**
a. Demographic trends of the aging population, including gender, racial, ethnic, and socioeconomic heterogeneity	
b. Resources to remain updated on the demographics of aging, including internet sites for US Census, Centers for Disease Control and Prevention, Social Security Administration, Bureau of Labor Statistics, National Institutes of Health, and World Health Organization	
3. Normal aging – biological, psychological, social aspects	**N I A P E**
a. Physical changes in later life	
b. Normal aging as distinct from disease, regarding both physical and mental health	
c. Interactions among physical changes, health behaviors, stress, personality, and mental health in older adults	
d. Aging-related changes in sensory processes including vision, hearing, touch, taste, and smell	
e. Aging-related changes in sexual functioning	
f. Aging-related changes in cognitive processes, including attention, memory, executive functioning, language, and intellectual functions	
g. Aging-related changes in personality	
h. Aging-related changes in emotional expression and coping mechanisms	
i. Factors that influence vocational satisfaction, job performance, leisure activities, retirement satisfaction, and volunteer participation	
j. Family dynamics and role changes in aging families	
k. Changing social networks in late life, and value of close friendships in later life	

4. Diversity in aging experience	NIAPE
a. The diversity of the older adult population, and that age alone is a poor predictor of an individual's functioning	
b. The unique experience of each individual – based on demographic, sociocultural, and life experiences – and that multiple factors interact over the lifespan to influence an older individual's patterns of behavior	
c. Historical influences affecting particular cohorts	

II. Foundations of professional geropsychology practice	
A. Knowledge base – the psychologist/trainee has *knowledge* of:	
1. Neuroscience of aging	**N I A P E**
a. The parameters of cognitive changes in normal aging, including their basis in age-related changes in the brain	
b. Factors that influence levels of cognitive performance in older adults (e.g., genetics, socioeconomic status, cohort effects, health status, mood, and medications or substances)	
c. Common types of dementia in terms of onset, etiology, risk factors, clinical course, associated behavioral features, and medical management of these disorders	
d. Characteristics and causes of mild cognitive impairment and reversible cognitive impairment, including delirium, and the pathway to their management or reversal	
e. Characteristics and causes of mild cognitive impairment and reversible cognitive impairment, including delirium, and the pathway to their management or reversal	
2. Functional changes	**N I A P E**
a. Relationships between age, environment and functional level	
b. Definition and assessment of activities of daily living (ADLs) and instrumental activities of daily living (IADLs)	
d. Relationship between functional ability and psychopathology in older adults, including how functional ability of older persons affects family members	
e. Strategies commonly used by older adults to cope with functional limitations	
3. Person–environment interaction and adaptation	**N I A P E**
a. Interaction of an elder's abilities and needs with the demands and opportunities provided by various living and treatment environments (e.g., private homes, assisted living facilitates, nursing facilities)	
b. Impact of aging stereotypes on an older individual's functional status and self-efficacy	
c. Importance and complexities around issues of maintaining optimal independence and optimal safety, particularly when medical conditions and cognitive disorders impair the elder's functioning	
d. Ethical and legal issues which arise in the context of markedly impaired functional status and decision making capacity	
e. Situations and signs that suggest risk for abuse and neglect	

4. Psychopathology	**N I A P E**
a. Biopsychosocial etiological models, applied within a lifespan developmental and cohort relevant context, for major psychological disorders affecting older adults	
b. Differential presentation, associated features, age of onset, and course of common psychological disorders and syndromes in older adults (e.g., anxiety, depression, dementia, etc.)	
c. Variations in presentations of psychopathology in later life due to cohort, cognitive, medical and pharmacological issues, including lifelong mental illness and late onset mental illness	
d. Underrecognized aspects of psychopathology in late life which affect functional impairment and safety (e.g., suicide risk, substance use, complicated grief)	
e. Interaction of common mental illnesses with the more common medical illnesses and medications and implications involved for assessment and treatment	
f. Psychosocial, psychotherapeutic and psychopharmacological approaches to treating psychological disorders in older adults, as well as the health-related consequences of not treating and side effects of the possible treatments	
5. Medical illness	**N I A P E**
a. Common medical and neurological problems (e.g., cardiovascular and cerebrovascular disorders), syndromes (e.g., falls, incontinence), and substances or medications (e.g., alcohol, benzodiazepines, narcotics, over-the-counter remedies) associated with psychopathology in older adults	
b. Multiple pathways of interaction between medical illness and psychopathology in late life	
c. Common medical tests (e.g., thyroid function, urinalysis, CT or MRI scan) relevant to differentiating medical and psychological illness in late life	
d. Relationships between chronic pain, functioning, and mental health in older adults (e.g., relationship of depression to pain)	
6. End of life issues	**N I A P E**
a. Physical, cognitive, emotional, and spiritual components of advanced illness and the dying process	
b. Diversity in ethnic, cultural, and spiritual beliefs and rituals involved in death and the dying process	
c. Models of hospice and palliative care	
d. Impact of advanced illness, caregiving, dying and death on family members	
e. Differences between normal grief reactions and complicated grief	

B. Professional geropsychology functioning – foundational skills – the psychologist/trainee is *able to*:	
1. Neuroscience of aging	**N I A P E**
Identify complex ethical and legal issues that arise in the care of older adults, analyze them accurately, and proactively address them, including:	
a. Tension between sometimes competing goals of promoting autonomy and protecting safety of at-risk older adults	
b. Decision making capacity and strategies for optimizing older adults' participation in informed consent regarding a wide range of medical, residential, financial, and other life decisions	
c. Surrogate decision making as indicated regarding a wide range of medical, residential, financial, end-of-life, and other life decisions	
d. State and organizational laws and policies covering elder abuse, advance directives, conservatorship, guardianship, multiple relationships, and confidentiality	
2. Address cultural and individual diversity with older adults, families, communities, and systems/providers by being able to:	**N I A P E**
a. Recognize gender, age, cohort, ethnic and/or racial, cultural, linguistic, socioeconomic, religious, disability, sexual orientation, gender identity, and urban or rural residence variations in the aging process	
b. Articulate integrative conceptualizations of multiple aspects of diversity influencing older clients, psychologists, and systems of care	
c. Adapt professional behavior in a culturally sensitive manner, as appropriate to the needs of the older client	
d. Work effectively with diverse providers, staff, and students in care settings serving older adults	
e. Demonstrate self-awareness and ability to recognize differences between the clinician's and the patient's values, attitudes, assumptions, hopes and fears related to aging, caregiving, illness, disability, social supports, medical care, dying, grief	
f. Initiate consultation with appropriate sources as needed to address specific diversity issues	
3. Recognize importance of teams	**N I A P E**
a. Understand the theory and science of geriatric team building	
b. Value the role that other providers play in the assessment and treatment of older clients	
c. Demonstrate awareness, appreciation, and respect for team experiences, values, and discipline-specific conceptual models	
d. Understand the importance of teamwork in geriatric settings to address the varied bio-psycho-social needs of older adults	

4. Practice self-reflection	**N I A P E**
a. Demonstrate awareness of personal biases, assumptions, stereotypes, and potential discomfort in working with older adults, particularly those of backgrounds divergent from the psychologist	
b. Monitor internal thoughts and feelings that may influence professional behavior, and adjust behavior accordingly in order to focus on needs of the patient, family, and treatment team	
c. Demonstrate accurate self-evaluation of knowledge and skill competencies related to work with diverse older adults, including those with particular diagnoses, or in particular care settings	
d. Initiate consultation with or referral to appropriate providers when uncertain about one's own competence	
e. Seek continuing education, training, supervision, and consultation to enhance geropsychology competencies related to practice	
5. Relate effectively and empathically	**N I A P E**
a. Use rapport and empathy in verbal and nonverbal behaviors to facilitate interactions with older adults, families, and care teams	
b. Form effective working alliance with wide range of older clients, families, colleagues, and other stakeholders	
c. Communicate new knowledge to patients and families, adjusting language and complexity of concepts based on the patient and family's level of sensory and cognitive capabilities, educational background, knowledge, values, and developmental stage	
d. Demonstrate awareness, appreciation, and respect for older patient, family, and team experiences, values, and conceptual models	
e. Demonstrate appreciation of client and organizational strengths, as well as deficits and challenges, and capitalize on strengths in planning interventions	
f. Tolerate and understand interpersonal conflict and differences within or between older patients, families, and team members, and negotiate conflict effectively	
6. Apply scientific knowledge	**N I A P E**
a. Demonstrate awareness of scientific knowledge base in adult development and aging; biomedical, psychological, and social gerontology; and geriatric health and mental health care; incorporate this knowledge into geriatric health and mental health practice	
b. Apply review of available scientific literature to case conceptualization, treatment planning, and intervention	
c. Acknowledge strengths and limitations of knowledge base in application to individual case	
d. Demonstrate ability to cite scientific evidence on aging to support professional activities in academic, clinical, and policy settings	

7. Practice appropriate business of geropsychology	N I A P E
a. Demonstrate awareness of Medicare, Medicaid, and other insurance coverage for diagnostic conditions and health and mental health care services	
b. Demonstrate appropriate diagnostic and procedure coding for psychological services rendered	
c. Demonstrate medical record documentation that is consistent with Medicare, Medicaid, Health Insurance Portability and Accountability Act (HIPAA), and other federal, state, or local or organizational regulations, including appropriate documentation of medical necessity for services	
d. Remain updated on policy and regulatory changes that affect practice, such as through professional newsletters and email forums	
e. Demonstrate understanding of quality indicators for the care of older adults with mental disorders	
8. Advocate and provide care coordination	**N I A P E**
a. Demonstrate awareness of potential individual and psychosocial barriers to the ability of older adults to access and utilize health, mental health, or community services	
b. Collaborate with patients, families, and other organizational and community providers to improve older adults' access to needed health care, residential, transportation, social, or community services	
c. Advocate for clients' needs in interdisciplinary and organizational environments when appropriate	

III. Assessment	
A. Knowledge base – the psychologist/trainee has *knowledge* of:	
1. Geropsychology assessment methods	**N I A P E**
a. Current research and literature relevant to understanding theory and current trends in geropsychology assessment	
b. Assessment measures or techniques which have been developed, normed, validated and determined to be psychometrically suitable for use with older adults	
c. Importance of a comprehensive interdisciplinary assessment approach (e.g., including other health professionals' evaluations of medical or social issues)	
d. Multimethod approach to assessing older adults (including cognitive, psychological, personality, and behavioral assessments, drawn from self-report, interviews, and observational methods)	
e. Importance of integrating collateral information from family, friends, and caregivers, with appropriate consent, especially when cognitive impairment is suspected	
f. Need for baseline and repeated-measures assessments to understand complex diagnostic problems	
g. Assessment of domains unique to older adults (e.g., potential elder abuse)	
2. Limitations of assessment methods	**N I A P E**
a. Criterion and age requirements, as well as specific standard normative data, for testing instruments	
b. Limitations of testing instruments, including those validated in older samples, for assessing diverse older adults	
3. Contextual issues in geropsychology assessment	**N I A P E**
a. The range of potential individual factors that may affect assessment performance (e.g., medications, substance use, medical conditions, cultural, educational, language background)	
b. The potential impact of the assessment environment on test performance (e.g., noise, lighting, distractions)	
c. The older person's environmental context and resources in deriving recommendations from assessment data	
B. Skills – the psychologist/trainee is *able to*:	
1. Conduct clinical assessment and differential diagnosis	**N I A P E**
a. Distinguish between signs of normal aging versus pathology in making diagnoses	
b. Consider base rates, risk factors, and distinct symptom presentations of psychological disorders in older adults when making diagnoses	
c. Conduct differential diagnosis (e.g., dementia vs. depression), including consideration of comorbid medical issues that may influence an older adult's presentation	

d. Identify subsyndromal disorders and implications for treatment	
e. Assess older adult's motivation for treatment	
f. Utilize biopsychosocial case conceptualization based on clinical evaluation to inform initial treatment plan or recommendations	
2. Utilize screening instruments	**N I A P E**
a. Utilize screening tools for mood, cognition, substance use, personality, and other clinical issues to guide and inform comprehensive assessment	
b. Evaluate age, educational, and cultural appropriateness of assessment instruments	
c. Consider reliability and validity data in using standardized instruments with older adults	
d. Assess older adult's ability to provide informed consent for psychological evaluation	
e. Recognize sensory impairments and makes environmental modifications accordingly	
f. Consider impact of medical conditions and medications on test performance	
g. Make specific and appropriate recommendations, based on testing results, to inform treatment planning	
3. Refer for other evaluations as indicated	**N I A P E**
a. Acknowledge personal level of expertise regarding geriatric assessment and know when to refer or consult with other health care professionals	
b. Utilize screening data to inform need for more comprehensive, multidisciplinary assessment	
c. Recognize when a medical evaluation is indicated to rule out underlying medical or pharmacological causes of presenting symptoms	
4. Utilize cognitive assessments	**N I A P E**
a. Integrate knowledge of normal and pathological aging, including age-related changes in cognitive abilities, into geropsychological evaluations	
b. Interpret meaning and implications of cognitive testing data or reports for case conceptualization	
c. Demonstrate ability to translate cognitive testing results into practical conclusions and recommendations for patients, families, and other care providers	
5. Evaluate decision making and functional capacity	**N I A P E**
a. Evaluate older adults' understanding, appreciation, reasoning, and choice abilities with regards to capacity for decision making	
b. Utilize clinically specific assessment tools designed to aid evaluation of decision making and other functional capacities	

c. Integrate testing results with information from clinical interview with older adult and collateral sources, including behavioral observations and interviews with family members, to formulate impressions and recommendations	
d. Collaborate with professionals from other disciplines to assess specific functional capacities (e.g., independent living, driving)	
e. Appreciate legal and clinical contexts of capacity/competence evaluations (e.g., need for guardianship, loss of right to drive)	
6. Assess risk	**NIAPE**
a. Identify risk factors for harm to self or others	
b. Screen and comprehensively assesses suicide risk	
c. Screen and assesses capacity for self-care including ADLs and IADLs	
d. Screen and assesses risk of elder abuse in emotional, physical, sexual, financial, and neglect domains	
7. Communicate assessment results and recommendations	**NIAPE**
a. Communicate results within the confines of federal, state, local, and institutional privacy and confidentiality rules and regulations	
b. Translate assessment results into practical recommendations for patient, family, and team, providing written recommendations and relevant psychoeducational materials understandable to stakeholders	
c. Provide recommendations to other providers to assure that treatment plans are informed by assessment results	

IV. Intervention	
A. Knowledge base – the psychologist/trainee has *knowledge* of:	
1. Theory, research, and practice	**N I A P E**
a. Broad research findings regarding the effectiveness of psychological interventions with older adults (e.g., application of behavioral, cognitive, interpersonal, psychodynamic, family, environmental, psychoeducational, group interventions)	
b. Specialized interventions in working with older adults and how they evolve from and are consistent with theory in life span development (e.g., reminiscence therapy, validation techniques, behavioral interventions for disruptive behavior)	
c. Modifications of therapeutic techniques to address common aging changes (e.g., sensory difficulties, cognitive impairment), care setting (e.g., community, hospital, nursing home), education, and cultural background	
2. Health, illness, and pharmacology	**N I A P E**
a. The complexity and interplay of common late-life medical problems, sensory changes and their impact on treatment approaches	
b. The possible impact of medications and procedures for medical and psychiatric problems, including detrimental side effects, on symptom presentation, mental status, and treatment effectiveness in older adults	
c. The frequent comorbidity between chronic medical and psychiatric problems, and need to address both medical and mental health issues	
d. The importance of setting realistic treatment goals (neither too high nor too low) for older adults with severe, chronic medical and psychiatric problems (e.g., remission of symptoms or maintenance of current functioning rather than cure)	
3. Specific settings	**N I A P E**
a. The varied preferences older adults have in discussing emotional problems with family, primary care providers, spiritual advisors and, thus, the importance of allying with others, with appropriate consent, to assure proper psychological care is rendered	
b. The salience and presentation of ethical issues when employing interventions across varied care settings (e.g., confidentiality in context of team treatment planning; privacy constraints in institutional settings)	
c. Adaptations of interventions appropriate to particular settings (e.g., focus on staff education and behavioral, environmental interventions in long-term care settings)	

4. Aging services	**N I A P E**
a. Specific referral sources including facilities (e.g., day care, residential), transportation, legal and safety (e.g., protective services), health, multicultural, caregiver, and other support services	
b. Referral processes and procedures to local community resources (e.g., via phone, internet)	
c. Follow-up mechanism(s) regarding referrals	
5. Ethical and legal standards	**N I A P E**
a. Informed consent procedures for services to older adults, and challenges to some older adults' capacity to provide informed consent	
b. Indications for and role of surrogate decision makers in health and mental health treatment of older adults	
c. Older client's right to confidentiality and to be informed of limits of confidentiality	
d. State and organizational laws and policies covering elder abuse, advance directives, conservatorship, guardianship, restraints, multiple relationships, and confidentiality	
B. Skills – the psychologist/trainee is *able to*:	
1. Apply individual, group, and family interventions	**N I A P E**
a. Prioritize treatment goals as appropriate, taking into account multiple problem areas	
b. Integrate relevant treatment modalities	
c. Modify evidence-based and clinically informed intervention strategies to accommodate chronic and acute medical problems, sensory impairments, mobility limitations, cognitive abilities, generational and cultural factors, late-life developmental issues, and possible client–therapist age differences	
d. Provide psychoeducation as needed to help the older adult client understand the therapeutic process	
2. Base interventions on empirical research, theory, and clinical judgment	**N I A P E**
a. Articulate theoretical case conceptualization and empirical support guiding choice of intervention strategies	
b. Describe the integration or adaptation of various strategies to meet the needs of particular older clients	
c. Measure the effectiveness of intervention	
d. Make appropriate adjustments to treatment based on client response	

3. Use available evidence-based treatments for older adults	**N I A P E**
a. Choose evidence-based treatment for older adult clients based on diagnosis and other relevant client characteristics	
b. Choose and implement intervention strategies based on available evidence for effectiveness with older adults	
c. Measure the effectiveness of intervention	
d. Make appropriate adjustments to treatment based on client response	
4. Use late-life interventions – provide effective, evidence-based interventions for particular issues affecting older adults, including:	**N I A P E**
a. For older adults with dementia (and other disabling illnesses) and their family caregivers	
b. For patients and families facing advanced illness, dying, and death	
c. For adjustment difficulties secondary to bereavement	
d. Inclusion of reminiscence and life review into psychotherapeutic interventions	
e. Psychoeducation for patients and families regarding normal aging and a range of medical and mental health concerns	
f. Group interventions for a range of aging-related health, mental health, and adjustment concerns	
g. For older adults adjusting to age-related changes in relationships and sexuality	
5. Use health-enhancing interventions	**N I A P E**
a. Determine which aspects of physical, mental and behavioral health can be improved in older clients via available psychological interventions	
b. Prioritize health issues to be addressed when multiple targets are possible	
c. Effectively intervene regarding health issues as part of overall mental health treatment plan, recognizing close link between medical and mental health and related disability in older adults	
d. Monitor impact of intervention on health behaviors and evaluates outcomes	
6. Intervene across settings	**N I A P E**
a. Intervene in common geriatric settings (e.g., home, community centers, nursing homes, assisted living facilities, retirement communities, medical clinics, medical and psychiatric hospitals)	
b. Intervene at the level appropriate to older adult client's needs, ranging from individual to family, systemic, and environmental contexts	
c. Modify interventions to adapt to the setting's particular environmental and social characteristics	

N. A. Pachana et al.: *Psychological Assessment and Treatment of Older Adults* © 2021 Hogrefe Publishing

V. Consultation	
A. Knowledge base – the psychologist/trainee has *knowledge of*:	
1. Prevention and health promotion	**N I A P E**
a. Incidence and prevalence rates of health problems in the older adult population	
b. How to partner with family and local community resources for health promotion	
c. Strategies for community-based training/education for promoting preventive interventions	
2. Diverse clientele and contexts	**N I A P E**
a. Multiple levels of geropsychological intervention and consultation, including individuals, families, health care professionals, organizations, and community leaders	
b. Systems-based consultative and intervention models and their use with appropriate modifications in different geriatric settings	
c. Strategies and methods for collaboration to address individual- and organizational-based needs	
3. Interdisciplinary collaboration	**N I A P E**
a. The distinction between types of treatment teams (e.g., multidisciplinary and interdisciplinary)	
b. The roles, and potential contributions, of a wide range of health care professionals in the assessment and treatment of older adult with mental disorders	
c. How team composition and functioning may differ across settings of care	
B. Skills – the psychologist/trainee is *able to*:	
1. Provide geropsychological advice	**N I A P E**
a. Recognize situations in which geropsychological consultation is appropriate	
b. Demonstrate ability to clarify and refine a referral question	
c. Demonstrate ability to gather information necessary to answer referral question	
d. Advocate for quality care for older adults with their families, professionals, programs, health care facilities, legal systems, and other agencies or organizations	
2. Provide training	**N I A P E**
a. Assess learning needs of trainees related to varying levels of training and amount of experience within and across disciplines	
b. Define learning goals and objectives as a basis for developing educational sessions	
c. Provide clear, concise education that is appropriate for the level and learning needs of the trainees	

3. Participate in interprofessional teams	N I A P E
a. Work with professionals in other disciplines to incorporate geropsychological information into team treatment planning and implementation	
b. Communicate psychological conceptualizations clearly and respectfully to other providers	
c. Appreciate and integrate feedback from interdisciplinary team members into case conceptualizations	
d. Work to build consensus on treatment plans and goals of care, to invite various perspectives, and to negotiate conflict constructively	
e. Demonstrate ability to work with diverse team structures (e.g., hierarchical, lateral, virtual) and team members (e.g., including the ethics board, chaplains, and families in palliative care teams)	
4. Communicate geropsychological conceptualizations	**N I A P E**
a. Provide clear and concise written communication of geropsychological conceptualizations and recommendations	
b. Provide clear and concise oral communication of geropsychological conceptualizations and recommendations	
c. Uses appropriate language and level of detail for the target audience of the communication	
5. Implement organizational change	**N I A P E**
a. Conduct needs assessment for service delivery within the setting or program that serves older adults	
b. Develop policies and procedures for service delivery that involve all appropriate disciplines and staff members	
c. Evaluate effectiveness of service delivery model or program	
6. Participate in a variety of models of aging services delivery	**N I A P E**
a. Differentiate goals and models of care in long-term, rehabilitation, acute, primary, home, assisted living, hospice, and other care settings	
b. Appreciate a variety of models of geriatric mental health care , including integrated mental health services in primary care, specialty consultation, and home- or community-based services	
c. Demonstrate awareness of strengths and constraints of various care models	
d. Demonstrate flexibility in professional roles to adapt to the realities of work in a variety of aging or health care delivery systems	

7. Collaborate and coordinate with other agencies and professionals	NIAPE
a. Work with team members to create smooth and efficient transitions across health care settings for older adults and their families	
b. Demonstrate respect for confidentiality and informed consent, as well as continuity of care, in coordinating with family members, other professionals, and agencies regarding care of an older client	
c. Establish working relationships with local and national agencies and organizations, such as elder services, Alzheimer's Association, and hospice	
8. Identify the client and explicate the expectations of the relationship at the outset of the consultation	**NIAPE**
a. Identify the client and explicate the expectations of the relationship at the outset of the consultation	
b. Advocate on behalf of the well-being of older adults within each professional role, including when the individual or group of older adults is not the direct client	
c. Discuss potential conflicts of interest with colleagues and teams as indicated	
b. Discuss financial arrangements with all stakeholders	

Summary

It may help learners and/or supervisors to summarize the geropsychology knowledge and skill strengths, and areas for growth, based on this assessment. Areas for growth may then be linked to further goals for education and training.

Strengths: Knowledge and skill domains in which the learner feels most confident and competent in geropsychology practice.

Areas for growth: Knowledge and skill domains in which the learner wishes to develop further competency.

Education and training goals (within a practicum, internship rotation, fellowship, or postlicensure program of self-study).

References

Hatcher, R. L., & Lassiter, K. D. (2007). Initial training in professional psychology: The practicum competencies outline. *Training and education in professional psychology, 1*(1), 49–63. https://doi.org/10.1037/1931-3918.1.1.49

Karel, M., Emery, E., & Molinari, V. (2010). Development of a tool to evaluate geropsychology knowledge and skill competencies. *International Psychogeriatrics, 22*(6), 886–896. https://doi.org/10.1017/S1041610209991736

Knight, B. G., Karel, M. J., Hinrichsen, G. A., Qualls, S. H., & Duffy, M. (2009). Pikes Peak model for training in professional geropsychology. *American Psychologist, 64*(3), 205–214. https://doi.org/10.1037/a0015059

Peer Commentaries

The editors of this important and timely book are leaders in the field of professional geropsychology, and they have assembled a stellar roster of contributors to address key topics regarding mental health practice with older adults. With its inclusion of a wide range of settings, assessment approaches, interventions, and disorders, this book offers a wealth of practical guidance for those new to professional geropsychology and to seasoned clinicians who want to increase their competencies in geropsychology. This book is an invaluable read and a superb addition to the field. Highly recommended!

Daniel L. Segal, PhD, Professor, Department of Psychology at the University of Colorado at Colorado Springs, CO, USA

Psychological Assessment and Treatment of Older Adults is a well written, needed book with up to date information on traditional and newer topics. One of the strengths of this book is the attention paid to cultural influences on both the assessment and treatment process. In addition, the book covers both traditional topics for assessment and treatment (i.e. depression, cognition) and cutting edge newer approaches with older adults such as elder abuse detection, treatment for those in palliative care. This valuable book will help geropsychologists update their knowledge and improve their practice.

Peter A. Lichtenberg, PhD, ABPP, Director Institute of Gerontology and Merrill, Palmer Skillman Institute, WSU Distinguished Service Professor, Professor of Psychology, Wayne State University, Detroit, MI, USA

This volume provides an engaging, evidence-based, culturally-informed, and practice-focused overview of psychological practice with older adults. With contributions from leading academic and clinical geropsychologists, its eleven chapters convey the richness of this growing and important field. Readers will learn about a wide range of assessment and therapeutic approaches for addressing mental health concerns common among older adults and their families. Chapters include timely references to the existing evidence base, links to practical tools, helpful case illustrations with older adults from diverse backgrounds, and recommended resources for those who are intrigued to learn more. This book offers a great introduction to the field, or a useful resource for those already doing this meaningful work!

Michele J. Karel, PhD, ABPP, Board Certified in Geropsychology